Cryosurgical Advances
in Dermatology and
Tumors of the Head and Neck

The continual ascent of man is inevitably traced to his predecessors who indelibly left their imprint upon the earth's crust. The advancement of science, throughout recorded history of time, has been achieved because one man stood upon the shoulders of giants who came before him.

S. A. Zacarian

Cryosurgical Advances in Dermatology and Tumors of the Head and Neck

Edited by

SETRAG A. ZACARIAN, M.D., F.A.C.P.

Assistant Clinical Professor of Dermatology
Boston University School of Medicine

Lecturer, Tufts University School of Medicine
Boston, Massachusetts

Director of Dermatology Service
Bay State Medical Center
Springfield, Massachusetts

Member, Board of Governors of the American Society for
Contemporary Medicine and Surgery
Editorial Board of the Journal of Comprehensive Therapy
Contributing Editor and
Member of the Editorial Advisory Board of
The Journal of Dermatologic Surgery
Diplomate of the American Board of Dermatology

Forewords by:

JOHN G. BELLOWS, M.D., Ph.D.

EDWARD A. KRULL, M.D.

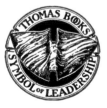

CHARLES C THOMAS · PUBLISHER
Springfield · Illinois · U.S.A.

Published and Distributed Throughout the World by
CHARLES C THOMAS • PUBLISHER
Bannerstone House
301-327 East Lawrence Avenue, Springfield, Illinois, U.S.A.

© *1977, by* CHARLES C THOMAS • PUBLISHER
ISBN 0-398-03597-0
Library of Congress Catalog Card Number: 76-27252

*With THOMAS BOOKS careful attention is given to all details of
manufacturing and design. It is the Publisher's desire to present books that
are satisfactory as to their physical qualities and artistic possibilities and
appropriate for their particular use. THOMAS BOOKS will be true to those
laws of quality that assure a good name and good will.*

Library of Congress Cataloging in Publication Data

Main entry under title:
Cryosurgical advances in dermatology and tumors of
  the head and neck.

  Bibliography: p.
  Includes index.
    1. Cryosurgery. 2. Skin—Surgery. 3. Head—
Tumors—Surgery. 4. Neck—Tumors—Surgery.
I. Zacarian, Setrag A., 1921-   [DNLM:
1. Cryogenic surgery. 2. Head and neck neoplasms—
Surgery. 3. Skin neoplasms—Surgery. WR500 C957]
RD33.4.C79   617'.477'05   76-27252
ISBN 0-398-03597-0

Printed in the United States of America
C-1

I dedicate this book to my parents who early in my childhood nurtured my interest in medicine.

Contributing Authors

Crowell Beard, M.D.

Clinical Professor of Ophthalmology, University of California Medical School, San Francisco, California.

Richard F. Elton, M.D.

Clinical Assistant Professor, Department of Dermatology, Wayne State University, Detroit, Michigan.

Andrew A. Gage, M.D.

Professor of Surgery, State University of New York at Buffalo, School of Medicine.
Chief Surgical Service and Chief of Staff, Veterans Hospital, Buffalo, New York.

Robert M. Goldwyn, M.D.

Associate Clinical Professor of Surgery, Harvard Medical School.
Head of Plastic Surgery, Beth Israel Hospital.
Surgeon, Peter Bent Brigham Hospital, Boston, Massachusetts.

Gloria F. Graham, M.D.

Assistant Clinical Professor of Dermatology, University of North Carolina Medical School at Chapel Hill, North Carolina.

Alfred S. Ketcham, M.D.

Professor of Surgery, Chief, Division of Surgical Oncology; University of Miami, School of Medicine, Miami, Florida.
Thomas Raffington Memorial Professor in Clinical Oncology, American Cancer Society and formerly Surgeon-in-Chief, National Cancer Institute of Health, Bethesda, Maryland.

Ronald R. Lubritz, M.D., F.A.C.P.

Clinical Associate Professor of Medicine (Dermatology), Tulane University School of Medicine, New Orleans, Louisiana.

Daniel Miller, M.D., F.A.C.S.

Associate Clinical Professor in Otolaryngology, Harvard Medical School.
Director of Ear, Nose and Throat Tumor Clinic, Massachusetts Eye and Ear Infirmary at Massachusetts General Hospital (1947-1974).
President, American Society for Head and Neck Surgery, 1974-75.

II. Bryan Neel, III, M.D., Ph.D.

Consultant, Department of Otolaryngology and Microbiology, Mayo Clinic and Mayo Foundation, Instructor Mayo Medical School and Mayo Graduate School of Medicine.

John H. Sullivan, M.D.

Assistant Clinical Professor of Ophthalmology, University of California Medical School, San Francisco, California.

Douglas Torre, M.D.

Clinical Professor of Medicine (Dermatology), Cornell University Medical College, New York.
Attending Dermatologist at Memorial Hospital for Cancer and Allied Disease, New York City.

FOREWORDS

Cryosurgical Advances in Dermatology and Tumors of the Head and Neck, the author's third book, is further proof that Doctor Setrag Zacarian is a leading expert on cryosurgery of the skin. Physicians, and especially cryosurgeons, are greatly indebted to Doctor Zacarian who was instrumental in developing the basic principles of cryosurgery. He was a pioneer in establishing the relationship of the freezing temperature, the length of time of the application, and the resulting cellular and tissue reactions. Before this, skin lesions that were destroyed by freezing depended upon the application to the skin of cotton swabs dipped into a cryogen.

Dr. Zacarian is not only preeminent in clinical cryosurgery of skin lesions, but also has contributed much to our knowledge through his work in experimental cryosurgery. Using his great energy and talents unsparingly, he has become the established leader in cryosurgery of the skin. In his classic studies of the cryolesion, he described the thermal gradients that exist in deepfreezing of biological systems; using thermocouples, he developed means of monitoring the temperature in the evolving cryolesion and demonstrated that the lowest temperatures occur near the heat sink. He emphasized that treating a skin malignancy without using thermocouple needles is unsatisfactory because the surgeon does not know the varying freezing temperatures of different parts of the tumor. Thus, many cancer cells can escape destruction. The author also demonstrated clinically the superiority of the wound healing which follows cryosurgery, in contrast to that which follows other methods of tumor removal.

Zacarian and his co-authors, who individually are experts in various scientific disciplines, in updating cryosurgery for head and neck tumors, oral tumors as well as eyelid neoplasms, have rendered a great service to patients and physicians alike.

JOHN G. BELLOWS, M.D., PH.D.
Editor-in-Chief:
Annals of Ophthalmology;
Comprehensive Therapy
Director of The American Society of
   Contemporary Medicine and Surgery

Doctor Setrag Zacarian is one of the foremost leaders in cryosurgery of skin tumors. His two previous books on cryosurgery have served both as a foundation for and major stimulus to the increasing scientific development and use of cryosurgery for cutaneous lesions. This book brings together the advances in the biology and techniques of cryosurgery, new instrumentation, and an in-depth study of the role and effectiveness of cryosurgery that have evolved in the intervening years since his last text. It is significantly different from his other books and is an important contribution to our knowledge of cryosurgery of skin tumors.

Cryosurgery has been used by dermatologists for many years in a variety of benign cutaneous lesions without much concern about cryogenics and cryobiology. This knowledge seemed unnecessary when treating warts and seborrheic and actinic keratoses. The end result of the destruction of the lesion was obvious. However, the employment of cryosurgery in the treatment of malignant lesions has necessitated the investigation of cryobiology and its careful application and evaluation in clinical situations. Thus concepts of the cryolesion, critical temperatures for normal and malignant cell destruction, thermal gradients, freeze-thaw cycles, double freeze-thaw cycles have been of necessity studied in great detail. Doctor Zacarian has presented the fundamentals of cryobiology in a fascinating and clinically relevant manner.

The very simplicity of cryosurgical technique creates inherent problems of failing to utilize appropriate control systems. I think it is very important that Doctor Zacarian has stressed the necessity of thermocouple monitoring of tumor treatment by measuring the temperatures within the tissue to be certain that the critical levels necessary for tumor destruction are attained. Without the establishment of specific methods and temperature monitoring systems the interpretation of results would have much less scientific value and might be more variable and unpredictable.

Cryosurgery is one of a number of physical modalities that is successfully used in the treatment of skin malignancies. Simplicity of techniques, possible better cosmetic results, relative preservation of the lacrimal duct system, avoidance of chondronecrosis and perforation of the ear and nose are some of the benefits of this treatment method.

But there has been some question about cure rates of basal cell and squamous cell carcinoma treated with cryosurgery. Doctor Zacarian's long-term statistics have established that cryosurgery, if properly used in appropriate circumstances, has a cure rate equal to that of x-ray, electrosurgery, and excision surgery.

The most frequent use and perhaps the main application of cryosurgery is for benign skin lesions such as warts, actinic and seborrheic keratoses, sebaceous hyperplasia, dermatofibromas, and acne. All physicians treating skin lesions should become familiar with the indications and use of cryosurgery for these lesions.

Cryosurgery knows no specialty restriction. Any tissue that is accessible to cryosurgical application may be amenable to this treatment. Doctor Zacarian has drawn together contributors from surgery, plastic surgery, otolaryngology, and ophthalmology, as well as dermatology to present the scope of current cryosurgical usage and to stress its potential value for other specialties.

Doctor Zacarian continues with this book his important contribution to cryosurgery. It is very well written, with a broad scope and a meaningful organization of material. It combines in a most understandable and interesting fashion the biology and techniques of cryosurgery, thus affording a guide to practical treatment and development of the foundations from which future investigations and new clinical application may be derived.

I strongly recommend Doctor Zacarian's excellent new book to all physicians treating skin and oral lesions—the family practitioner, surgeon, plastic surgeon, otolaryngologist, oral surgeon, ophthalmologist, gynecologist and the dermatologist—and to those who might conceive of even other roles in medicine for cryosurgery.

Doctor Zacarian is to be congratulated on his outstanding book and his abiding scientific endeavors in cryosurgery.

EDWARD A. KRULL, M.D.
Chairman, Department of Dermatology
Henry Ford Hospital, Detroit, Michigan

Preface

CRYOSURGERY IS NOT ONLY an established technical procedure but also an accepted medical discipline for the effective treatment of benign and malignant neoplasia. In some instances freezing or cryogenics has replaced the traditional scalpel, irradiation and other conventional modalities for the ablation of unwanted tumors. The therapeutic effects of subzero temperatures for various medical disorders was known to Hippocrates and his followers. However, it was not until the turn of the century that the use of extremely cold refrigerants became available to the physician and were enthusiastically explored by the dermatologists. The application of liquid nitrogen with a cotton swab upon benign and precancerous growths of the skin was passed on from one generation of dermatologists to another for almost sixty years.

During this same period of time, cryobiologists diligently investigated and observed the effects of subzero temperatures upon plant and animal cells. Subsequently, the new science of cryopreservation of living cells, tissues, and organ systems was evolved. Indirectly they paved the way and contributed to our own divergent specific interests in cryogenics, not to preserve tissues but to destroy them.

Fifteen years ago there emerged an imaginative clinician and investigator, Doctor Irving S. Cooper, who employed a sophisticated cryogenic instrument which delivered liquid nitrogen to freeze a specific focal area of the basal ganglia, to relieve the symptoms of Parkinson's Disease and other neurological disorders. Through his pioneering research and extensive clinical studies, he promulgated the modern science of cryogenic surgery. This new technical skill very rapidly made inroads to almost all of our surgical specialties, including dermatology. The cotton swab was soon replaced by various sophisticated instruments which delivered liquid nitrogen with greater precision and offered a sustained heat sink to eradicate malignant tumors of the skin, the oral cavity, and selected head and neck tumors. The high cure rate, simplicity of application, and superb cosmetic end results from freezing, and the added role as a useful modality for palliation of external neoplasms, has brought cryogenic surgery into the forefront with other contemporary medical disciplines.

You may well ask, why then have I authored and helped edit a third book? The desire to familiarize the physician and the clinical investigator with the fundamental pathogenesis of freezing temperatures upon normal and malignant tissue was foremost in my mind. I want to stir his imagination to explore and elucidate the enigmas of superb wound healing following cryogenic surgery and to make him aware of the specific selectivity of various cells to freezing temperature.

It is extremely important to understand the development of the cryolesion, temperature gradients, and the importance of freeze-thaw cycles. The clinician should not embark upon cryogenic surgery if he does not understand these important parameters clearly outlined in the first chapter.

The need to learn from each other and share our experiences in diverse medical and surgical disciplines is extremely important if medicine is to advance. In this monograph I have brought together the expertise of not only the dermatologist, but also the general surgeon, the plastic surgeon, the ophthalmologist, and the head and neck surgeon. We have described the various cryosurgical instrumentations that have evolved in the past fifteen years as well as their specific use in various medical disorders. Some of the complications and limitations of cryogenic surgery have not been deleted. Since my two monographs in 1969 and 1973, a larger number of patients with skin cancers have been cryosurgically treated by this author and others. The follow-ups and cure rates, therefore, are more meaningful now and give further impetus to this new technology. This treatise also presents the effects of freezing through the tarsal plate of dogs and lacrimal duct with preservation of these vital structures. Freeze-thaw cycles have been further defined both upon canine skin and HeLa cells as they would relate to human experience. Several authors present their experience in cryosurgery for lentigo maligna which appears to be very promising.

We have touched upon the possible implications of cryoimmunology, a fertile field, yet unexplored and unchartered in the management of human malignancy. Cryogenic surgery is still in its infancy, but it has already proven its usefulness as a therapeutic regimen for most primary neoplasia of the skin and selected lesions of the oral cavity. It has its place as an adjunctive modality for advanced carcinomas when there is no other recourse. The cryosurgical approach for the management of eyelid cancers is both provocative and promising. Throughout the chapters there may be some differences among the authors as to critical temperatures, single versus double freeze-thaw cycles, as well as success and failure of specific malignant tumors of the skin and their location. These divergent views need not necessarily confuse the reader but may clarify the dynamic phase of this new burgeoning technology.

The future of cryosurgery is as limited as the myoptic vision of the physician and as unlimited as his imagination, curiosity and clinical investigation. I am reminded of Edgar Allan Poe who said, "Those who dream by day are cognizant of many things which escape those who dream only by night."

If this monograph stimulates and inspires others in the pursuit of truth and advancement of this new technique for the benefit of mankind, this alone will have sufficed to fulfill my goal and purpose and that of the contributing authors.

Our ultimate desire is for the physician who is unacquainted with cryogenic surgery to consider its usefulness in the management of human malignancy. Was it not Alexander Pope who said, "Be not the first by whom the new attract, nor yet the last to lay the old aside."

SAZ

Acknowledgments

Wᴡʀɪᴛɪɴɢ ᴀ ʙᴏᴏᴋ is a prodigious undertaking, particularly in a field of medicine where changes and innovations are capricious and concepts and therapeutic indications are so ephemeral. Cryogenic surgery, an established medical and surgical discipline, is very much alive. Clinical investigators are developing new ideas and exploring fertile fields in our struggle against human disorders. I am indeed fortunate and most grateful to the contributing authors, who have kindly consented to share their expertise in cryogenic surgery to make this monograph the most complete and contemporary in its field. Each author has been a pioneer in this new technology and has authored many papers and promulgated important principles in cryosurgery.

The invaluable help and advice of Dr. Charles D. Cox, Chairman of the Department of Microbiology at the University of Massachusetts at Amherst is herein acknowledged and much appreciated. I also thank Miss Ann Progluske and Mary Lee Noden at the University of Massachusetts for their technical assistance.

The first chapter would have been totally incomplete and inadequate without the help and contributions of Dr. Joseph T. Giammalvo, Pathologist-in-Chief of the Providence Hospital in Holyoke, Massachusetts. His meticulous interpretations in the pathogenesis of human carcinoma of the skin and specimens of in vivo freezing of dog integument with variant cryogenic techniques was both informative and stimulating. I am genuinely indebted to him.

Dr. Joseph M. Stoyak, a veterinarian in Springfield, Massachusetts, worked diligently with me to help with the experimental studies on freeze-thaw cycles and the effects of freezing upon the eyelids and lacrimal apparatus of dogs. He has contributed much to elucidate the effects of cryogenic surgery as it may relate to humans. In his own right, Dr. Stoyak is a pioneer in veterinary cryogenic surgery in the United States.

I acknowledge with thanks the help of Mrs. Jean E. Scougall and the library staff of the Bay State Medical Center. The assistance offered by Mr. Joseph Stumpf, Joseph Andera, and Robert Eisenberg from the Engineering Department of Frigitronics, Inc. of Shelton, Connecticut were invaluable in the final modifications and implementations of the templates to measure central and peripheral depth of the cryolesion during freezing and also in the development of the new C-76 portable unit.

This author expresses his gratitude to the Zacarian Cancer Research Foundation for the financial support it has given to pursue the experimental studies at the University of Massachusetts, and the studies pertinent to the pathogenesis of cryonecrosis of malignant tumors of the skin and the canine experiments. This Foundation has also helped to defray the cost of many of the color plates in this monograph along with the Rudolph Ellender Medical Foundation through the efforts of Dr. Joseph A. Baldone, President. The following pharmaceutical companies have generously contributed toward the colored plates: Cooper Laboratories; Dermik Laboratories; Dome Laboratories, Division of Miles Laboratories; Herbert Laboratories; Johnson & Johnson; Lederle Laboratories, Division of American Cyanamid; Owen Laboratories; Pfizer Laboratories, Inc.; J. B. Roerig; Reed and Carnrick; Schering Corporation; E. R. Squibb and Sons, Inc.; Stiefel Laboratories; Syntex Laboratories; Texas Pharmacal, Division of Warner Lambert; and Westwood Pharmaceuticals, Inc. to each, I express my sincere thanks.

The commercial art work of Patricia Dupont and the excellent reproduction of many prints rendered by Armen Tashjian are herein acknowledged with appreciation. I also want to thank the staff of Charles C Thomas, Publisher, in particular, William H. Bried who worked diligently in the preparation of this treatise and made special efforts to reproduce the excellent quality of the color plates which have enhanced this monograph. I thank Miss Teresa C. Boylam for the preparation of the subject and author indices.

Last but not least, I am grateful to my wife, Rocky, who not only served as my sounding board, but also tolerated my incessant long hours, the cluttered study, and reediting and retyping the mountainous hand-scribbled notes of my manuscript to its final revision.

SAZ

Contents

Cryosurgical Advances
in Dermatology and
Tumors of the Head and Neck

CHAPTER ONE

Cryogenics, the Cryolesion and the Pathogenesis of Cryonecrosis

SETRAG A. ZACARIAN, M.D., F.A.C.P.

I. CRYOGENICS

WHILE CRYOBIOLOGY RELATES to the effects of subzero temperatures upon a living system, cryogenics primarily concerns itself in the development of freezing temperatures within a biological system. The physical basis by which freezing is accomplished within a living tissue or a cell is essentially the withdrawal of heat from that medium. This heat exchange is dependent in part upon the underlying tissue environment, its water content and the degree of its vascularity. Equally important is the type of refrigerant or cryogen employed. The lower the boiling point of refrigerant, greater is its capacity to freeze in both depth and volume; for example, Freon 12® with a boiling point of $-29.8°C$ is not cold enough to freeze malignant tumors of the skin, yet is quite effective for freezing the lens of patients with cataracts, referred to as cryoextraction. Liquid nitrogen, on the other hand, with a lower boiling point of $-195.6°C$ has the capacity to freeze not only benign but malignant neoplasia of the skin, oral cavity and bone as well.

The birth of modern cryogenics, interestingly enough, came on Christmas Eve in the year 1877. Two papers were delivered before the French Academy of Sciences, one by the French scientist Louis Cailletet and the second by the Swiss engineer Raul Pictet. Cailletet had liquefied small quantities of oxygen and carbon monoxide by expansion of the gases from extremely high pressures.[1] Pictet demonstrated his experiments wherein he had liquefied oxygen by means of a mechanical refrigeration cascade, by employing sulfur dioxide and carbon dioxide, boiled under reduced pressures.[2] Two Polish scientists, Wroblewski and Olszewski, in 1883, successfully converted oxygen and nitrogen into a liquid state.[3] The commercial production of large quantities of liquid air and subsequent extraction of liquid nitrogen were the contributions of Linde in 1895.

II. DEVELOPMENT OF THE CRYOLESION

Refrigerants in current use today are essentially capable of producing cryolesions of varying magnitude. However, the rapidity of its formation, its volume, depth, and the intensity of achieving subzero temperatures below the skin and neoplasia vary with the refrigerant selected and its boiling point. Insofar as the following chapter discusses at length various cryogens and instrumentations, the author will confine his remarks to the capacitance of liquid nitrogen.

The development of the cryolesion is interdependent upon the applicator used and probe size (Figures 1-1 and 1-2). If one

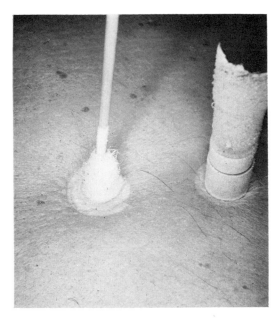

Figure 1-1. The extent and depth of the cryolesion is dependent upon the refrigerant and composition of the heat sink. Liquid nitrogen chilled copper disc will offer a greater degree of conduction and retention of the cryogen than cotton swab. From S. Zacarian, *Cryosurgery of Skin Cancer,* 1969. Courtesy of Charles C Thomas, Publisher, Springfield, Illinois.

employs an open system, the aperture size of the interchangeable plastic needle for the refrigerant spray is to be considered. The duration of freeze time (Figures 1-3 and 1-4), thermal conductivity, cellular composition and osmolality, and the underlying vascularity of the given tissue subjected to freezing will govern the extent of the cryolesion. The velocity of cooling inevitably closely correlates with the degree and depth of cryonecrosis which subsequently follows. The more rapid the rate of cooling, more profound is the underlying tissue destruction.[4-6] The heat generated during the cooling process with conversion of water to ice is referred to as the *latent heat of fusion.* As water is transformed into ice, one can measure

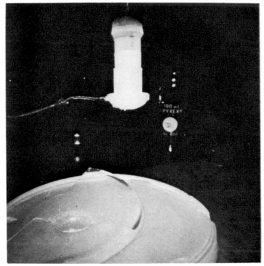

Figure 1-2. The classic hemisphere of a cryolesion produced in a gelatin mold as it would evolve in vivo. From S. Zacarian, *Cryosurgery of Skin Cancer,* 1969. Courtesy of Charles C Thomas, Publisher, Springfield, Illinois.

the production of heat equivalent to eighty calories per gram of water.

The survival or demise of normal or malignant cells is closely related to the velocity of the cooling experience to which they are subjected. Among cryobiologists there is no uniformity of opinion as to what constitutes rapid, moderately rapid,

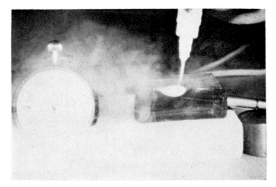

Figure 1-3. The early development of a cryolesion within thirty seconds of liquid nitrogen spray upon a gelatin mold with an open spray unit.

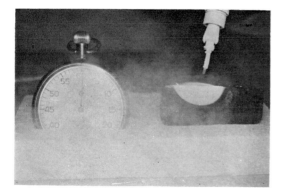

Figure 1-4. One minute of liquid nitrogen spray produces an extensive spread of the ice front both in surface and in depth.

and extremely rapid freezing rates.[7-10] The author believes the cooling rate as monitored during the clinical application of cryosurgery would be uniformally accepted as rapid. Certainly the lethality of freezing and subsequent elimination of malignant tumors ascertain that the rate of cooling is optimum for its destruction. Bear in mind that even with the most extremely rapid rate of cooling, there will always be some survival of both normal and malignant cells, however small their numbers.[11, 12]

III. MEASUREMENT OF TEMPERATURE PROFILE WITHIN THE CRYOLESION (THERMAL GRADIENTS)

It is extremely difficult to establish a specific rate of cooling within tissue in vivo during the evolvement of the cryolesion as compared to a homogeneous cell suspension immersed in liquid nitrogen. In vivo experimental studies upon canine skin with liquid nitrogen spray show that within sixty seconds the temperature at 2 mm depth dropped to −90°C. This represents a precipitous drop of temperature from +37°C to −90°C, an increment of 2.1 degrees per second. Monitored temperatures

in 90 seconds at −120°C at the same depth reflects an increment of 1.7 degree temperature drop per second. In contrast at 5 mm depth wherein the temperature was monitored at −40°C the rate of cooling appeared to be 1.3 degrees per second. Undoubtedly cells and tissue in closest proximity to the heat sink or the source of the cryogen at −196°C manifest an increment of rate of cooling or velocity ten to one hundred times that observed at levels of 2 and 5 mm deep within the neoplasia. It is quite clear then that a specific rate of cooling cannot be really established in tissue, for it is neither homogeneous nor confluent as in cell suspension. The true ingredient of freezing in depth is the function of time.[14]

It is extremely important to appreciate the thermal profile and the temperature differential within the cryolesion as it de-

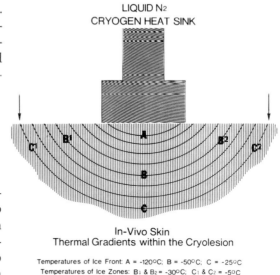

LIQUID N2
CRYOGEN HEAT SINK

In-Vivo Skin
Thermal Gradients within the Cryolesion

Temperatures of Ice Front: A = -120ºC; B = -50ºC; C = -25ºC
Temperatures of Ice Zones: B₁ & B₂ = -30ºC; C₁ & C₂ = -5ºC

Figure 1-5. It is important to consider temperature gradients within the cryolesion during freezing. Also note that the center depth of the ice front below the heat sink approximates the surface spread of the ice front from the edge of the heat sink to the outer margin of the surface freeze.

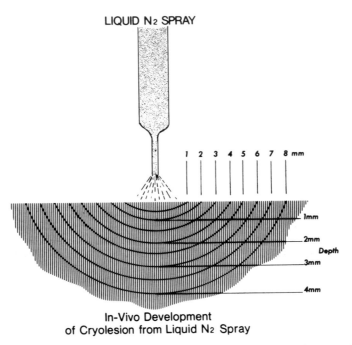

**In-Vivo Development
of Cryolesion from Liquid N₂ Spray**

Figure 1-6. In using a spray to deliver liquid nitrogen, providing it is an intermittent spray of the refrigerant, the measurement of one half the radius of the surface ice front is approximately equivalent to the central depth of the cryolesion.

velops within a given biological system when subjected to freezing temperatures. We refer to this temperature difference as thermal gradients (Figure 1-5). With the employment of multiple thermocouple needles, the thermal history within the evolving cryolesion in vivo can be clearly monitored. Temperatures nearest to the heat sink are coldest while peripherally and at the lowest depth are considerably warmer. It is also important to note that the marginal measurement of the surface extension of the ice front from the edge of the liquid nitrogen probe approximates the central depth of extension of the cryolesion below the skin or neoplasia subjected to freezing (Figure 1-5). When using a spray delivery of liquid nitrogen, the extent of one half the radius of the surface ice front approximates the depth of the cryolesion (Figure 1-6), providing an *intermit-*

tent spray technique is directed to the center of the tumor. These are simply rules of thumb to serve as a clinical guide should you not choose to employ microthermocouple needles to specifically measure the depth and extent of the cryolesion.

For the clinician who initially employs cryosurgery for the destruction of skin cancer, the use of thermocouple needles is most essential. Not taking initial measurements and monitoring tissue depth of freezing is similar to setting sail without a compass and exploring an unchartered sea without a sextant. The ideal monitoring device would be a simple multisensoring thermocouple needle to record thermal gradients at various depths of the cryolesion.[15–18] We have shown that during the application of a cryosurgical probe, the cellular population of both normal and

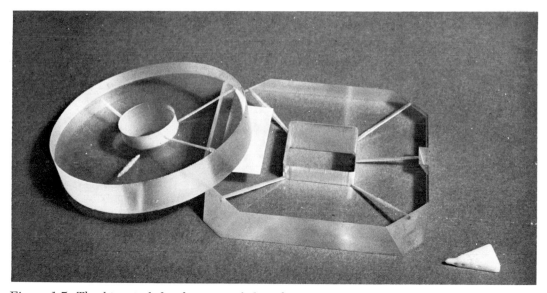

Figure 1-7. The historical development of the original acrylic jigs or templates of Brodthagen to the smaller clinically applicable modification by Zacarian. From S. A. Zacarian, *Cutis, 16:* Sept. 1975. Courtesy of Yorke Medical Journals, Dun Donnelley Publishing Corp.

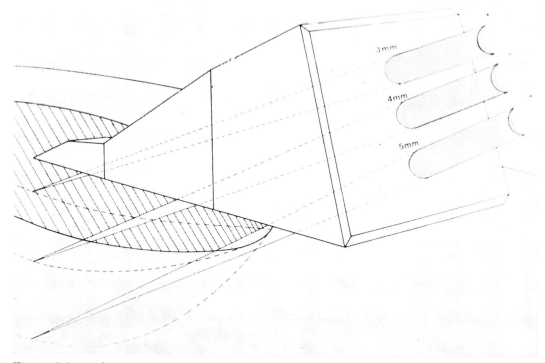

3 mm

4 mm

5 mm

Figure 1-8. A diagramatic sketch of a small template with three separate tracks which allow for the accurate measurements of 3, 4, and 5 mm below the skin surface. From S. A. Zacarian, *Cutis, 16:* Sept. 1975. Courtesy of Yorke Medical Journals, Dun Donnelley Publishing Corp.

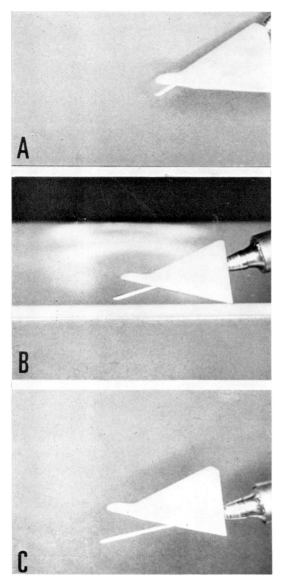

Experimentally a multisensoring needle is ideal and clinically very applicable but reportedly the manufacturing costs and feasibility of such a thermocouple needle are extremely expensive.

An adequate compromise is to effectively monitor the extent and central depth of the cryolesion. This can be accomplished with the miniature template devised by this author and engineered by Frigitronics, Inc., from the original Brodthagan jig® (Figure 1-7). This small template has 3,

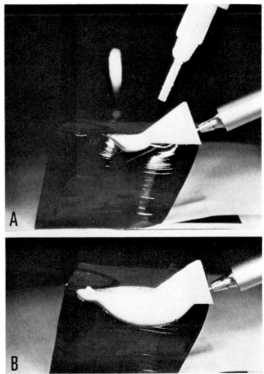

Figure 1-9. A serial view of the microthermocouple needle passed through the (a) 3 mm track; (b) 4 mm track; (c) 5 mm track, as it would relate in vivo, below the skin. From S. A. Zacarian, *Cutis, 16:* Sept. 1975. Courtesy of Yorke Medical Journals, Dun Donnelley Publishing Corp.

cancerous cells are exposed to widely divergent temperature and cooling rates and indeed are not uniformly exposed to the same damaging conditions (Figure 1-5).

Figure 1-10. (a) A gelatin mold to represent the placement of the template and the passage of the microthermocouple needle through the 5 mm track while freezing on the surface. (b) With continuous spray of liquid nitrogen, the ice front has extended deep below the surface of the mold and *conducted through the plastic jig* to the depth beyond the tip of the microthermocouple needle. From S. A. Zacarian, *Cutis, 16:* Sept. 1975. Courtesy of Yorke Medical Journals, Dun Donnelley Publishing Corp.

4, and 5 mm tracks to determine depth of the cryolesion (Figure 1-8). It is further clarified in Figure 1-9a, b, and c, with each track individually positioned. A gelatin mold serves as a model to demonstrate the placement of the template. The microthermocouple is passed through the 5 mm track (Figure 1-10a). As the freezing continues, the ice front enlarges until the base of the cryolesion touches and envelopes the thermocouple needle and its tip registers the temperature at that level upon the pyrometer (Figure 1-10b). The *plastic template will not serve* as a barrier for the extension of the ice front.

Insofar as most recurrences of skin cancers appear to be at the margins, it is extremely important that freezing be adequately extended to the periphery of the tumor edge and beyond. The surface may appear frozen, but its depth and more important, its temperature, is usually undetermined. With this in mind, the template was further modified to sensor a secondary area within the evolving cryolesion, namely at its margin. The clinician can now select the central depth of ice front which he wishes to monitor below the tumor and with a second thermocouple needle passed vertically through the same template, will now measure 2 or 3 mm at a specified margin (Figure 1-11). You may well ask what about measurements of the ice front on the opposing edges of the tumor? The ice front developed from the liquid nitrogen probe will extend equally in all directions and its temperature at the peripheral margins will be circumferentially uniform. When using a spray, if one *intermittently* directs the liquid nitrogen to the *center of the tumor*, he will achieve the same temperature gradients in the margins as mentioned above with the probe. With the employment of two thermocouple needles, the clinician will need to simply turn the

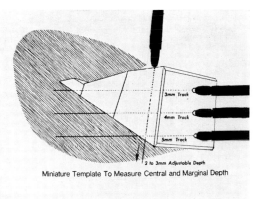

Figure 1-11. With further modification of the template, one can measure two parameters of the cryolesion, its central depth and its margin.

knob of the pyrometer from one direction to the other and quickly observe the advancing ice front temperatures below the tumor as well as its margin. In chapter five, the author will clinically demonstrate the application of this modified template.

Many of the newer instruments now available do not include either microthermocouple needles or a pyrometer. The author is deeply concerned that the inexperienced clinician will freeze malignant tumors without monitoring and thereby experience a high recurrence rate from cryosurgery. After over a decade of work by the early pioneers in cryogenic surgery in establishing this technique with guidelines and measurements, this modality may fall by the wayside and even retrogress. Even today with lesions situated upon the nasolabial fold, the cheeks, and in particular the area of the face anterior to the tragus of the ear, the author monitors freezing depth.

IV. THE IMPORTANCE OF FREEZE-THAW CYCLES

The period of freezing is but one phase of cryogenesis which leads to cellular and tissue death. The pathogenesis of hypo-thermia will be further discussed in this chapter. Equally important, however, is the period of thawing. Cryobiologists consider this phase to be even more lethal than the freezing cycle.[19] Rapid thawing will enhance more survival in both plant and animal cells. It is during the thaw period that recrystallization of ice develops, particularly intracellularly, which proves to be more lethal and further enhances the electrolyte concentration and dehydration within the cells.

In the laboratory, working with animal or plant cells, freezing rates as well as thawing rates can be controlled and regulated at will; this however is not possible in vivo. In a clinical setting, we can somewhat alter the rate and depth of freezing dependent upon the cryogen we select. For example, nitrous oxide, with a boiling point temperature of $-89.5°C$, will render considerably slower rates of freezing as compared to liquid nitrogen with a lower boiling temperature of $-195.6°C$. With liquid nitrogen, the velocity of freezing and depth of the ice front far exceeds that of nitrous oxide at the same interval of time.

Thawing period on the other hand is not entirely within our control. We do know, however, that the thawing period is usually one and a half times the duration of freezing time. Its duration therefore is interdependent upon the length of freezing. If for example the freezing period of a given tumor is achieved within sixty seconds, the complete thaw period will terminate approximately ninety seconds after cessation of freezing. Thawing period can be slightly altered, and indeed prolonged, by the vascularity of the tissue subjected to freezing if one were to place an ice pack over the frozen tumor site. It is also somewhat abbreviated if the local anesthesia used contains epinephrine.

In cryosurgery of malignant tumors, the author insists on a double freeze-thaw cycle. There is both clinical and laboratory documented evidence that a second freeze-thaw cycle enhances the lethal effects of freezing temperatures upon cells and tissues.[20] It is also apparent that a third freeze-thaw cycle is even more destructive and will produce higher cure rates in transplanted mouse mammary adenocarcinoma.[21, 22] In the past year, cancers of the skin situated in critical areas of the eyelid, ala nasi- and nasolabial fold, have been subjected to a triple freeze-thaw cycle by this author.

It is extremely important that, following the freezing cycle, one waits until thawing is complete, i.e. clinically the surface ice front has virtually disappeared, before a second freeze or the third is initiated. A contemporary thought is that a half-thaw (or waiting for the thawing to approximate the edge of the tumor site), referred to as "Halo-thaw-time," is adequate to start to freeze again. The author takes exception to this view because he feels strongly that the total sum of the thawing period is essential to enhance further cell destruction. There is indirect evidence to support the view that maximum damage to cells may well occur between $-10°$ to $0°C$.[23, 24] During the incomplete thaw period the temperature range within the cryolesion may well vary from $-20°C$ to $-10°C$ and it has not even approached the phase change of $-5°C$. Is it not during this interval of thawing that we observe the regrowth of ice crystals within the cells which is so destructive for their survival?

V. EXPERIMENTAL EVIDENCE TO SUPPORT THE IMPORTANCE OF COMPLETE THAW CYCLE

A. Freeze-thaw Cycles Upon HeLa Cells

With the assistance of Dr. Charles D. Cox, head of Microbiology at the University of Massachusetts at Amherst, the author conducted the following experiments with the help of his research assistant, Ann Progluske. A HeLa cell line in BME medium supplemented with 10 percent fetal calf serum was obtained from the Flow Laboratories, Rockville, Maryland. The cells were harvested with trypsin and were counted on the hemocytometer. Suspensions of the HeLa cells, approximating 2000 cells per 0.25 ml, were then placed in a plastic tube within a teflon sleeve in preparation for freezing (Figure 1-12). A microthermocouple wire was inserted within the column of the cell suspension to monitor the temperature upon the pyrometer. To determine the viability of cells before and after freezing, trypan blue staining technique was employed. Cell staining with the vital dye trypan blue has been shown to occur in dead cells, while membranes of viable cells are impermeable to this stain. Generally in the studies described, the trypan blue method has been employed to assay viability.[25]

Control HeLa cells showed a viability of 97 percent. Three separate experiments were carried out to determine the ratio between viable and killed cells following a single freeze-thaw cycle, double freeze-thaw cycle, and a single freeze, half-thaw, and freeze-thaw cycles. The HeLa cell suspension in the plastic tubing enveloped within the teflon sleeve was immersed in liquid nitrogen to a temperature range between −35 to −40°C and then quickly immersed in a warm water bath whose temperature was controlled at +37°C. Freezing and thawing cycles were timed and closely correlated to human experiences in cryogenic surgery. Immediately after thawing, a 0.1 ml aliquot of cell suspension was mixed with 0.02 ml of 0.4 percent aqueous trypan blue and after standing for approximately five minutes, a small amount was pipetted into a hemocytometer. A

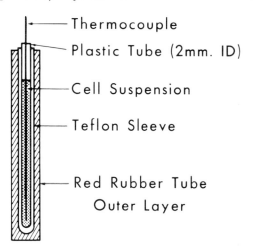

Figure 1-12. HeLa cells in BME medium prepared for freezing experiment.

count of total cells and of the strained cells were then recorded. The percentage of unstained cells gave the percentage of viable cells in the cell population. Viability studies were carried out at five minutes and were also repeated two hours forty-five minutes following freezing.

The composite of several experiments was averaged and recorded in Table 1-I. It is quite evident that the higher kill ratio following a double freeze-thaw cycle far exceeded that of a single freeze-thaw experience. On the other hand, *the partial thaw* in the third experiment yielded a viable population of 25 percent, as compared to the *complete thaw cycle* in the second experiment that yielded a 15 percent viable cell population. These studies were carried on for their qualitative value. Even though a 10 percent disparity between a partial thaw and complete thaw may appear small in a laboratory setting, *clinically it merits serious consideration.* The percentage of killed versus viable cell population increased with each of the three experiments two hours forty-five minutes following freezing. A diminished number of viable cells was noted in the

TABLE 1-I

HeLa CELL STUDIES

Experiment I	Freeze	Thaw		
Temperature	−35° to −40°C	+37°C		
Time	60″	90″		
Killed Cells—55 percent				
Viable Cells—45 percent				
Experiment II	Freeze	Thaw	Freeze	Thaw
Temperature	−35° to −40°C	+37°C	−35° to −40°C	+37°C
Time	60″	90″	60″	90″
Killed Cells—85 percent				
Viable Cells—15 percent				
Experiment III	Freeze	Partial Thaw	Freeze	Thaw
Temperature	−35° to −40°C	−5° to −10°C	−35° to −40°C	+37°C
Time	60″	30″	35″	90″
Killed Cells—75 percent				
Viable Cells—25 percent				
Control HeLa Cells (Viable)—97 percent				

interim, but the disparity between completely thawed cells and partially thawed cells remained constant. There were 10 percent more killed cells with the former technique than the latter.

B. Canine Studies Following Freeze-Thaw Cycles

With the assistance of Joseph M. Stoyak, D.V.M., a dog was anesthetized and a portion of his fur was shaved and the underlying skin exposed. Three distinct and separate areas of his back were subjected to freezing with liquid nitrogen. An area of 1.0 cm was pencilled and an added margin of 0.5 cm outside this area was secondarily outlined (Figure 1-13). The freezing time was kept uniform at 60 seconds upon each of the three designated areas (Figure 1-14). A liquid nitrogen delivery system was employed directing the refrigerant onto the center with intermittent spray.

The first area of canine skin was frozen

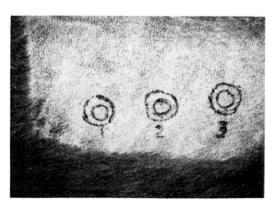

Figure 1-13. Three distinct areas of canine skin outlined prior to freezing. The inner circle measures 1 cm in diameter with a peripheral margin of 0.5 cm.

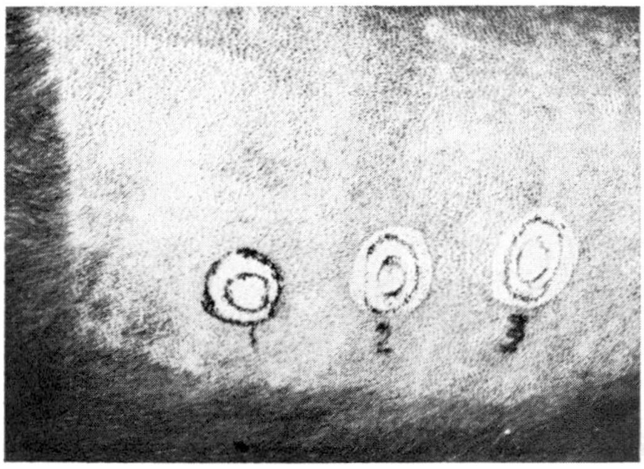

Figure 1-14. Experimental site one, received a single freeze; site two a double freeze-thaw cycle, while site three was subjected to a single freeze, partial thaw (Halo-thaw-time) and subsequent freeze.

and allowed to thaw. The freeze time was sixty seconds and complete thaw period was ninety seconds. The second designated area of canine skin was frozen and allowed to *completely* thaw and was frozen again, essentially a double freeze-thaw cycle. The third area of skin was frozen with freezing time of sixty seconds. Thawing proceeded up to the outer margin of the 1 cm pencilled outline. In other words a *partial thaw*, or what is referred to as "Halo-thaw time," was undertaken which involved thawing only up to the 0.5 cm peripheral margin outside the initially delineated 1.0 cm site. The partial thaw time was approximately thirty seconds, or sixty seconds short of the complete thaw period measured in the first experiments. Each of the frozen sites were carefully examined for several days.

At the end of sixty-two hours (Figure 1-15), Dr. Stoyak totally excised each frozen site with a wide margin and depth and marked the specimens 1, 2, and 3, placing them in formalin for histological examination. The specimens were submitted to Dr. Joseph T. Giammalvo, Pathologist-

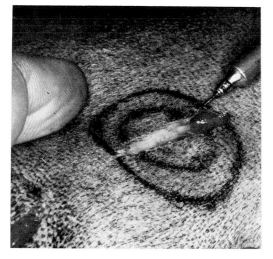

Figure 1-16. Immediately following disappearance of the surface freeze upon the canine skin, an incision at this site still demonstrates the underlying frozen integument.

in-Chief of the Providence Hospital, Holyoke. Without giving him a protocol of the experiments, he was asked to section them thoroughly and carefully measure and evaluate the *degree* and *depth* of cryonecrosis of each specimen of canine frozen skin. Microscopically each of the specimens showed a *surface* area of cryonecrosis of 1.5 cm. The depth and invasion of cryonecrosis in specimen 1 extended 0.3 cm; in specimen 2, 0.5 cm; while in specimen 3, the invasion was 0.4 cm.

The degree of hemorrhagic necrosis and involvement of underlying subcutaneous tissue and skeletal muscle was greatest in specimen 2 which had sustained a double freeze-thaw cycle. That extra depth of freezing of 2 mm following a double freeze-thaw cycle is clinically very important when it comes to effectiveness of cryosurgery of malignant tumors in man.

These two sets of laboratory experiments are quite documentary and certainly convincing to the author that a complete thaw is absolutely essential between freez-

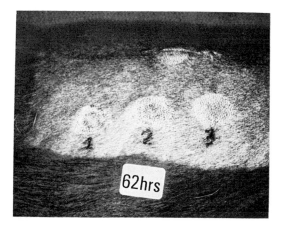

62hrs

Figure 1-15. At sixty-two hours, the three frozen sites of canine skin showed considerable edema and each site was widely excised and submitted for histological examination.

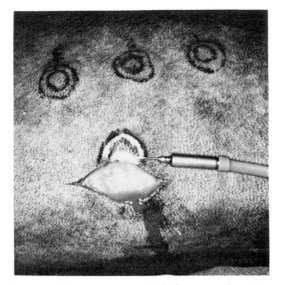

Figure 1-17. During partial thawing of canine skin, one observes the depth of the ice front below which is being monitored.

ing cycles to promulgate the greatest potential to kill cells and extend the depth and intensity of cryonecrosis.

When the surface of the canine skin appeared completely thawed following freezing, the author made an immediate incision through the center of the experimental skin site and observed a white sheet

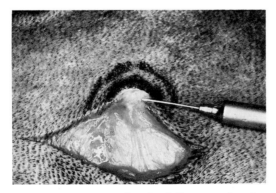

Figure 1-18. Immediately following thawing of the surface integument, one can still demonstrate and measure a frozen ice front within the epidermal-dermal plate at −10°C.

of frozen integument just beneath the surface (Figure 1-16). These observations were repeated several times with monitored temperatures below the surface of the skin (Figure 1-17), and it was noted after *complete surface* thawing that there was an underlying ice front measuring 4 mm in depth, monitored at −10°C (Figure 1-18).

This clearly indicates that even though the surface appears thawed, there is still some underlying frozen tissue which has not yet reached the phase change of −5°C.

VI. THE EFFECTS OF CRYOGENESIS OR HYPOTHERMIA

Scientists have known for three hundred years that many cells are killed when they are frozen. The effects of extremely cold temperatures upon plant and animal cells as well as cancer cells have been under investigation since the turn of the century.[26] With the use of a compound microscope and micromanipulating pipettes, Chambers and Hale[27] observed the formation of ice crystals within amoebae and the fibers of frog leg muscles. Father Luyet was an astute scientist and pioneer who may well be regarded as the founder of the modern science of cryobiology. One of his earliest writings, "Life and Death at Low Temperatures"[28] still remains a classic. The lethal effects of subzero temperatures upon erythrocytes have been extensively studied.[29, 30] More recently, electron microscopy has shed much light on the subtle changes within plant and animal cells from hypothermia.[31-35] For the serious investigator of cryobiology, the author recommends the classic text by Meryman.[36]

A. Cellular Response to Subzero Temperatures

The fundamental change in a freezing experience is the conversion of the liquid content of a cell and its interspaces into a solid state, namely ice. This phase change takes place during the period of heat exchange between the living cellular structure and the cold heat sink to which it is suddenly exposed. The more rapid the fluctuation of temperature to hypothermia, the more deleterious it is upon living cells. Also the period of thawing is extremely important. Rapid thawing, as has been pointed out earlier, will produce more survival, while slow thawing will induce a higher kill ratio.[37] Animal and plant cells undergo profound physical and chemical alterations when subjected to cryogenic temperatures. Some of the recognized and documented changes are as follows:

1. Development of extracellular ice formation.
2. Development of intracellular ice formation.
3. Cell dehydration with cell shrinkage.
4. Abnormal concentration of electrolytes within the cell.
5. Thermal shock.
6. Denaturation of lipid-protein complexes.

When plant or mammalian cells are subjected to a slow rate of cooling, ice crystals develop between cells in their interspaces. On the other hand, rapid cooling produces intracellular ice crystals and has been proven to be more lethal to the cell and far less favorable to survival. The rate of freezing in cryosurgery would be considered moderately rapid. Bear in mind that a given tissue is not homogeneous and freezing temperatures are at various temperature gradients. The surface cells are almost instantly frozen and brought to temperatures approximating that of your refrigerant, namely liquid nitrogen, −196°C, while deeper layers of cells within the given tissue reach freezing temperatures at a less rapid interval of time, and indeed do not experience the extremely low temperatures as on the surface. The extracellular ice which forms is nevertheless not innocuous, for it causes the withdrawal of water across the cell membrane contributing to cell dehydration. This phenomenon subsequently permits the marked and toxic increase of electrolytes within the cell leading to final shrinkage and collapse of its vital cell membrane. These events are incompatible with cell life.[38, 39] The entire volume or content of water within a given cell is not totally freezable. The small amount of unfrozen water, referred to as "bound water," constitutes as much as 8 to 10 percent and is

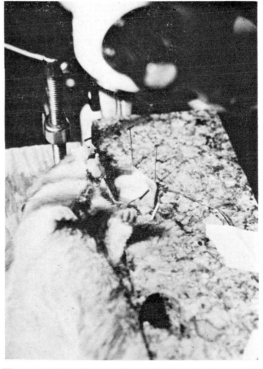

Figure 1-19. Preparation of the cheek pouch of Syrian golden hamster under a moat of a dissecting microscope with a microthermocouple needle placed within the pouch prior to freezing.

held tightly in the protein complex within the cell.[40, 41] No matter how rapid or profound the hypothermia, this bound water remains in liquid state. At temperatures below $-20°C$, approximately 90 percent of available water is totally frozen.

At this point it is important to discuss the term *eutectic freezing*. The lowest temperature at which a solution remains in a liquid state is referred to as the eutectic temperature.[10] For instance the eutectic temperature of a solution of KNO_3 is $-2.9°C$ while NaCl is $-21.8°C$. Various electrolyte solutions have varied eutectic temperatures. This is an important and a very meaningful datum. Tissues and organs have a varied mixture and content of electrolytes and therefore their eutectic zone will vary considerably. It is safe to freeze to at least $-20°C$ in order to achieve a total phase change, that is, convert most of the available water to ice. Only then can you be certain that your hypothermia will be effectual and lethal. It is interesting to note

that liquid water which has a high content of magnesium and calcium has been detected in animal tissue down to about $-70°C$.[42]

The phenomenon of sudden and profound temperature change in a biological system is referred to as thermal shock.[43] This precipitous chilling has been theorized to be incompatible to maintain the homeostasis of a living system, and thereby incompatible with life. Cryobiologists have varied opinions regarding the lethality of thermal shock. Another concept that is not too well understood is the manner by which subzero temperatures will produce denaturation of lipid-protein complexes. Lovelock[44, 45] interprets the detachment of lipids and lipid proteins from cell membranes as a consequence of the solvent action of the toxic electrolyte concentration within the cell. There is no evidence to support that enzyme activity is altered during freezing but DNA synthesis is inhibited.[46]

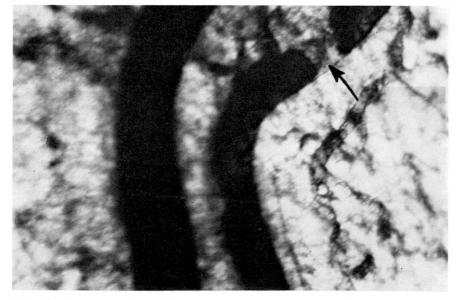

Figure 1-20. The formation of a white thrombus (blood cells and fibrin) within a venule thirty minutes after freezing the hamster cheek pouch to a temperature of $-25°C$.

B. Vascular Response to Subzero Temperatures

The continuous flow of circulation with sustained integrity of the blood vasculature is synonymous with life itself. The microvessels (the arterioles, capillaries and venules—the terminal vascular components of the circulatory system) comprise over 90 percent of blood vessels in the mammalian organism. Capillaries traverse within 25 to 50 microns from any cellular component[47] and, with this intimacy, any disturbance or impairment of its integrity will determine the survival or demise of its immediate biological milieu. In the Twentieth Century Krogh and Lewis con-

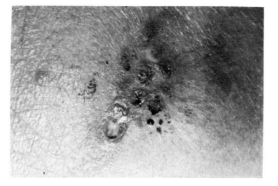

Figure 1-22. Carcinoma in situ, Bowen's disease upon the back of an eighty-year-old female patient, measuring 5 × 7 cm.

tributed much to our understanding and significance of the microcirculation.[48, 49]

Experimental evidence supports the view that some 62 percent of the capillary circulation will cease in the temperature range between +11 and +3°C, while 35 to 40 percent of blood flow will cease in arterioles and venules respectively.[50] Tissue injury secondary to vascular stasis leads to inevitable anoxemia with resulting ischemic necrosis.[51, 52]

An excellent laboratory model to study in vivo microcirculation is the cheek pouch of the golden Syrian hamster.[59] Dr. David Stone, Senior Scientist of the Worcester Foundation for Experimental Biology, and this author carried out one year's investigative study to elucidate the effects of subzero temperatures upon the microvessels of thirty-six hamster cheek pouches (Figure 1-19). Cinephotomicroscopy was employed along with careful postfreeze histological examination of the pouch at the site of direct freeze. The temperatures were carefully monitored and hypothermia was carried to various degrees ranging from 0°C to −100°C. The concentrated range, pertinent and consistent with the usual clinical setting of −20° to −30°C, were execut-

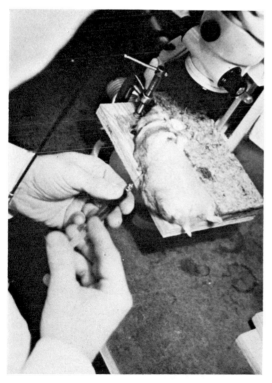

Figure 1-21. Intravenous injection of Evans blue, a vital dye of colloidal particle, to demonstrate the integrity and pathogenesis of the microvessels of the hamster cheek pouch following freezing.

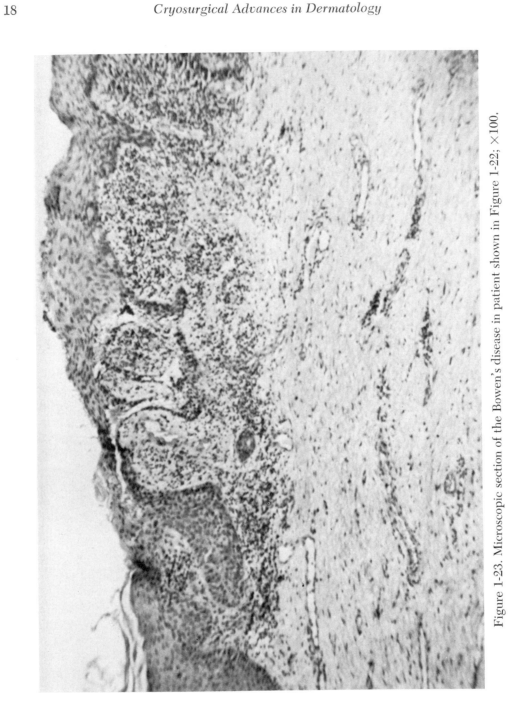

Figure 1-23. Microscopic section of the Bowen's disease in patient shown in Figure 1-22; ×100.

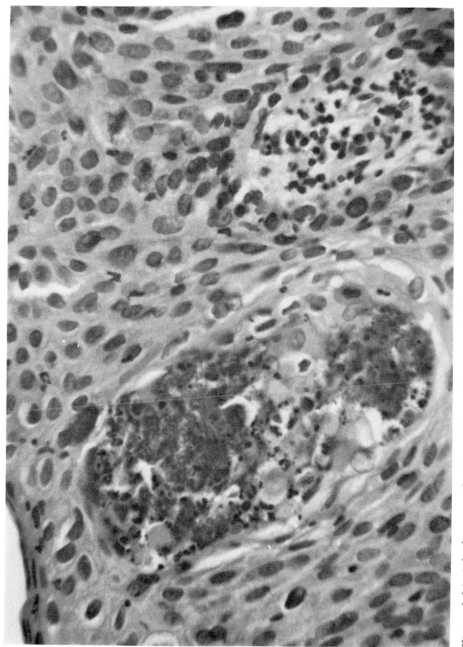

Figure 1-24. A higher magnification of the carcinoma-in-situ demonstrates marked anaplasia and hyperchromasia of the Bowenoid cells. ×430.

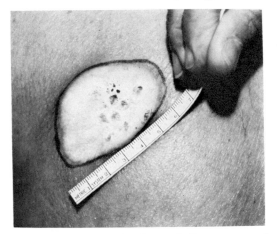

Figure 1-25. Two and one-half minutes of freezing of the carcinoma with a safe margin of 1 cm beyond its visible margin. The thaw period was three and one-half minutes.

ed. A single and double freeze-thaw cycle were also carried out. Within fifteen to twenty seconds of freezing time with a copper disc, cooled in liquid nitrogen, a temperature drop from ambient +37°C to −25°C was observed. The thaw period lasted from twenty to thirty seconds. Immediately after thawing, three concurrent and almost simultaneous phenomena were observed: (1) the momentary and initial vasoconstriction of the arterioles and venules, (2) the resumption of circulation and blood flow, (3) instantaneous and continued shower of emboli coursing through the microvessels. Within minutes vasodilation was noted which continued and progressed to its peak, forty-five minutes following the freeze-thaw experience.

Hypothermic injury appears to be greatest upon the venules, due in part to slower circulation present in their vasculature. The arterioles, whose rate of flow of blood is more rapid (almost twice that of venules), are less damaged by freezing and develop stasis a little later than venules. Capillaries manifest the least direct effects from thermal injury, but because they are

in essence the communicating bridge between arterioles and venules, their flow very quickly is arrested. Generalized stasis of all microvessels and cessation of circulation at the frozen site of the pouch were observed within twenty minutes. Platelet thrombi were later followed by white thrombi (blood cells and fibrin) (Figure 1-20) as blood flow progressively slowed with progressive attempts to adhere to the wall of the vessels. Sludging and final stasis were accomplished when a definitive thrombus had permanently occluded the vascular lumen.

In subsequent experiments, the author injected 1 percent Evans blue, a colloidal particle, into the circulation of the hamster (Figure 1-21) and observed how quickly the dye leaked out from the damaged endothelial walls of the microvessels following a freeze-thaw cycle. Formed elements of the blood and plasma proteins are confined within the blood vessels. Substances with a molecular weight of over

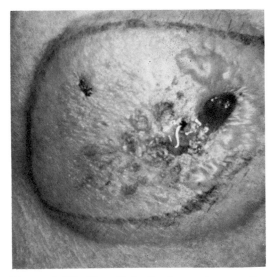

Figure 1-26. The clinically frozen tumor site, forty-five minutes following cryosurgery, demonstrates a marked degree of edema and vesicle formation.

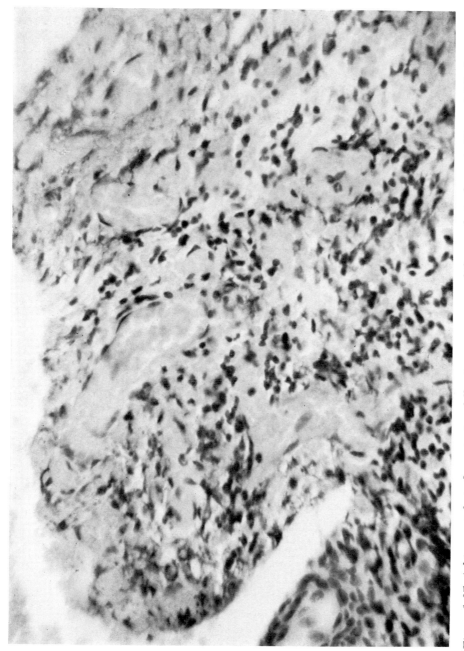
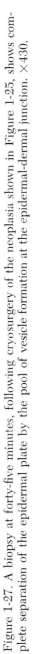

Figure 1-27. A biopsy at forty-five minutes, following cryosurgery of the neoplasia shown in Figure 1-25, shows complete separation of the epidermal plate by the pool of vesicle formation at the epidermal-dermal junction. ×430.

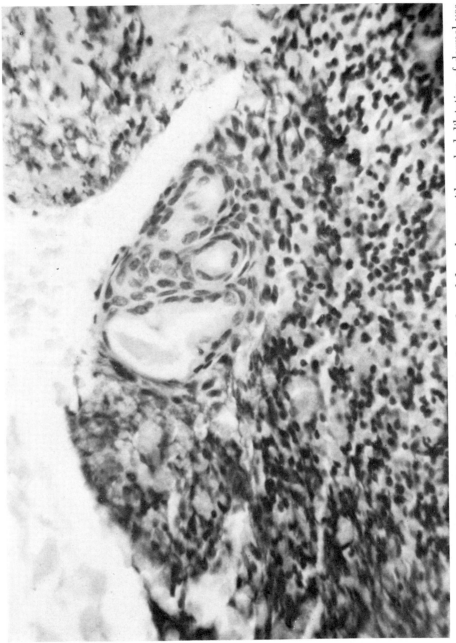

Figure 1-28. Observe the frank hemorrhage within the epidermal-dermal zone with marked dilatation of dermal vessels within forty-five minutes following cryosurgery. ×430.

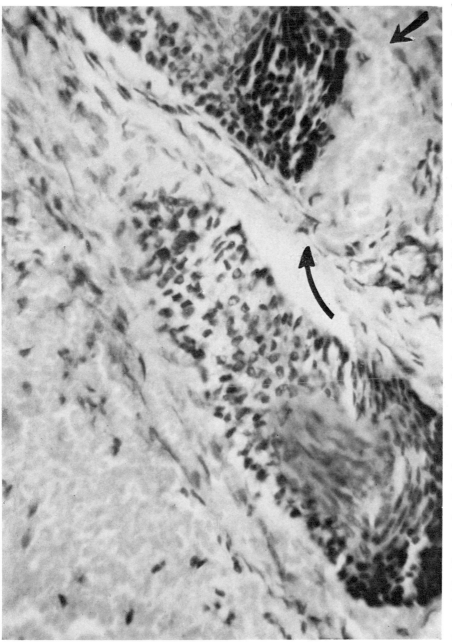

Figure 1-29. Observe the frank hemorrhage at the base of the hair follicle due to freezing; note the extravasation of red blood cells in the dermis in the upper left area of the photograph. ×430.

5000 are also confined within the vessels and only upon injury to their wall will they leak out. As in the case of the vital stain used, it was observed that prior to freezing the dye was confined within the intact circulation and only following freezing and thawing did the dye find its way through the damaged wall and leak out. With severe trauma, as with freezing, the endothelial cells of the vascular walls begin to swell and protrude inward into the lumen and finally undergo lysis.

Similar freezing studies upon hamster cheek pouch circulation have been carried out since the author's work, namely that of Dr. Herman Lenz of West Berlin.[61] Rabb and his associates[62] used electronmicroscopy to show the effects of freezing and the early damage sustained by the endothelium of the capillaries of the hamster cheek pouch following subzero temperatures. They observed ultrastructural derangement of the endothelial cells following the thaw period and progressing after one hour of observation.

The author has considered the effects of cryogenic temperatures upon the microvessels and will further discuss it later in this chapter under histopathological changes following freezing of a carcinoma in situ. Suffice to say that the blood vessel endothelium holds the key to the lethal effects of hypothermia as with frost bites and the consequences of cryosurgery resulting in cryonecrosis of benign and malignant tissues. The larger blood vessels defy freezing damage, but arterioles, venules and capillaries, which comprise 90 percent of blood vessels in the mammalian,[47] cannot escape cold injury.

VII. PATHOGENESIS OF CRYONECROSIS

The salient indication for cryosurgery is the eradication and ablation of unwant-

ed neoplasia of the skin, head and neck and the oral cavity. It is extremely important to understand the effects of subzero temperatures upon cells and tissues and most imperative to comprehend the pathogenesis upon the vasculature from which the neoplasia[13] is nurtured and proliferates.

An eighty-year-old female patient presented a malignant growth of the back of four years' duration. This tumor measured 5 x 7 cm in size (Figure 1-22), and is a recurrent growth treated earlier by a surgeon with electrocautery with repeated satellite recurrences. A skin biopsy revealed a carcinoma in situ (Bowen's Disease) (Figure 1-23). Under higher magnification one notes the nest of malignant cells with increased nuclear size and hyperchromasia close to the maturing Bowenoid cells. There is an abundance of mitotic atypical cells (Figure 1-24).

A safe margin of one cm of normal skin is outlined beyond the visible margins of the carcinoma and the tumor is frozen

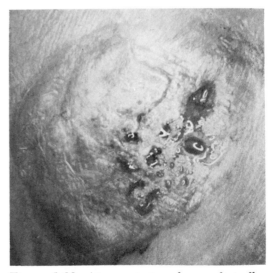

Figure 1-30. At seventy-two hours clinically, the patient exhibits a tumor site following freezing which is markedly edematous, with confluent hemorrhagic vesicles and bullae.

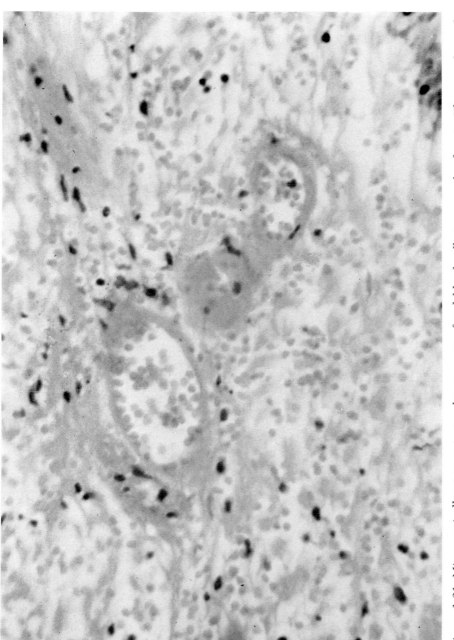

Figure 1-31. Microscopically at seventy-two hours, a sea of red blood cells traverse the dermis. The vascular endothelium of the microvessels are damaged and early formation of thrombus within the lumen is observed. ×430.

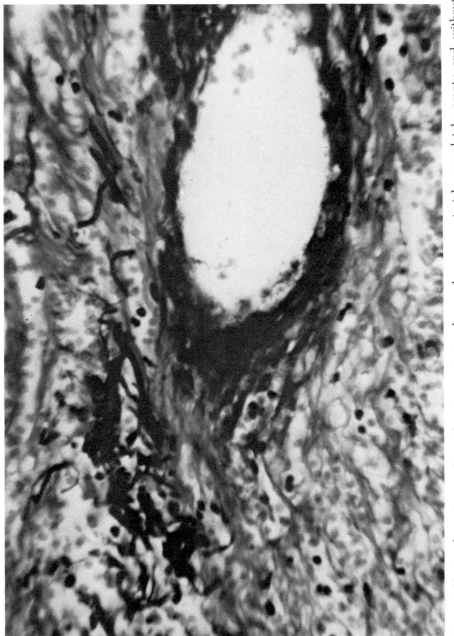

Figure 1-32. Another microscopic section at seventy-two hours shows an arteriole completely empty and without circulation with heavy deposition of fibrin within its wall.×430.

(Figure 1-25). The initial freeze time was two and one-half minutes and the complete thaw period was three and one-half minutes. A second freeze was accomplished which lasted two minutes and the final thaw time was timed at four minutes.

Within forty-five minutes, the frozen tumor site shows marked urticarial edema with serous exudation (Figure 1-26). A biopsy at this time revealed complete separation and denudation of the surface epithelium from its underlying supportive corium (Figure 1-27). The very site of the carcinoma in situ is totally ablated by means of freezing from its underlying dermal support, which now demonstrates markedly dilated and congested arterioles and venules. There is present early inflammatory response. Another section of the biopsy forty-five minutes following freezing exhibits the marked dilatation of the microvessels within the corium and extravasated red blood cells from hemorrhage at the epidermal-dermal junction of separation of the integument (Figure 1-28).

Deep within the dermis at the level of the underlying hair follicle, one observes the marked degree of edema and distortion of cells following freezing. The hair follicle architecture (Figure 1-29) shows a marked degree of hemorrhage at its base. The effects of cryogenic temperatures upon neoplasia is quite rapid and one can readily appreciate that within a period of less than one hour, marked and profound cellular and vascular alterations take place to destroy both malignant and normal tissue.

At seventy-two hours the clinical appearance of the carcinoma in situ (Figure 1-30) shows a marked degree of edema and exudation of blood from the frozen tumor site. Microscopically at this time, one notes extensive dermal hemorrhagic ne-

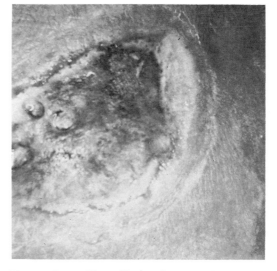

Figure 1-33. Clinically on the seventh day following cryosurgery, the frozen site of the tumor shows the early formation of an eschar.

crosis. There is a loss of vascular endothelium in the capillary walls giving the appearance of being smudged due to deposition of fibrin (Figure 1-31). Another section of dermis (Figure 1-32) shows a necrotic arteriole. Its endothelium is totally destroyed and the fibrin is saturating its wall. The vessel itself is empty and free of circulating blood and for all purposes nonfunctioning.

On the seventh day following cryosurgery, clinically (Figure 1-33) the tumor shows moderate edema with early formation of an eschar. There is still a moderate degree of blood oozing from the wound site. Microscopically, the epidermis is entirely void, having been detached as early as forty-five minutes after freezing. One observes a heavy growth of bacterial colonies upon papillary corium (Figure 1-34). Another section of the underlying dermis (Figure 1-35) shows the marked degree of hemorrhagic necrosis with extravasation of red blood cells throughout. One vessel

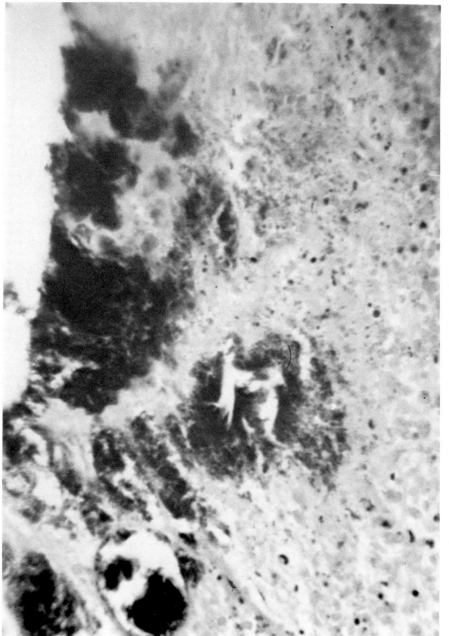

Figure 1-34. On the seventh day, histologically the dermal surface is populated with islands of bacterial colonies. ×430.

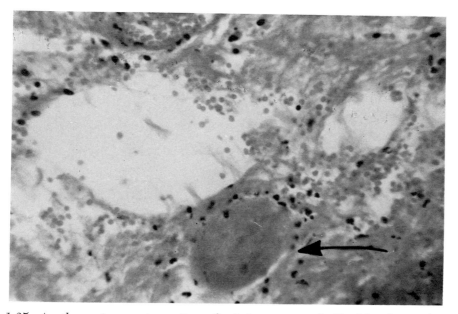
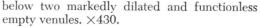

Figure 1-35. Another microscopic section of the dermis on the seventh day shows a completely hyalinized blood vessel situated just below two markedly dilated and functionless empty venules. ×430.

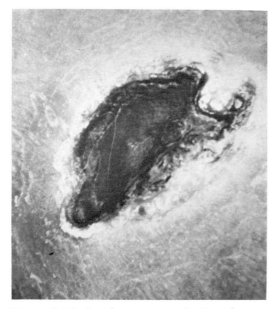

Figure 1-36. On the seventeenth day, the patient presents a thick, black adherent eschar at the site of the previously frozen carcinoma-in-situ.

shows stasis while another a hyaline thrombus which totally occludes the arteriole.

On the seventeenth day following cryosurgery, the patient presents a tumor site completely covered with an eschar (Figure 1-36). A biopsy at this time reveals a totally necrotic tissue (Figure 1-37). The dermis, void of any architecture, shows no identifiable cells nor blood vessels in this section. The pathology is one of profound ischemic gangrenous necrosis. Another microscopic section in this same period (Figure 1-38) shows a hyaline thrombus of a small artery at the junction between the corium and subcutaneous tissue. The fat cells also show damage with macrophages. There is no evidence of a reparative process on the seventeenth day following freezing, as evidenced by a total lack of circulation. A further section of the biopsy specimen demonstrates a hyaline

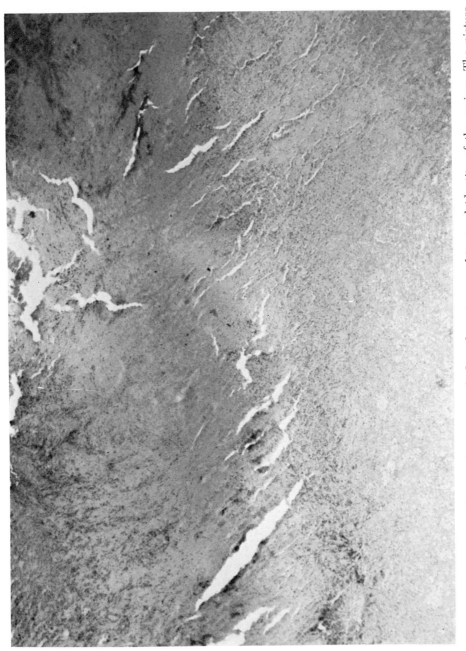

Figure 1-37. Microscopically, on the seventeenth day, there is no architectural identity of the corium. The picture is one of total and complete gangrenous necrosis. ×430.

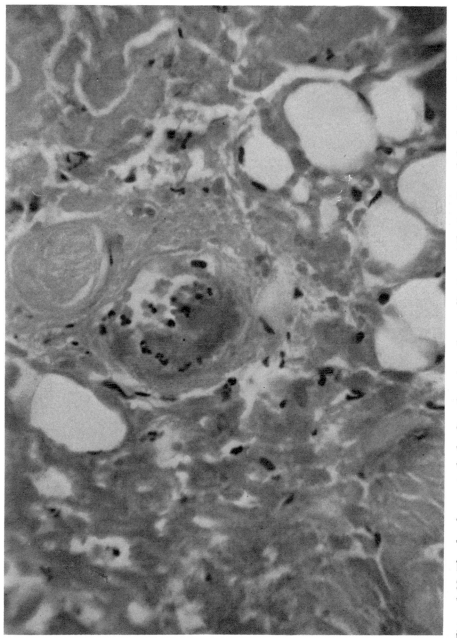

Figure 1-38. The development of a hyaline thrombus of a small artery at the junction of the dermis and subcutaneous tissue on the seventeenth day. ×430.

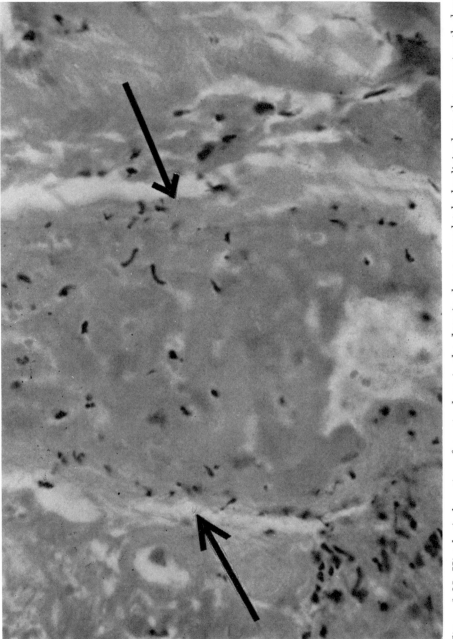

Figure 1-39. Histological section of a vein deep in the dermis almost completely hyalinized on the seventeenth day following freezing. ×430.

thrombus occluding a deep dermal vein longitudinally cut (Figure 1-39).

On the twenty-seventh day the patient presents a wound site that is partially granulating and also an area with an adherent thick black eschar (Figure 1-40). The edges of the eschar are curled up and irregular as it is being pushed upward by a wall of granulating tissue which is migrating inward from all sides. From a biopsy taken on this same day, one notes the extensive inflammatory granulation tissue repair (Figure 1-41). The collagen is well established along with elastic fibers, and throughout the granulation tissue an abundance of well-formed and well-developed blood vessels exists. There is a conspicuous cellular infiltrate with cells migrating from the vessels into the newly-formed connective tissue. The epidermis is absent in this section but is migrating centrally from the far edge of the wound site. Complete healing of the wound site is clinically observed in two months (Figure 1-42). There is some residual erythema which may well persist for six months.

In summary the effect of freezing temperatures upon normal skin and upon a malignant tumor of the skin is one of marked hemorrhagic infarction and pyknotic changes in both normal and malignant cells. As early as forty-five minutes following freezing, the epidermis bearing the carcinoma is totally detached. This immediate detachment at the dermal-epidermal junction is undoubtedly due to the large pools of vesicles developing into bullae which form soon after freezing. The transudation of fluid from the damaged microvessels and injury to the vascular endothelium due to the marked degree of hypothermia is complete and irreversible. Ischemic necrosis is then the *initial and inevitable hallmark* from hypother-

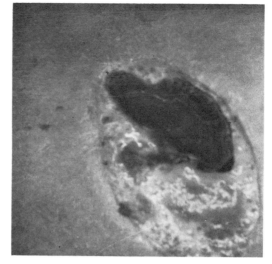

Figure 1-40. On the twenty-seventh day, the patient shows a partially adherent eschar at the frozen tumor site.

mia commencing soon after thawing. The vascular changes which then follow are stasis and development of hyaline thrombi. The gangrenous necrosis is at its peak in seventeen days leaving behind total disintegration of the frozen site with the absence of tumor, cutaneous appendages and blood vessels.

The hemorrhagic eschar which surfaces the wound site acts as a dressing to keep the underlying tissue moist. This explains why healing following cryonecrosis is superior to other methods of destruction. As granulation tissue migrates inward from the periphery of the cryonecrotic tissue, the degenerated and gangrenous center is sloughed off in degrees. Needless to mention, macrophages do their part during the period of wound healing. The cryonecrosis in this tumor site extended down to the subcutaneous tissue. This is an important consideration, particularly if one has to freeze an invasive basal cell carcinoma or an epidermoid which may infrequently ex-

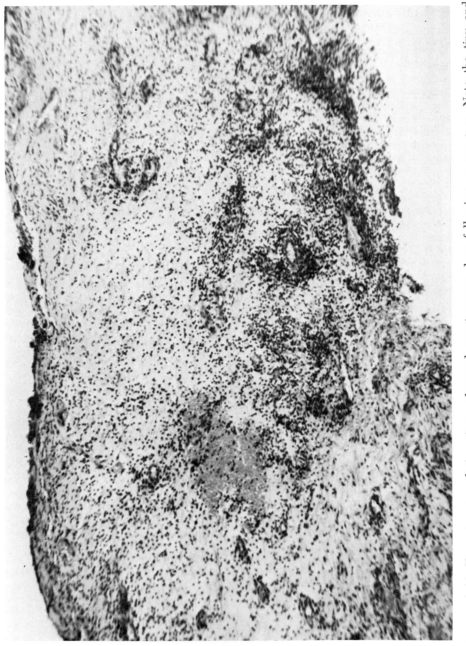

Figure 1-41. Extensive granulation tissue observed twenty-seven days following cryosurgery. Note the tiny and abundant islands of new vascular components. ×100.

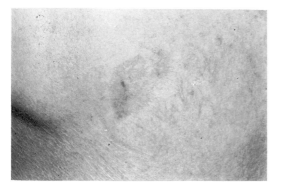

Figure 1-42. Two months following cryosurgery, the patient presents complete healing of her cutaneous carcinoma. The residual macular erythema will resolve within six months.

tend to the subcutaneous level. Although the thermal gradients or degree of hypothermia induced throughout the frozen tumor undoubtedly varies, the hemorrhagic necrosis seems microscopically quite uniform and universal.

Even nominal subzero temperatures are quite lethal to the microvessels of the skin and quickly injure their endothelium. It is for this reason then that the fundamental key to cryonecrosis as a result of hypothermia is upon the tiny blood vessels. Once damaged (as they invariably are), ruptured, and thrombosed, cancer cells, which would otherwise survive hypothermia, will undergo death from ischemic necrosis.

REFERENCES

1. Cailletet, L.: *Annales de Chemie et de Physique, XV* (5):113, 1878.
2. Pictet, R.: *Annales de Chemie et de Physique, XIII* (5):145, 1878.
3. Wroblewski, S. U. and Olszewski, K. S.: *Wiedemann's Annalen der Physik, XX:* 256, 1883.
4. Gill, W., DaCosta, J. and Fraser, J.: The control and predictability of the cryolesion. *Cryobiology,* 6 (4):342-353, 1970.
5. Henriques, F. J.: Studies of thermal injury; Automatic recording caloric applicator and skin tissue and skin surface. *Rev Sci Instrum,* 18:673-676, 1947.
6. Poppendiek, H. F., Randall, R., Bredden, J. A., Chambers, J. E. and Murphy, J. R.: Thermal conductivity measurements and predictions for biological fluids and tissues. *Cryobiology,* 3 (4): 318-327, 1967.
7. Cooper, I. S.: Cryogenic cooling or freezing of basal ganglia. *Clin Neurol,* 22: 336-339, 1962.
8. Smith, A. U.: In Harris, R. J. C. (Ed.): *Biological Applications of Freezing and Drying.* New York, Academic Press, 1954.
9. Meryman, H. T.: Personal communication from the Naval Medical Research Institute, Bethesda, Md. October 13, 1966.
10. Meryman, H. T.: The interpretation of freezing rates in biological materials. *Cryobiology,* 2 (4):165-170, 1966.
11. Farrant, J.: Some mechanisms of freezing injury. *Proc Int Congress of Cryosurgery,* 23-32, 1972.
12. Shimada, K. and Asahina, E.: Visualization of intracellular ice crystals formed in very rapid frozen cells at $-27°C$. *Cryobiology,* 12:209-218, 1975.
13. Zacarian, S. A.: *Cryosurgery of Tumors of the Skin and Oral Cavity.* Springfield, Thomas, 1973, p. 8.
14. Cowley, C. W.: Cryobiology as viewed by the engineer. *Cryobiology,* 1 (1):40-43, 1964.
15. Jagodinsky, R. V., Soanes, W. A. and Gonder, M. J. A.: Multisensor temperature probe for cryosurgery. *J Cryosurgery,* 1:222-223, 1968.
16. Benn, D. N. and Merry, J. J.: A multisensor cryogenic temperature probe. *Proc Int Cryog Eng Conf* 4:375-376, 1973.
17. Smith, J. J. and Fraser, J.: An estimation tissue damage and thermal history in the cryolesion. *Cryobiology,* 11:139-147, 1974.
18. Cooper, I. S. and Gionino, G.: In Von Leden, H. and Cahan, W. (Ed.), *Cryogenics in Surgery,* Flushing, N.Y., Med Exam, 1971.
19. Leibo, S. P., Farrant, J., Mazur, P., Hanna, M. G., Jr. and Smith, L. H.: The effects of freezing in marrow stem cell

suspensions; Interactions of cooling and warming rates in the presence of PVP, sucrose or glycerol. *Cryobiology, 6 (1)*:315-332, 1970.

20. Stone, D., Zacarian, S. A. and DiPeri, C.: Comparative studies of mammalian normal and cancer cell subjected to cryogenic temperatures in vitro. *J of Cryosurgery, 2 (1)*:43-52, 1969.

21. Myers, R. S., Hammond, W. G. and Ketcham, A. S.: Cryosurgery of Experimental Tumors. *J of Cryosurgery, 2 (5)*:225-228, 1969.

22. Neel, B. H., III, Ketcham, A. S. and Hammond, W. B.: Requisites for successful cryogenic surgery of cancer. *Arch Surg, 102*:45-48, 1971.

23. Mazur, P.: Personal communication. October 13, 1975 and December 10, 1975.

24. Leibo, S. P., Mazur, P. and Jackowski, S. C.: Factors affecting survival of mouse embryos during freezing and thawing. *Exp Cell Res, 89*:79-88, 1974.

25. Merchant, D. J., Kahn, R. H. and Murphy, H. W.: *Handbook of Cell and Organ Culture.* Minneapolis, Burgess, 1960, p. 120.

26. Molisch, H.: Unter Suchungen uber der pflanzen, Jene, Fisher, 1897, pp. 73-78.

27. Chambers, R. and Hale, H. P.: The formation of ice in protoplasm. *Proc Royal Soc Biol, 110*:336-352, 1932.

28. Luyet, B. J. and Gehinio, P. M.: Life and death at low temperatures. *Biodynamica, 3 (60)*:1945.

29. Smith, A. U., Polge, C. C. and Smiles, J.: Microscopic observations of living cells during freezing and thawing. *J Royal Micro Soc, 71*:186-195, 1951.

30. Rinfret, A. P.: In Vance, R. W. (Ed.) *Cryogenic Technology.* New York, Wiley, 1963, pp. 528-577.

31. Stowell, R. E., Young, D. E., Arnold, E. A. and Trump, B. F.: Structural, chemical, physical and functional alterations in mammalian nucleus following different conditions of freezing, storage and thawing. *Fed Proc, 24 (2)* Part III Supp (15): S115-S141, 1965.

32. Trump, B. F., Young, D. E., Arnold, E. A. and Stowell, R. E.: Effects of freezing and thawing in the structure, chemical constitution and function of cytoplasmic structures. *Fed Proc, 24 (2)*, Part III Supp (15): S144-S168, 1965.

33. Menz, L. and Luyet, B.: An electron microscope study of the distribution of ice in single muscle fibers frozen rapidly. *Biodynamica,* 8:261-294, 1961.

34. Luyet, B.: Some aspects of the process of freezing as seen at the molecular level. *J of Cryosurgery, 2 (5)*:249-256, 1969.

35. Sherman, J. K.: Freeze-thaw induced structural changes in cells. *J of Cryosurgery,* Part I, *2 (2)*:123-134, 1969; Part II, *2 (3)*:156-177, 1969; Part III, *2 (4)*:189-205, 1969.

36. Meryman, H. T. (Ed.): *Cryobiology,* New York, Acad Pr, 1966.

37. Mazur, P., Rhian, M. A. and Mahlandt, B. G.: Survival of Pasteurella Tularensis in gelatin-saline after cooling and warming at subzero temperatures. *Arch of Biochem and Biophysics, 71*: 31-51, 1957.

38. Mazur, P.: Theoretical and experimental effects of cooling and warming velocity in the survival of frozen and thawed cells. *Cryobiology, 2 (4)*:181-192, 1966.

39. Meryman, H. T.: Mechanics of freezing in living cells and tissues. *Science, 124*:124-129, 1956.

40. Meryman, H. T.: General principles of freezing and freezing injury in cellular materials, *Ann NY Acad Sci,* 85:503-509, 1960.

41. Love, M. R.: The freezing of animal tissue. In Meryman, H. T. (Ed.), *Cryobiology,* New York, Acad Pr, 1966, pp. 317-405.

42. Mazur, P. and Harkrider, M. T.: Flow of water in multicompartmented cells and tissues during freezing. *Abstracts of the Biophysical Society Meeting,* Nov., 1974, TE 2.

43. Greenfield, A. D. M. and Shepherd, J. T. and Whelan, R. F.: Cold vaso-constriction and vasodilation. *Irish J Med Sci, 309*:415-419, 1951.

44. Lovelock, J. E.: The denaturation of lipid-protein complexes as a cause of dam-

age by freezing. *Proc Royal Soc Biol,* *147*:427-433, 1957.

45. Lovelock, J. E.: Physical instability in thermal shock in red blood cells. *Nature, 173*:659-661, 1954.
46. Johnson, B. E. and Daniels, F., Jr.: Enzyme studies in experimental cryosurgery of the skin. *Cryobiology, 11*:22-232, 1974.
47. Zweifach, B. W.: *Functional Behaviour of the Microcirculation.* Springfield, Thomas, 1961.
48. Krogh, A.: *Anatomy and Physiology of the Capillaries.* New Haven, Yale, 1922.
49. Lewis, T.: *Blood Vessels of the Human Skin and Their Responses.* London, Shaw and Sons, 1947.
50. Rinfret, A. P.: Cryobiology. In R. W. Vance (Ed.), *Cryogenic Technology.* New York, Wiley, 1962, pp. 528-577.
51. Kreyberg, L.: Local freezing. *Proc Royal Soc Biol, 147*:427-439, 1957.
52. Kreyberg, L.: Stasis and Necrosis. *Scand J Clin Lab Invest,* 15 (Suppl. 71):1-9, 1936.
53. Kulka, J. P.: Experimental injuries produced by prolonged exposure to cold air. In Viereck, E. (Ed.), *Proc of the Symposia in Arctic Medicine and Biology, IV Frostbite,* Washington, Office of Technical Services, U.S. Dept of Commerce, 1964, pp. 13-31.
54. Lange, K., Weiner, D. and Boyd, L. J.: Frostbite, physiology, pathology and therapy. *N Engl J Med,* 237:383-390, 1947.
55. Mundt, E. D.: Studies in the pathogenesis of cold injury: Microcirculatory changes in tissue injured by freezing.

In Viereck, E. (Ed.), *Proc of the Symposia in Arctic Medicine and Biology, IV Frostbite.* Washington, Office of Technical Services, U.S. Dept of Commerce, 1964, pp. 51-69.
56. Quintanilla, R., Krussen, F. H. and Essex, H. E.: Studies in frostbite with special references to treatment and effect on minute vessels. *Am J Physiol,* 149-169, 1947.
57. Weatherley-White, R. C. A., Sgostrom, and Paton, V. C.: Experimental studies in cold injury, II. Pathogenesis of frostbite. *J Surg Research, 4 (1)*:17-22, 1964.
58. Zacarian, S. A.: Histopathology of skin cancer following cryosurgery. *Int Surg, 54 (4)*:255-263, 1970
59. Fulton, G. P., Jackson, R. G. and Lutz, B. R.: Cinephotomicroscopy of the normal blood circulation in the cheek pouch of the hamster. *Anat Rec, 96*:532-541, 1946.
60. Zacarian, S. A., Stone, D. and Clater, M.: Effects of cryogenic temperatures on the microcirculation in the golden hamster cheek pouch. *Cryobiology, 7 (1)*:27-39, 1970.
61. Lenz, H.: Cryosurgery of the cheek pouch of the golden syrian hamster: physical, vascular, microscopical and histological observations. *J Int Surgery, 57*:223-228, 1972.
62. Raab, J. M., Renand, M. L., Brandt, P. A. and Witt, C. W. Effect of freezing and thawing on the microcirculation and capillary endothelium of the hamster cheek pouch. *Cryobiology, 11*:508-518, 1974.

CHAPTER TWO

Cryosurgical Instrumentation

Douglas Torre, M.D.

IN INSTRUMENTATION, the trend in the past few years has been toward hand-held liquid nitrogen units build on a small vacuum insulated Dewar. A variety of units are now commercially available. No new or revolutionary principle has been involved since A. Campbell White devised a similar basic unit before 1900.[1, 2] Whitehouse described this apparatus in 1907:[3]

Liquid air is kept in what is called a "Dewar" bulb which is a double bulb of glass, one blown inside the other, the space intervening being a vacuum. The surfaces of these bulbs are silvered, and this together with the separating vacuum, retards the radiation of heat: the whole is enclosed in cotton-wool or thick felt to prevent further radiation. These retainers are made in various sizes, but for office use one containing a liter is most convenient, and this amount will last six days in ordinary room temperature during the winter. In summer it will not keep so long, unless it can be kept in an ice chest. A loose wad of

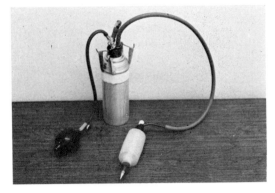

Figure 2-1b. Early model (circa 1967) portable liquid nitrogen unit built by author on vacuum insulated reservoir (Thermos).

absorbent cotton constitutes the cork. The spray is obtained by inserting a rubber cork pierced by two glass tubes in the manner employed in the ordinary laboratory wash-bottle, the mouth of the entering tube being closed by the finger.

The author has used small units built on glass of steel Thermos® Dewars since 1967. In 1972 Tromovitch devised a modification of the author's design which is being produced as the TT 32® (Physicians Products, Co.).[4] This is a portable spray unit which uses a flexible plastic tube to deliver the liquid nitrogen from the 500 cc steel Dewar to a Luer-Lok® type nozzle. The plastic tube acts as a heat exchanger, converting a portion of the liquid nitrogen to a gas phase and thus delivering to the skin lesion a liquid-gas phase combination which has less tendency to drip, run or spatter than pure droplets of liquid nitro-

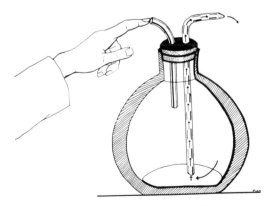

Figure 2-1a. White's "Wash Bottle" spray—circa 1900. From *J Cryosurgery*, 1:202, 1968.

gen. The unit is pressurized by repeatedly squeezing a sphygmomanometer type rubber bulb with a one-way valve with thumb-forefinger control. This is a two-hand operation and does not permit instant intermittent flow. It does act as its own reservoir and will maintain liquid nitrogen for at least eight hours, thus many patients can be treated between fillings.

The first hand-held unit clinically in-

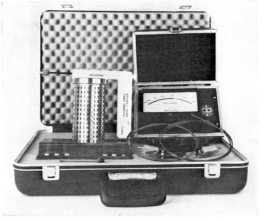

Figure 2-3. Kryospray®—Brymill Corporation, 30 Lafayette Square, Vernon, CT 06066
Type of unit—one-hand portable
Reservoir—250 cc stainless steel cannister
Holding time—less than fifteen minutes
Pressurization—self-pressurizing
Intermittent spray control—trigger type instantaneous
Luer-Lok fittings—no
Heat exchanger—metal tube between reservoir and nozzle
Other equipment available—pyrometers (single or double) usually sold with unit; cryoprobes optional
Cost—

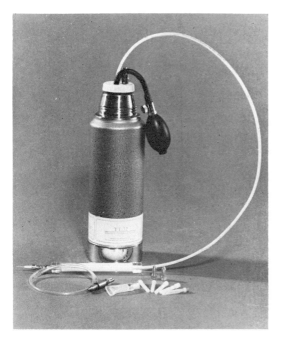

Figure 2-2. TT 32®—Physicians Products, Inc., Box 44, Milbrae, CA 94030.
Type of unit—two-hand portable
Reservoir—500 cc stainless steel vacuum Dewar
Holding time—8+ hours
Pressurization—self-pressurizing + bulb
Intermittent spray control—not instantaneous; lag time on-off by "sphygmomanometer" type valve
Luer-Lok fittings—yes
Heat exchanger—plastic tube from reservoir to handle
Other equipment available—optional cryoprobes and acne spray tip
Cost—approximately $200.00 for basic unit

vestigated by Zacarian and commercially available (1967) is the Brymill Kryospray.®[5] This is built on a noninsulated metal reservoir and has to be filled shortly before use as the liquid nitrogen evaporates in a short time following filling. The only heat exchanger in the delivery system is the short metal line between the intake tube and the nozzle, so almost pure nitrogen is delivered through the nozzle. Drip and spatter is minimized by selecting the smallest size nozzle opening (several size interchangeable tips are provided) and intermittent spray. A trigger type control makes intermittent spray easy for this one-hand type instrument.

The Zacarian C 21® unit manufactured

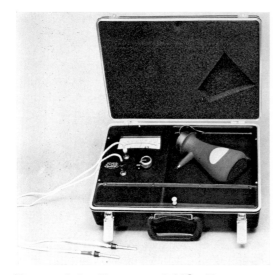

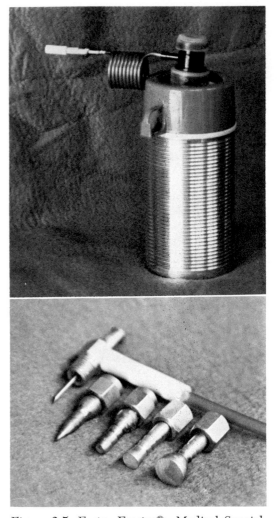

Figure 2-4. Zacarian C-21®—Frigitronics, Inc., 770 River Road, Shelton, CT 06484
Type of unit—one-hand portable
Reservoir—250 cc plastic flask
Holding time—less than thirty minutes
Pressurization—self-pressurized
Intermittent spray control—trigger type instantaneous
Luer-Lok fittings—yes
Heat exchanger—coil in base of unit
Other equipment available—usually sold as fitted kit which includes pyrometer and two thermocouple-tipped needle assemblies; jig template for desired depth insertion of thermocouples optional; cryoprobes also optional
Cost—approximately $800.00 for kit

by Frigitronics since 1969 is a one-hand portable trigger-activated unit built with a semi-insulated plastic reservoir allowing for only short term storage (less than thirty minutes). This unit has a built-in heat exchanger and has proved excellent in treating skin malignancies.[6]

The Foster Froster® designed by Dr. Ronald Lubritz and Foster Johns in 1974 and manufactured by Medical Specialties Company[7] is a light one-hand unit built on a 250 cc glass vacuum-insulated Dewar. A copper-coil heat exchanger in the delivery

Figure 2-5. Foster Froster®—Medical Specialties, Inc., 3214 Howard Avenue, New Orleans, LA 70113
a. Unit with "No Drip" tip attached
b. Cryoprobes
Type of unit—one-hand portable
Reservoir—250 cc glass vacuum Dewar
Holding time—8+ hours
Pressurization—self-pressurizing
Intermittent spray control—instantaneous by finger over exhaust in cap
Luer-Lok fittings—yes
Heat exchanger—copper coil
Other equipment available—set of 2, 5, 7, 9 mm cryoprobes optional
Cost—less than $100.00 for basic unit

system produces a gas-liquid mixture at the nozzle with minimal drip or spatter. This unit reverts back to the original White concept of using the finger to occlude the vent from the liquid cryogen reservoir so that pressure produced by the gas from the liquid "boiling" will force liquid through the nozzle. "Boiling" of the liquid is speeded up by tilting the reservoir so that liquid contacts the warmer wall of the Dewar above the liquid level. Easy intermittent control is attained with this simplest and least expensive apparatus. Careful handling is a must as the reservoir is glass and thus fragile, and the finger which is used to occlude the vent may be frozen if the unit is carelessly tilted too far lat-

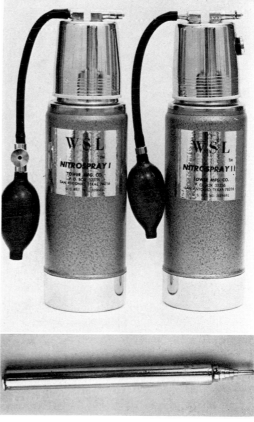

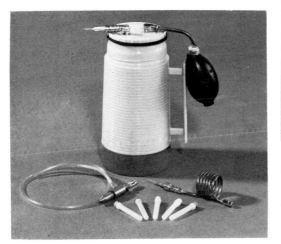

Figure 2-6. MMFI®—Physicians Products Inc., Box 44, Milbrae, CA 94030
Type of unit—one-hand portable
Reservoir—250 cc glass vacuum Dewar
Holding time—8+ hours
Pressurization—self-pressurized + bulb
Intermittent spray control—instantaneous by thumb of vent in bulb
Luer-Lok fittings—yes
Heat exchanger—copper coil which fits into Luer-Lok nozzle
Other equipment available—acne spray tip + cryoprobes optional
Cost—$100.00 for basic unit

Figure 2-7. WSL-Nitrospray I and II®— Tower Manufacturing Company, P.O. Box 32336, San Antonio, TX 78216
a. Nitrospray I: two-hand model; Nitrospray II: two-hand model
b. Heat exchanger nozzle
Type of unit—hand-held portables
Reservoir—500 cc stainless steel vacuum Dewar
Holding time—8+ hours
Pressurization—self-pressurizing + bulb
Intermittent spray control—instantaneous by finger occlusion of opening near bulb (Nitrospray I) or on head (Nitrospray II)
Luer-Lok fittings—yes
Heat exchanger—metal tubular insert at nozzle
Other equipment available—acne spray tip optional
Cost—approximately $150.00

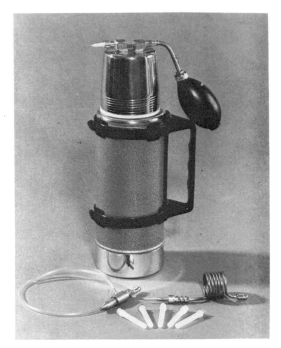

Figure 2-8. MMF II®—Physicians Products Inc., Box 44, Milbrae, CA 94030
Type of unit—one-hand portable
Reservoir—500 cc stainless steel vacuum Dewar
Holding time—8+ hours
Pressurization—self-pressurizing + bulb
Intermittent spray control—instantaneous by thumb control of vent in bulb
Luer-Lok fittings—yes
Heat exchanger—copper coil which fits into Luer-Lok nozzle
Other equipment available—acne spray tip and cryoprobe
Cost—$200.00 for basic unit

erally in an attempt to build up more pressure.

The MFF I® manufactured by Physicians Products, Inc. and designed by Tromovitch is another inexpensive hand-held model built on a 250 cc glass Dewar base. Cryoprobes are optional for this unit as well as the Foster Froster.

The WSL Nitrospray I® unit made by Tower Manufacturing Co. is based on a

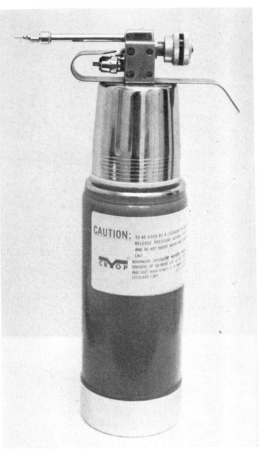

Figure 2-9. Cryop GCS-72®—Gilmore Liquid Air Company, 9503 East Rush Street, S. El Monte, CA 91733
Type of unit—hand-held unit
Reservoir—500 cc stainless steel vacuum Dewar
Holding time—8+ hours
Pressurization—self-pressurized to operating pressure of 10 PSI
Intermittent spray control—levered "clarinet" type valve independent of main screw type throttle valve
Luer-Lok fittings—yes
Heat exchanger—metal tube between reservoir and nozzle
Other equipment available—6 RWS-LR 10 liquid nitrogen withdrawal system (a 10 liter Dewar with withdrawal device) optional
Cost—$300.00 for basic unit

500 cc steel Dewar and delivers a liquid nitrogen spray when the vent near an attached rubber bulb is closed off with the finger. Intermittent spray is readily obtained. It is used as a two-hand unit, with the bulb and cut-off vent being operated by one hand and the unit held with the other. A modification, Nitrospray II®, has the vent on the cap so that the unit can be operated as a one-hand unit. When introduced no heat exchanger was provided, so the liquid was delivered to the skin in droplets which ran and spattered. A heat-exchanger spray tip is now available and can be inserted in the Luer-Lok fitting. This has improved performance in regard to spatter and drip.

The MMF II® produced by Physicians Products, Inc. is quite similar but provides an insertable copper coil heat exchanger and has its vent located in the bulb.

The Cryop GCS 73® apparatus uses a 500 cc steel Dewar for a reservoir and is the only hand-held unit which depends on constant pressure within the system to force out the liquid nitrogen on demand when the valve is turned on. Therefore a few minutes waiting period is necessary between filling the reservoir and self-pressurization to occur so that the 10 PSI operating pressure is attained. At this pressure the boiling point of nitrogen in the tank is at a temperature warmer than the one atmosphere boiling point of liquid nitrogen. Thus when the liquid is sprayed on the skin at one atmosphere it vaporizes more readily, so that drip and spatter are greatly lessened. This PSI pressure allows use of smaller caliber nozzles, with 19 and 22 gauge needle openings being used for most procedures. A clarinet-type rocker valve allows finger tip control for intermittent spray, but the cut off is not as instantaneous or reliable as with the other non-pressurized units, and the valve is somewhat awkward to use. Another minor drawback is that this apparatus becomes quite cold on continuous use. It is a more complicated apparatus to master than the other units and more subject to malfunction, such as freeze-up. The relative absence of

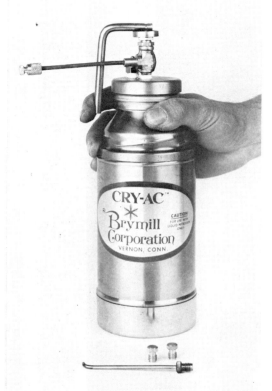

Figure 2-10. Cry-Ac®—Brymill Corporation, 30 Lafayette Square, Vernon, CT 06066
Type of unit—one-hand portable
Reservoir—stainless steel vacuum Dewar
Holding time—information not obtainable at time of publication
Pressurization—self-pressurizing
Intermittent spray—instantaneous by trigger-like finger control
Luer-Lok fittings—no
Heat exchanger—metal tube from reservoir to nozzle
Other equipment available—extension nozzle
Cost—not rendered

Figure 2-11. CE 8®—Frigitronics, Inc., 770 River Road, Shelton, CT 06484

a. Floor standing unit

b. Cryoprobes and intermittent spray tips

c. Luer-Lok adapter and spray tips

Type of unit—table or floor standing unit with handle connected to reservoir by flexible tube

Reservoir—17, 25, 31 liter steel or aluminum vacuum Dewar

Holding time—two to eight weeks

Pressurization—immersion heater

Intermittent spray control—levered "ethyl chloride" type nozzles (optional equipment)

Luer-Lok fittings—yes

Heat exchanger—plastic tube between reservoir and handle

Other equipment available—"Dermatology Kit" cryoprobes consist of 12.7 mm round tip, pointed tip and 3 and 5 mm flat; other size probes including a "door knob" type and insulated extension type also available; acne spray tip, pyrometer, and special wheeled carrier optional

Cost—approximately $1000.00 for basic unit

From *J Cryosurgery*, 1:206, 1968.

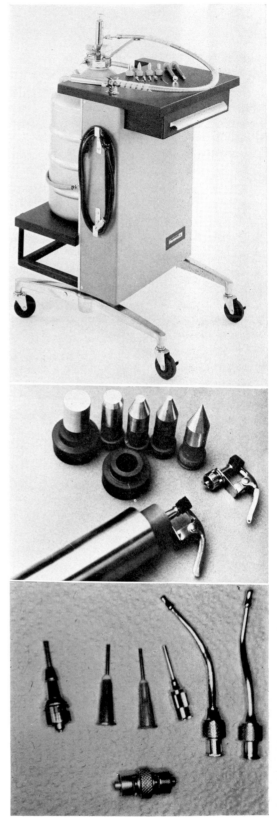

drip and spatter and the steady pressure however, are definite assets.

A more recent model introduced is the Cry-Ac® by Brymill which is a one-hand trigger-operated unit built on a stainless steel vacuum reservoir.

The Frigitronics CE 8® is the standard unit for dermatological use. It is the present successor of the original liquid nitrogen spray-cryoprobe unit, the Cryoderm® system which the author built in 1965.[8, 9] It has the distinct advantage of an incorporated long term storage system for liquid nitrogen so that it has to be refilled only at two to six week intervals (depending on type and size of reservoir and frequency of use). The liquid nitrogen is held in 17, 25, or 31 liter Dewars which can be free standing or mounted on a cart or caster apparatus for mobility. The liquid nitrogen is kept under approximately 8-10 PSI pressure and is delivered to the skin through a hand piece which accepts sprays nozzles (Luer-Lok fittings) or cryoprobes. The hand piece is connected to the tank by a flexible plastic hose, which acts as a heat exchanger. Intermittent spray is obtained only by use of special levered nozzles (similar to those on the old style ethyl chloride spray bottles). This intermittent spray system is not as satisfactory as those employed by the new hand-held units. Using cryoprobes with this unit, however, is more convenient than with the hand-held units.

The Frigitronics CE 4® unit is a closed system liquid nitrogen apparatus with cryoprobes that can be chilled to any temperature down to −195°C. This is a direct lineal descendent of the original liquid nitrogen apparatus devised by Dr. Irving Cooper and first described in 1961.[10] It is expensive and more suitable to the major surgical specialties but is used by some noted cryosurgeons including Dr. Andrew Gage for treatment of malignant skin tumors.

Brymill also makes a heavy duty liquid nitrogen unit (Model SP-5®) for general surgical use.

The most recent portable cryosurgical unit, the C-76 is described by Zacarian in this volume, end of Chapter 5.

Liquid Nitrogen Storage Devices

Liquid nitrogen can be stored in any size vacuum-insulated Dewar. A wide choice is available. Small (under 10 liters) portable Dewars are satisfactory if a supply source is close by and available (as at university centers). However for most office use, where the liquid nitrogen is delivered by commercial companies (usually welding supply outfits), larger tanks are advised.

Storage vessels of 15 to 35 liter capacity are the most practical as these can be refilled economically at two to six week intervals. Storage Dewars are rated by the daily evaporation rate (the rate at which the liquid nitrogen vaporizes without being used). A daily evaporation rate of a 25 liter tank having an evaporation of 0.25 liters per day would thus evaporate the entire 25 liters in one hundred days or have a "holding time" of one hundred days. In general the lower the evaporation rate the more expensive the initial cost but the less expensive the yearly cost of liquid nitrogen.

For example, Minnesota Valley Engineering supplies a 34 liter (Apollo S × 34®) Dewar for approximately $350.00 and a cheaper 30 liter laboratory model (Lab 30®) for $250.00. The more expensive model has a static evaporation rate of 0.18 liters per day and the cheaper model a rate of 0.32 liters per day. The more expensive unit would lose 66 liters per year and the cheaper unit 117 liters. At $1.00 a liter cost, this difference would be $50.00 a year. At the end of the two year warranty period costs would be equal. If the Dewars were used over a longer period (as expected) the *more expensive* unit would be the better buy.

Ice (sometimes in chunks as large as hail) can form from water vapor entering storage Dewars during refills so that from time to time they should be completely emptied and turned upside down before filling.

Withdrawal Devices

Transferring liquid nitrogen from a storage facility to a treatment unit can be accomplished by manual pouring from the storage device to the treatment unit, by dipping into the storage unit or by a "withdrawal device." These withdrawal devices work on the principle of nitrogen gas pressure within the system forcing liquid nitrogen through the nozzle (withdrawal tube). Some are self-pressurizing and one must wait after insertion of the device for continual evaporation to build up sufficient pressure to cause liquid flow.

Some devices make allowance for a hand or foot pump to be used to force atmospheric air into the device and increase the pressure. Attaching a nitrogen gas tank to the device will also solve the pressure problem.

Another solution for pressure on demand is to include a small immersion heater in the system. When pressure is needed the heater is turned on and liquid nitrogen is vaporized.

Pyrometers

For measuring temperatures beneath the skin surface during the cryosurgical procedure, it is necessary to have thermocouple-tipped hypodermic needles and a pyrometer. The needle probe assemblies should be capable of sterilization by autoclave or dry heat so that they be sterilized before use on each patient protecting not only against transfer of pyogenic organisms but also viral agents including the one responsible for hepatitis. These needle probes may be obtained in several diameters and lengths. For use with the Frigitronics template a one inch length #24 gauge needle is used, and this is the usual size for clinical dermatological use.

In research it is usual to calibrate the pryometer before each use, and in clinical practice periodic calibration is recommended, although it does not have to be done with each use.

With pyrometers having a range from $-200°C$ to $+50°C$ calibration is simple. Inserting the needle into liquid nitrogen checks the down side at $-196°C$, into ice/water mixture checks the $0°C$ point, and normal body temperature ($37°C$) can be used for an approximate upside check. With a pyrometer having a range of $-75°C$ to $+95°C$, a down side check has to be made with fluorocarbon liquids such as Freon 12.[11] This liquid is available in 1 pound cans with dispensing kits from auto supply stores (used for car air conditioners) or as Cryokwik® in 12 ounce siphon dispenser

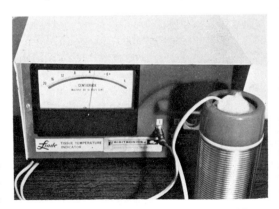

Figure 2-12. Using Freon 12 to calibrate pyrometer.

cans. A small amount of the freon is sprayed into the bottom of a small Dewar (250 cc glass thermos is satisfactory) and the thermocouple needle inserted into the liquid. A cotton ball is placed in the neck of the Dewar and the liquid is allowed to boil until a stable temperature is reached. This is to ensure that the liquid will reach its listed boiling point, which is approximately $-30°C$ at one atmosphere pressure of the pure gas overlying the liquid. The boiling point will be lower (due to Dalton's Law of partial pressures) if air or another gas is mixed with the freon vapor. With a pyrometer having a range to $-100°C$ the downside check can be made with alcohol-solid carbon dioxide mixture (temperature approximately $-80°C$) as well as freons.

Jigs (Templates)

Brodthagen described devices for emplacing thermocouple tipped hypodermic needles at specific depths beneath the skin in 1961,[12] and the author has been using circular nylon jigs for this purpose since 1966,[9] but the only device commercially available is the template modified by Zacarian[6] and manufactured by Frigitronics. This is a small plastic triangular device with three tubular channels allowing placement of the thermocouple at 3, 4, and 5

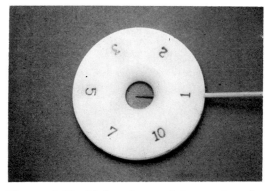

Figure 2-13. Nylon jig used by author for monitoring subsurface temperatures.

mm beneath the center of the lesion being treated.

Alternate Cyrogens

Liquid nitrogen has become the standard cryogen in dermatology because it is efficient, relatively inexpensive, nontoxic, and nonflammable, and because of its low temperature is capable of treating *all* dermatological lesions satisfactorily. *Liquid air* has properties almost identical to liquid nitrogen and was the original dermatological cryogen used by Dr. White in 1899.[1] However it is not as easily available at this time as liquid nitrogen, so is not used. *Liquid oxygen* also has similar characteristics to liquid nitrogen and was used in the 1920's, '30's and '40's,[14] but although readily available at this time is not used because of its flammability.

The chief drawback to liquid nitrogen, liquid air and liquid oxygen is lack of "storability." These cryogens continually evaporate and must be replaced even if not used for treating skin lesions. *Liquid helium*, the coldest of available cryogens (and from this standpoint the ideal cryogen) also shares this drawback, and is also much more expensive, more difficult to handle and not as efficient a cryogen as liquid nitrogen.

Storable cryogens are available. *Carbon dioxide* has been used since about 1905.[15] It is a limited cryogen as its coldest obtainable temperature is $-79°C$. This is used as a solid "stick" or mixed with alcohol, ether, or acetone as a "slush." Solid carbon dioxide can be purchased as nonstorable slabs and fashioned by the user to forms suitable for treatment, or purchased in storable carbon dioxide liquid-containing cylinders yielding particles which are compressed into proper form just before use. Many devices have been invented producing these "forms."[16] The most commonly

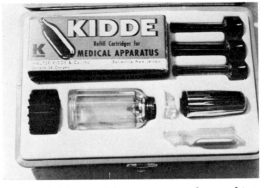

Figure 2-14a. Kidde apparatus for making carbon dioxide pencils.

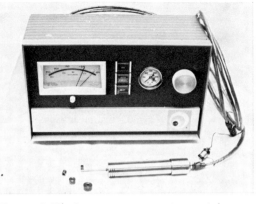

Figure 2-15. Argon gas apparatus, not in production. From *J Cryosurgery*, 1:205, 1968.

used apparatus is that manufactured by Kidde® which uses small disposable cylinders of CO_2.[17] Carbon dioxide is suitable for treating benign lesions but not malignancies as the cold produced ($-79°C$) is incapable of producing a $-25°C$ isotherm more than 2-3 mm deep using the usual treatment techniques.

Utilizing the Joule-Thompson effect, *nitrogen gas* and *argon gas* (which are storable) are capable of producing cold comparable to liquid nitrogen and the author has experimented with such apparatus both in cryoprobe and spray form.[9] However these pieces of equipment were never marketed because of the inefficiency of the cooling capacity compared to liquid nitrogen. The unit cost per minute of freezing was comparable only when a few cases per week were treated, which is not the case in the usual dermatological office where cryo-

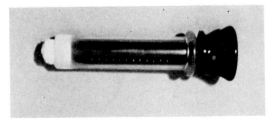

Figure 2-14b. Carbon dioxide pencil made with Kidde apparatus.

surgery is the treatment of choice for many patients daily.

Nitrous oxide is a storable cryogen used by several manufacturers in producing cryosurgical apparatus for use by physicians other than dermatologists. Several of these machines can be used for treating a limited range of skin lesions, and at least one apparatus (manufactured by Dynatech) has been marketed as being designed specifically for dermatological use. One limiting factor with nitrous oxide is that the coldest temperature attainable is about $-89°C$. Cryoprobes furnished with the systems are capable of treating many benign skin lesions. The pointed probe is very handy for treating small flat warts, milia and sebaceous hyperplasia. Using nitrous oxide in a spray technique, however, has a serious drawback. Due to the nature of this cryogen, while spraying the liquid forms small crystals of solid nitrous oxide, which either pile up on the treated site like a white "snow cone" or fly off in all directions with the secondary hazard of freezing areas outside of the target zone. With spraying, the depth of penetration of cold is also limited so that only a superficial effect can be obtained. Use of this spray should be limited to very superficial le-

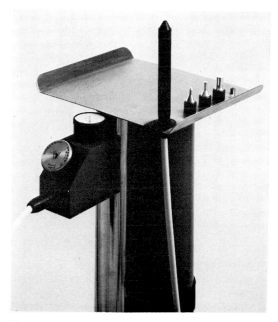

Figure 2-16. Dermadyne DNB-6510®—Dynatech Cryomedical Company, 90 Cambridge Street, Burlington, MA 01803

Type of unit—floor model portable nitrous oxide apparatus

Reservoir—6 lb 7 oz refillable "E" bottles

Holding time—indefinite

Intermittent spray control—special handle with lever control

Other equipment available—2, 5, and 10 mm cryoprobes are provided with unit

sions (such as thin actinic keratoses) or acne lesions.[17]

Fluorocarbon liquids have been used in dermatological practice since 1955 when Freon 114 was advocated by Wilson, Lui-

kart and Ayers for hardening the skin prior to dermabrasion.[18] These same authors also warned against using Freon 12 for this use because of the possibility of deep necrosis with use of this cryogen.[19]

Fluorocarbons have been utilized in cryoprobe type equipment used in other medical specialties (particularly ophthalmology),[20] but use as a spray-on cryogen instead of liquid nitrogen was not advocated until the author's publications in 1975.[17, 21] Several fluorocarbon liquids (Freon 12, Freon 22, Freon 13 and combinations of these liquids with other fluorocarbons) are suitable for dermatological cryosurgery. They are inexpensive, storable and easily portable. Temperature ranges down to about $-90°C$ can be obtained by spraying these liquids on the skin (see Table 2-I). These temperatures obtained are lower than the listed boiling point of the liquid because of Dalton's Law, which states that in a mixture of gases the pressure of the mixture is the sum of the individual pressures (partial pressures) exerted by each gas. Each gas behaves independently as though it alone occupies the space. Sprayed on the skin surface the fluorocarbon gas is mixed with air—thus giving a fluorocarbon pressure less than one atmosphere and a boiling point lower than the listed value. Using a blower or vacuum system lowers the pressure (and working temperature) even more.

TABLE 2-I

FREON REFRIGERANTS

Freon	Chemical Name	Formula	Boiling Point at One Atmosphere	Low Temp. by Spraying (Approx.)
114	Dichlorotrifluoroethane	$C_2Cl_2F_2$	$+ 3.8°C$	$-33°C$
12	Dichlorodifluoromethane	CCl_2F_2	$-27.8°C$	$-60°C$
22	Chlorodifluoromethane	$CHCl_2F_2$	$-40.8°C$	$-70°C$
13	Chlorotrifluoromethane	$CClF_3$	$-81.5°C$	$-90°C$

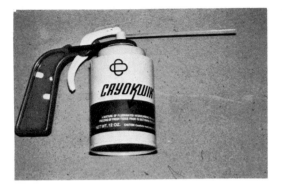

Figure 2-17. Freon 12 siphon dispenser can: Cryokwik.

With fluorocarbon cryogens the great majority of benign skin lesions can be treated as effectively if not as efficiently or as safely as with liquid nitrogen.

Freon 114 is suitable for hardening the skin for dermabrasion and for superficial "peeling" of the skin. Freons 12 and 22 seem to have the highest cryosurgical potential as to cost, availability and freezing efficiency.

Freon 12 is suitable for treating acne pits and various superficial lesions. Freon 22 is suitable for treating all types of lesions except deep, malignant tumors. Freon 13 has the coldest temperature and fastest freezing time of the fluorocarbons tested but technical and cost drawbacks are present.

Freon 114 is available as Frigiderm® in 14 oz push-button cans. Freon 12 is available in 1 lb can and 30 lb disposable cannister, and as Cryokwik in a 12 oz syphon can with push-button dispenser. Freon 22 is available in 1 and 2 lb cans and a 25 lb disposable dispenser. Freon 13 is available only in heavy refillable cyclinders containing 9 or 25 lbs.

Instrumentation, except for the push-button type can dispensers of Freon 114 (Frigiderm) and Freon 12 (Cryokwik), is "do-it-yourself." Some equipment including hoses can be obtained from refrigeration supply or repair shops. The liquid must be valved down to a fine spray equivalent to that obtained by use of a #30 hypodermic needle.

Freons are not "inert" in the true sense and their potential toxicity (particularly cardiac toxicity) should be considered before they are used. Fluorocarbons are currently under study for their possible depletion of our atmospheric ozone layer.

"Do-It-Yourself-Equipment"

For limiting the lateral spread of cryogens sprayed on the skin surface, collimating devices are sometimes necessary. Metal, plastic, rubber, or wood in the shape of funnels, cones, collars, tubes or fenestrated spoons may be used.[22] Some that the author has found useful are: (1) neoprene cones, (2) pressure rings, and (3) tubular constricting devices.

Neoprene Cones

For confining surface spray area, hollow truncated neoprene cones originally designed as filter adapters are quite useful. These come in six sizes (see Table 2-II), and additional sizes can be easily made by cutting off or grinding the available cones to different inner diameters. An inner diameter cone of 8 mm is particularly useful in treating epitheliomas. This cone is made by shortening a #1 cone which has an original inner diameter of 5 mm. When these cones are used with liquid nitrogen spray for treatment of epitheliomas, the cone which most closely surrounds the epithelioma is selected, the edge is moistened with water or water soluble sterile lubricating jelly (KY jelly) and firmly applied to the skin. Spray is directed into the cone and continued intermittently, until a frozen

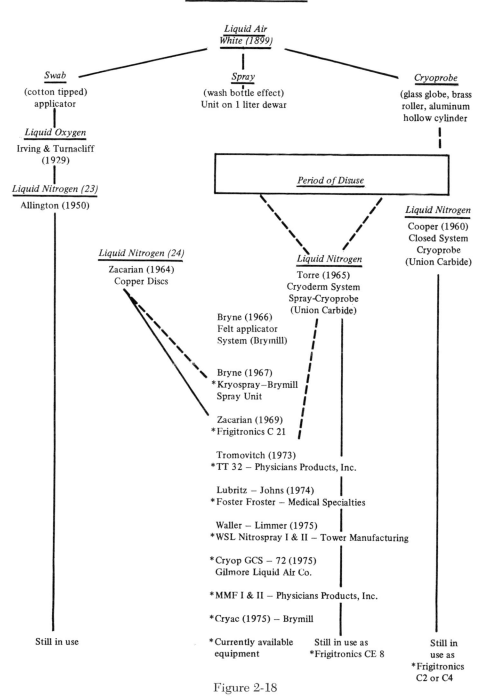

GENEALOGY OF CRYOSURGICAL DEVICES

USING LIQUID NITROGEN

Figure 2-18

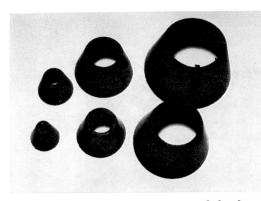

Figure 2-19a. Neoprene cones used for limiting surface application of spray.

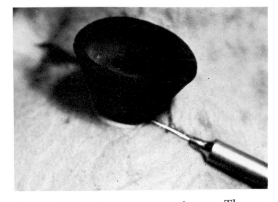

Figure 2-19c. Neoprene cone in use. Thermocouple needle inserted to correlate depth temperature with lateral spread of ice ball.

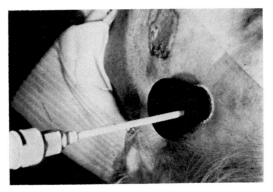

Figure 2-19b. Spraying into neoprene cone.

collar appears on the skin surface outside the cone. This will produce an ice ball surrounding the epithelioma sufficient to treat those of usual depth.

Using #1 and #2 cones (2.5 mm thick walls) with a lateral spread of freeze of 3 to 3½ mm the central depth of the ice ball will be about 5 mm and the depth of the −25°C isotherm at approximately the 3 mm level. For deeper lesions continued spraying until a greater lateral spread of freeze (and consequently deeper ice ball) is attained is recommended.

Pressure Ring

The Walsh pressure ring which is available in 8, 10, and 12 mm size, either in

bare or insulated form, has several uses. When freezing a lesion which has been biopsied prior to the freezing, it is useful to compress the surrounding tissue to (1) stop bleeding, or (2) prevent nitrogen gas from spreading subcutaneously. This is particularly helpful in treating epitheliomas around the eyes and on the forehead or nose. Another use of this instrument is as a collimating device to limit lateral spray. Disposable foam rubber Dr. Scholl's® pads can be used with the 8 mm ring to limit the surface application to 5 mm when treating small lesions. If openings smaller than 5 mm are desired, small

TABLE 2-II

NEOPRENE (FILTER ADAPTERS) CONES
Thomas # 4584—To5*

Size	Inner Diameter	Outer Diameter	Wall Thickness
1	5 mm	10 mm	2.5 mm
2	11 mm	16 mm	2.5 mm
3	16 mm	22 mm	3 mm
4	22 mm	28 mm	3 mm
5	31 mm	37 mm	3 mm
6	38 mm	46 mm	4 mm

Taper angle is 17°.
* Arthur H. Thomas, P.O. Box 779, Philadelphia, Pennsylvania.

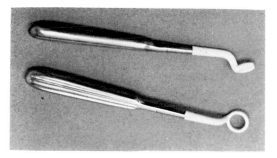

Figure 2-20a. Walsh pressure rings.

rubber or neoprcne "washers" can be used with the 8 mm ring.

Tubular Constricting Devices

Disposable syringe barrels make simple lateral limiting devices for surface application of sprayed cryogens. This type of device is particularly useful with the hand-held devices (such as the Foster Froster) which offer easy intermittent flow-control and a Luer-Lok nozzle. The barrel is sawed off near the plunger insertion end. A 16 or 17 gauge 1½ inch needle is inserted in reverse through the needle attachment end and fixed with quick acting adhesive (or rubber piece which fits the plungcr of the tuberlin syringe into the barrel). Holes for dissipation of the gas are punctured

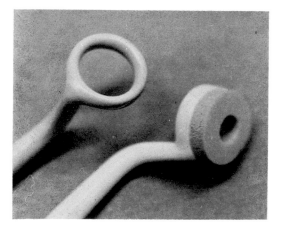

Figure 2-20b. Disposable foam rubber ring (Dr. Scholls) attached to pressure ring.

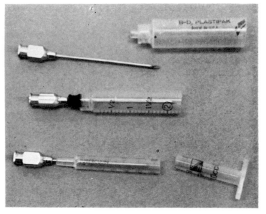

Figure 2-21. Tubular constricting devices made from disposable syringes.

into the syringe surrounding the needle attachment tip.

The device is then attached to the female Luer-Lok nozzle. Liquid nitrogen flows through the needle lumen to be sprayed on the skin where it vaporizes. The vapor exhausts to the outside atmosphere through the holes around the former needle attachment end piece. Such a device is particularly useful in treating lesions in the oral cavity because without such a device the vapor produced during the spraying process frequently obscures the treatment site.

The disposable tuberculin syringe barrel has a 5 mm inner diameter, the 3 cc syringe and 8 mm diameter and the 5 cc syringe a 12 mm inner diameter.

REFERENCES

1. White, A. C.: Liquid air in medicine and surgery. *Med Rec*, 56:109, 1899.
2. White, A. C.: Possibilities of liquid air to the physician. *JAMA, 36:*426, 1901.
3. Whitehouse, H. H.: Liquid air in dermatology: Its indications and limitations. *JAMA,* 49:371, 1907.
4. Tromovitch, T.: An Intermediate Cryosurgical Unit: The TT32. *Cutis, 16:*502, 1975.

5. Zacarian, S. A.: *Cryosurgery of Skin Cancer.* Springfield, Thomas, 1969.

6. Zacarian, S. A.: *Cryosurgery of Tumors of the Skin and Oral Cavity.* Springfield, Thomas, 1973.

7. Lubritz, R. R. and Johns, F. III: A new simplified cryosurgical instrument— The Foster Froster. *J Derm Surg, 1:* 59, 1975.

8. Torre, D.: New York: Cradle of cryosurgery. *NY State J Med, 67:*465-667, 1967.

9. Torre, D.: Cutaneous cryosurgery. *J Cryosurgery, 1:*202-209, Oct., 1968.

10. Cooper, I. S. and Lee, A. S.: Cryostatic congelation: a system for producing a limited controlled region of cooling or freezing of biologic tissues. *J Nerv Ment Dis, 133:*259, 1961.

11. Gage, A.: Cryosurgery for difficult problems in cutaneous cancer. *Cutis, 16:* 465.

12. Brodthagen, Holger: *Local Freezing of the Skin by Carbon Dioxide Snow.* Copenhagen, Munksgaard, 1961.

13. Torre, D.: Cryosurgery in Dermatology. In Von Leden, H. and Cahan, W. G. (Eds.): *Cryogenics in Surgery.* Flushing, NY, Med Exam, 1971.

14. Irvine, H. G. and Turnacliff, D. D.: Liquid Oxygen in Dermatology. *Arch Dermat and Syph, 19:*270, 1929.

15. Pusey, W. A.: The use of carbon dioxide snow in treatment of nevi and other skin lesions. *JAMA, 49:*1354, 1907.

16. Low, R. Cranston: *Carbonic Acid Snow.* New York, Wm Wood and Co, 1911.

17. Torre, D.: Alternate cryogens for cryosurgery. *J Derm Surg, 1:*56, 1975.

18. Wilson, J. W., Luikart, R., II and Ayers, S. W., III: Dichlorotetrafluoroethane for surgical planning. *Arch Derm, 71:* 523, 1955.

19. Wilson, J. W., Ayers, S. W., III and Luikart, R., II: Mixtures of fluorinated hydrocarbon as refrigerant anaesthetic. *Arch Derm, 74:*310, 1956.

20. Barron, R. F.: Cryoinstrumentation. In Von Leder, H. and Cahan, W. G. (Eds.): *Cryogenics in Surgery.* Flushing, NY, Med Exam, 1971.

21. Torre, D.: Freezing with freons. *Cutis, 16:*437, 1975.

22. Torre, D. and Torre, S.: Gadgets and gimmicks. *Cutis, 12:*93, 1973.

23. Allington, H. V.: Liquid nitrogen in the treatment of skin diseases. *Calif Med, 72:*153, 1950.

24. Zacarian, S. W. and Adham, M. I.: Cryotherapy of cutaneous malignancy. *Cryobiology, 2:*212-218, 1966.

CHAPTER THREE

Cryosurgery of Benign and Premalignant Cutaneous Lesions

RONALD R. LUBRITZ, M.D., F.A.C.P.

CRYOSURGERY HAS BEEN reported to be a rational therapeutic modality for a variety of benign and premalignant conditions.[1-4] However, the cryosurgical management of these diseases demands a different philosophy on the part of the clinician than that for malignant lesions. The objectives for which treatment is instituted preclude using the same standards which apply to malignancies.

The overriding objective in treating cancerous lesions is cure. This is not necessarily true in all benign conditions. While ideally always wishing to achieve this aim, many times a more pragmatic goal is amelioration or improvement. As an example, lesions of sebaceous hyperplasia can be reduced in size and gross appearance in many cases. The patient is satisfied with this in most instances, but to seek complete eradication is an impractical desire.

Benign and premalignant lesions require more relative attention paid to cosmetic after-appearance. Since many of these conditions will not affect the general health of the individual there is need to make, insofar as possible, the best cosmetic result one of the integral aims of the treatment plan. In general, better cosmetic results can be expected in treating benign rather than malignant tumors. This is in part due to the facts that the depth of freezing is deeper and the duration of freezing is usually much longer in treating malignant processes. Cosmetic appearance depends to no little degree on these two factors.

Certain complications seen when treating cancerous tumors are much less frequent concerns in benign lesions. Again, this is due to shorter and more superficial freezing techniques used. Nix[5] reported nerve damage to the finger as a postfreezing complication for warts. This can be a potential hazard. But for the reasons listed above, it is usually less so with benign or premalignant conditions. The same might be said for Gage's[6] reports of damage to the postauricular, mandibular, inferior alveolar, and lingual nerves. Greer and Bishop[7] have reported the development of a benign tumor (pyogenic granuloma) with a routine deep freezing for basal cell carcinoma. Both hypertrophic scars and pigmentation problems are occasionally seen, but do not occur often.

Indeed, it is fair to say that far fewer complications of most types are seen in cryosurgical therapy of benign and premalignant tumors. Freezing is so rapid and the actual time involved so short that pain, postoperative infections, and debilitating edema are only infrequently encountered. Nevertheless, there are certain complications inherent to the freezing process itself which may or may not be related to time and depth of freeze. Bullae, especially on the hands and arms, are frequent occurrences in some patients even with short freezing times (Plate 1). These can be hemorrhagic on occasion (Plate 2). Insufflation of soft tissues by cryogen vapor has been reported. This can occur when any opening in the target site communicates with deeper soft tissues in the skin. This is seen only with spray procedures in lesions where morphology (ulcer, sinus tract, etc.) or manipulation (biopsy, probing, I&D, etc.) predisposes to communicative tracts. One should also be aware that when working around the nostrils or mouth the theoretical possibility of nitrogen hypoxia can exist.

The rule that fewer complications are seen in treating benign diseases is not completely hard and fast. For example, pain is very frequent around the periungual areas when treating warts. Pigmentation problems, although reversible, are seen in treating dermatofibromas.

The thermocouple is hardly, if ever, used for benign and precancerous lesions. This is in contrast to its use in malignancies of at least some degree as reported by several major workers in the field.[8] Freezing and thaw times are adequate clinical measures and when coupled with palpation and ballottement form sufficient parameters of adequacy of freezing in the vast majority of cases.

Preoperative anesthesia is rarely necessary. In many instances the pain of the needle is more than the total freezing procedure. In some cases it can serve a useful purpose: It lifts the lesion away from cartilage or bone so freezing can proceed in a more efficient fashion.

Perhaps one of the major differences in approach when treating benign versus malignant tumors is that it is better, when in doubt, to undertreat rather than overtreat. This might, at first glance, be somewhat risky to say. On reflection there is merit in this proposition. First, one is not concerned with complete cure in many types of benign lesions. As has been mentioned, improvement rather than cure may be the primary objective. The degree of cosmetic results can in large measure be controlled by the degree of freezing. Similarly, certain complications can be kept to a minimum. Lastly, the nature of the conditions themselves allow more time and flexibility in adjusting the treatment regimen.

Selection of instruments permits wide ranges of choice. Both liquid nitrogen and nitrous oxide units may be used for benign and premalignant therapies. Even freon apparatuses have recently been shown to have possibilities.[9, 10] Devices limiting the lateral spread of freeze lend further flexibility to some of these.[11, 12]

A previous report states what the author considers to be the major advantages of a nearly ideal cryosurgical unit.[13] To summarize, it should be:

1. Capable of producing freezing to any depth sufficient to treat all skin lesions.
2. Simple to operate with adjustments that can provide varying control of the applied refrigerant.
3. Light and portable.
4. Uncomplicated to produce and manufacture and therefore inexpensive.
5. Able to provide long term storage of the unused refrigerant.

One might add the factors of safety and freedom from malfunction to these criteria.

There is no ideal cryosurgical instrument yet on the market. Each has its own set of advantages and disadvantages. Regardless, most units have no major disadvantages which would preclude their use for benign and premalignant therapy. The final choice depends primarily on individual experience and the degree of elaborateness and sophistication (and therefore

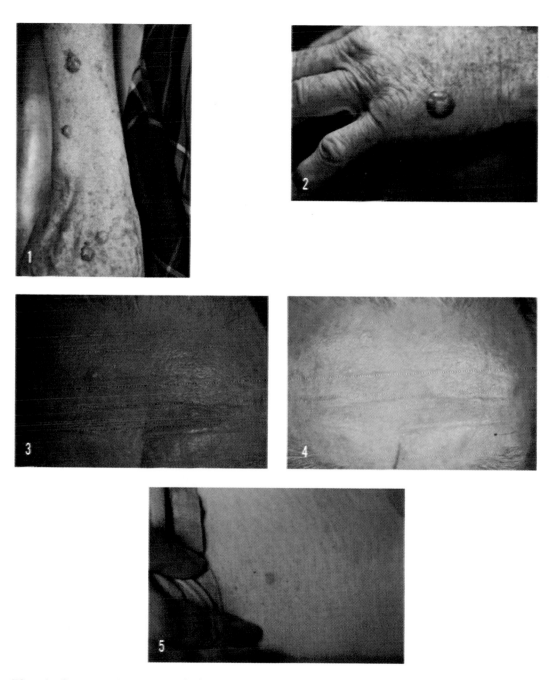

Plate 1. Crusts and hemorrhagic bullae one week postoperative for actinic keratoses.
Plate 2. Hemorrhagic bulla after freezing.
Plate 3. Adenoma sebaceum (sebaceous hyperplasia) forehead.
Plate 4. Sebaceous hyperplasia forehead after two probe treatment sessions. Despite camera exposure differences, marked improvement can be seen.
Plate 5. Dermatofibroma left upper inner thigh.

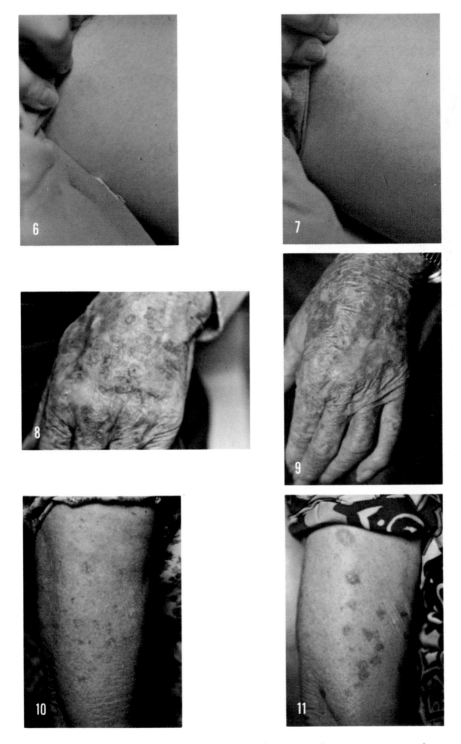

Plate 6. Dermatofibroma left upper inner thigh three months posttreatment by cryoprobe. Hyperpigmentation present in treated site.

Plate 7. Dermatofibroma left upper inner thigh approximately twelve months posttreatment. Hyperpigmentation has disappeared.

Plate 8. Large plaque actinic keratosis left dorsal hand. Focal areas of squamous cell carcinoma are present.

Plate 9. Same area eight weeks postoperative spray.

Plate 10. Multiple actinic keratoses upper arm.

Plate 11. Same area one week postfreezing by spray.

expense) one wishes to employ in his own practice set-up.

Both spray and cryoprobe techniques are used in treating benign and premalignant conditions. In following discussions, the method best suited to each condition will be commented upon. It might be wise to detail briefly the two procedures for guide reference.

Spray Technique

This method is used for the majority of lesions. Torre pioneered its development into an acceptable and successful modality.[14-17] It can be employed for lesions with irregular surfaces. Characteristically, it produces a more superficial depth of freeze in relation to lateral spread. In this process the cryogen is applied from an open spray tip directly onto the target site. The actual technique is as follows:

1. A needle size is selected which will apply the spray within the borders of the lesion when started at the center. This is not so much a problem with larger lesions than with smaller ones of less than ¼ or ½ inch. A needle-tip opening which is too large in these instances does not permit fine control.

2. Place the spray nozzle at the center of the lesion.

3. One may start at a distance of approximately 1 cm from spray tip to target site. The tip may then be adjusted toward or away from the target area as needed for control of the procedure.

4. In many instances the lateral spread of freeze is sufficient to adequately cover the peripheral areas and normal surrounding rim of the lesion. For larger lesions a small circular centrifugal motion may be necessary.

5. Freeze for the desired freeze time or expected thaw time. This is based primarily on experience and must be acquired. Estimates given in the following sections cannot be strictly adhered to in all instances. The operator must gain expertise in order to accurately judge when changes in these figures should be made.

6. If another cycle is desired this can be performed immediately after complete thaw of the frozen site. It should be stated here that multiple freeze-thaw cycles do not carry the same importance in treating benign and premalignant lesions as is the case with malignancies. With exceptions, most benign cases require only one cycle if adequate freezing has been accomplished the first time.

Cryoprobe Technique

Zacarian has made fundamental and important contributions in the development of this technique.[18, 19] This method can be used on regular-surfaced lesions. It is slower than spraying. A surface other than the actual cryogen apposes the area to be treated. Using the probe results in a deeper depth of freeze to lateral spread ratio than does the spray. The probe surface is cooled by previous immersion in the cryogen or by circulating the cryogen either inside or through it. A heat sink is thus created whereby heat is transferred from the treatment site to the probe.

The technique is as follows:

1. Select a probe type and size suitable to the lesion to be treated. These are described in the appropriate sections.

2. It is best to precool the probe before applying it to the surface of the lesion. This is particularly helpful in wet or mucous membrane tumors as it helps to prevent the tip from adhering to the site.

3. Apply the probe tip firmly to the target site.
4. Pressure in varying degree can influence depth of freeze.
5. Measure adequacy of freeze by extent of the frozen rim of normal tissue.
6. Allow the probe to thaw sufficiently before removing it from the treatment site.
7. A repeat cycle, if needed, should be commenced after allowing complete thaw of the lesion.

These techniques may require some degree of modification depending on the actual instruments used.

Cure rates when discussing cryosurgical therapies of benign/premalignant conditions are not as meaningful as in malignancies. As commented upon earlier in this section, cure may not be the practical objective in certain types of lesions. In others, actual cure versus recurrence or newly developing lesions may be difficult to assess. Cure rates for benign lesions are difficult to obtain and maintain especially in a private practice. Admittedly, true cure rates for all conditions are the ideals to be striven for. However, exact percentages cannot be given for many categories; it is hoped that the reader will understand this limit. The author has communicated with several colleagues who have large cryosurgical practices. None of us, either in our private work or in medical school affiliations, has completely accurate cure rates for benign tumors. Almost all have adopted the overall views of satisfactory or unsatisfactory management; that is, over a period of years and after treating many types and numbers of lesions, how well does cryosurgery in general compare to other treatment methods available. It is in this regard that the degree of therapeutic adequacy of certain type lesions will be presented.

Unlike benign lesions, premalignant tumors, because of their possible consequences, require very high actual cure rates. Thus, specific mention will be made in the appropriate sections on these tumors, to the extent where this is known.

In outlining the cryosurgical management of benign and premalignant conditions which follow, an attempt will be made to present them in groups of relative therapeutic success rates. For quick reference a table is presented at the end of this chapter. It provides a summary of each disease in alphabetical order with respect to therapy using cryosurgery.

The group headings are:

1. CONDITIONS MOST RESPONSIVE TO CRYOSURGERY

   Under this heading are those diseases or tumors where cryosurgery can be considered a primary or alternate primary treatment of choice. Included in this section are diseases with the highest cure rates. In addition, there are those which, where cure may not be practical, cryosurgery offers a primary or alternate form of management. This management will usually provide satisfactory improvement.

2. CONDITIONS VARIOUSLY RESPONSIVE TO CRYOSURGERY

   Conditions in this category will have varied results to cryosurgical methods. Nevertheless, they exhibit satisfactory response often enough to cryosurgery as to warrant consideration of these techniques alone or as adjunctive therapy in selected cases.

3. CONDITIONS UNDETERMINEDLY RESPONSIVE TO CRYOSURGERY

   Diseases or tumors listed in this section may show excellent initial results to cryosurgery. However, in most instances not enough cases have been treated and reported or have not been followed long enough to warrant inclusion in either of the first two categories.

Conditions Most Responsive to Cryosurgery

Adenoma Sebaceum (Sebaceous Hyperplasia)

Lesions of sebaceous hyperplasia are primarily cosmetic problems. Care should be taken, therefore, to insure that the cure is not worse than the disease. Noticeable scarring should be avoided in any treatment program. Cryosurgery can be well-suited for eradication or control of these lesions.

The patient is first told what these hamartomas really are and what results may be expected after treatment is employed. Many patients then elect not to be treated at all. Those who do elect to undergo therapy show very little discomfort to freezing. They are perhaps the most highly motivated, having passed the "elimination" test.

A point cryoprobe is selected. The point is placed directly into the central punctum. A steady hand is required. To avoid prolonged probing of the first lesions it is best to cool the probe first. The yellowish buds blanch after a few seconds. Freezing five to ten seconds or until a 1 mm rim is included is sufficient. Thaw time is not necessary. Larger lesions may require more freeze time. Re-treatments are frequently necessary and the patient should be told this. Treatment in this condition can be tedious but no more so than with other methods. As expected, small lesions seem to respond much better than larger ones. The author frequently asks the patient if there are any lesions in particular of concern, and is often surprised to find that instead of being asked to treat all the innumerable lesions sometimes present only several have been singled out. By this maneuver, much tedium can be avoided. This method compares favorably to insertion of a needle using the hyfrecator. It is not nearly as painful and healing appears to be faster. Probably two thirds of patients treated are satisfied with results. Some lesions, even after re-treatments, are not completely eliminated but are reduced in size. Being much less noticeable, this is acceptable to most (Plates 3 and 4).

Dermatofibromas

Using traditional surgical methods has resulted in singular problems for the dermatologist in treating dermatofibromas. Not the least of these is the amount of work which is frequently needed to adequately remove these lesions. The location of many dermatofibromas on the legs necessitates surgical techniques requiring resultant scars out of proportion to the type of lesion involved. Spreading atrophic scars are the usual end result of simple eliptical excision with suture closing.

Cryosurgical alternatives introduced by Torre[20] now prove this modality as one of the treatments of choice for this condition. He has reported a series of one hundren nine lesions treated in this manner. Seventy-nine lesions were followed after treatment. Sixty-one were no longer palpable. Fifty-five showed excellent cosmetic results. Re-treatments were required in some instances.

Spiller and Spiller[21] have also reported favorably on cryosurgical techniques for dermatofibroma. They achieved cure in forty out of forty-five lesions ranging in size from 4 to 15 mm and in lesion age four months to ten years.

The author's experiences have been similar. He was introduced to this method by Dr. Torre around 1970, and was so impressed with the simplicity of the procedure and the results obtained as compared to traditional surgical techniques that it rapidly became his therapy of choice. To date there has been no reason to regret this decision. Indeed, it has become distasteful to think of having to excise and suture a dermatofibroma when a simple alternative method is at hand on most occasions.

If biopsies are obtained a spray may be directed into the biopsy site and continued until the tumor is completely frozen. Total thaw times of around one minute are usually adequate. Multiple freeze-thaw cycles can be used, especially on larger lesions. The spray method is well suited to these.

Cryoprobes can also be used effectively. A flat-head type is selected which is approximately one half to two thirds the diameter of the lesion. Freezing depth should be gauged by the extent of the frozen rim rather than thaw time. This method is slower than using the spray but control of lateral spread of freeze is easier. Alternately, spraying into a lesion-size rubber cone will increase freezing depth while helping to limit lateral spread.

It is often necessary to repeat treatments. These can be done at six to eight week intervals.

A frequently seen temporary sequela is hyperpigmentation at the border of the lesion with occasional hypopigmentation in the center. (Plates 5, 6, and 7.) It is not necessarily related to the complexion of the individual, being seen in fair-skinned blondes as well as brunettes. Although usually temporary it may take months to fade out completely. Hyperpigmentation appears to be less common in proportion to thaw time. Thus several treatments with smaller thaw times may give better cosmetic results. The usual case, even when developing initial hyperpigmentation, gradually becomes flat or slightly atrophic with a normal or lightly hypopigmented color. Hypertrophic scars are rarely seen.

Keratoses, Actinic (Including Leukoplakias)

Perhaps the conditions for which cryosurgery is best suited are actinic keratoses and leukoplakia. If performed correctly the techniques used are extremely effective for the areas treated. Many lesions can be treated at one sitting and can be done in a short time. Complications are relatively lacking. Not the least important, cosmetic results can be most satisfactory.

The simplest way to treat these lesions is with the dip-stick. Certainly in many cases this is an adequate method of eradication. No great argument could be lodged against one adhering to this technique. Still, use of devices enabling the cryogen to be in controlled contact with the treated area offers advantages in certain instances.

Control of lateral spread of freeze can be accomplished more easily with instrumentation devices. This can be done both by changing various tips when using the spray and by varying spray pressure (on certain units only). Using a cotton-tip applicator does not allow lateral control as evenly.

In treating certain actinic keratoses one may be in doubt as to the presence of superficial carcinoma. In these instances a deeper freeze with corresponding increased thaw times might be valuable. This is not practical with cotton-tipped applicators. Grimmett[22] has shown that only with hemostatic pressure could simple applicators freeze lower than 2 mm. This is not deep enough for many carcinomas.

The drip problem is almost always an

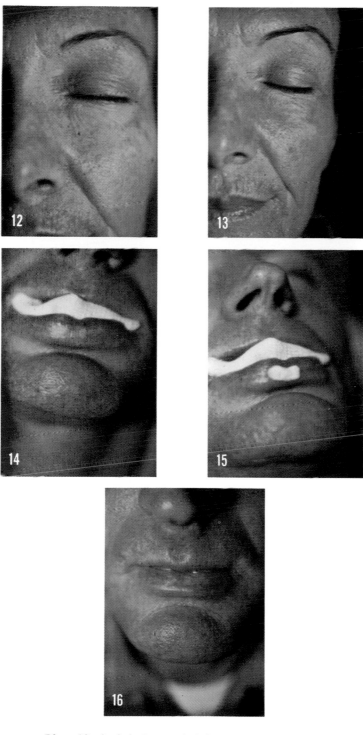

Plate 12. Actinic keratosis left upper medial eyelid.
Plate 13. Same area eight weeks postoperative spray.
Plate 14. Leukoplakia center lower lip.
Plate 15. Same area immediately postfreezing by spray.
Plate 16. Same area eight weeks postfreezing.

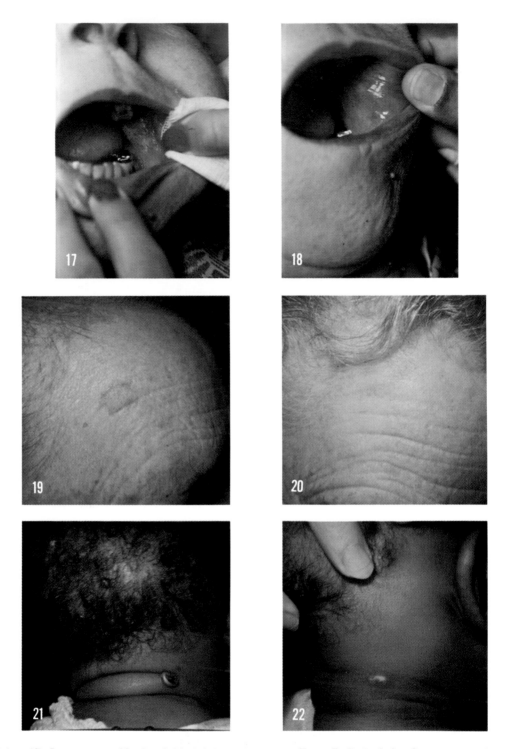

Plate 17. Large area of leukoplakia left buccal mucosa. From R. R. Lubritz, Cryosurgery of benign lesions, *Cutis, 16*:431, Sept. 1975. Courtesy of Yorke Medical Journals, Dun Donnelley Publishing Corp.

Plate 18. Same area twelve weeks postoperative. Site was divided into three sections and treated separately at different visits by spray. From R. R. Lubritz, Cryosurgery of benign lesions. *Cutis, 16*:431, Sept. 1975. Courtesy of Yorke Medical Journals, Dun Donnelley Publishing Corp.

Plate 19. Lentigo right forehead. (Courtesy Dr. G. Graham).

Plate 20. Same area at different camera angle four weeks postoperative. (Courtesy Dr. G. Graham)

Plate 21. Granuloma pyogenicum right posterior neck. (Courtesy Dr. G. Graham).

Plate 22. Same area six weeks postoperative. Note hypopigmentation. (Courtesy Dr. G. Graham).

inconvenient one when treating either a large keratosis or multiple lesions. It can be potentially serious when working around the eyes. The necessity of dipping the applicator back and forth in the liquid nitrogen reservoir creates this problem, which can be solved with proper instrumentation.

The next point is more a question of psychology than a problem. It is more delicate and subjective than previous discussions. In regards to using the cotton-tipped applicator the author has wondered many times what the patient thinks. He is first told that he has a potentially malignant lesion or lesions on the skin. Certainly to anyone this is an important condition to be reckoned with. After seeing all the gadgets and wondrous gleaming instruments around the dermatologist's treatment room, he is then treated with a Q-tip® dipped in a thermos bottle. Might an uneducated layman not wonder at the apparent disproportion between the diagnosis and therapy?

The spray technique is employed almost exclusively. No local anesthetic is necessary. When treating multiple lesions it is sometimes advisable to mark those for therapy. This is not to mark borders but rather to keep track of those frozen. Because of the short freeze and thaw times used, edema and erythema occasionally cannot be relied on to flag the treated sites. Usually a #16 or #17 spray tip is best suited for this work. The spray tip is placed at the center of the target site. For many lesions no movement is necessary. Otherwise a slight circular motion is used. The plaque is frozen just outside the border. Thaw times of twenty to thirty seconds are usually adequate.

Multiple or large lesions can be treated at one visit if this is desired (Plates 8 and 9). However the patient should be told of the normal sequence of events using cryosurgery. It is the author's policy not to treat more than three or four lesions on the first visit. Subsequently the patient is better able to understand the amount of discomfort (or lack of it) entailed with freezing multiple lesions (Plates 10 and 11).

Treating actinic keratoses in this manner involves little risk of complications. Bullae, even hemorrhagic, may form after treatment but these should not be described to the patient as complications. They resolve in the normal course of healing and occur most often on the hands and arms. They are seen occasionally on the ears and only rarely on the face.

Cryosurgical techniques allow treatment of keratoses in delicate or inaccessible locations (Plates 12 and 13). Lesions in areas such as the eyelids, eyebrows, ears, and ala nasi crease may become relatively easy to manage. One special location where good results are seen is above the upper lips. Less puckering results from spray-freezing this area.

Cure rates using these methods approach 100 percent. Occasionally large or hypertrophic sites need re-treatment, but this is not a frequent occurrence.

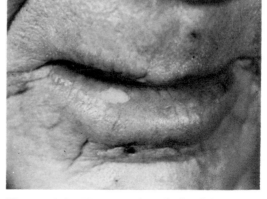

Figure 3-1. Hypertrophic leukoplakia right lower lip.

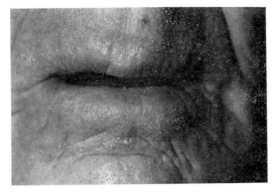

Figure 3-2. Same area eight weeks postoperative spray technique.

Leukoplakia of the lips and buccal cavity are particularly suited to instrumentational cryosurgical methods (Figures 3-1 and 3-2). On the lip after biopsy confirmation, a spray technique should be employed. Because the lesions are often linear, starting at one end and working toward the other may be easier than starting at the center and working out. The lesion is frozen solidly. Total thaw time can be one minute or more (Plates 14, 15, and 16). Ballottement is a valuable guide in this site. Often the spray tip can be used to "tap" the frozen area. This can give an idea of the solidness of the freeze. The vascularity of the lip sometimes requires more freezing than one estimates at the start; multiple freeze-thaw cycles might need to be used (Figures 3-3, 3-4, 3-5, and 3-6). If an entire lip needs to be treated, it is the author's policy to treat up to one-

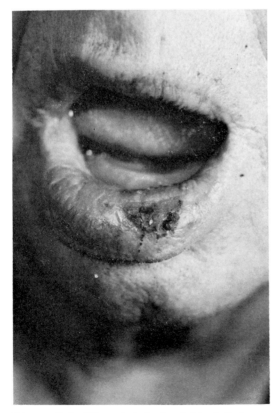

Figure 3-3. Ulcerated leukoplakia left lower lip.

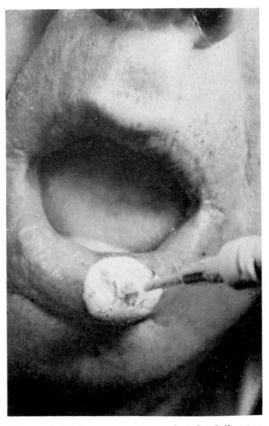

Figure 3-4. Same area immediately following freezing using spray.

half on any one visit. This provides the patient some degree of convenience and comfort.

Large plaques of leukoplakia in the mouth can be difficult management problems. Cryosurgery can effectively and relatively easily control many of these cases (Plates 17 and 18). Cryoprobes can be used on these plaques; they should be frozen just outside the active border. The lesions thaw quite rapidly and thaw times are difficult to judge in these areas. Probes will adhere to the mucous membranes when cold. This can be partially prevented by cooling the probe before applying it to the membrane surface and by moving it over the treatment area until the target site is slightly frozen.

Spray techniques can also be used quite effectively. A long curved adaptor is avail-

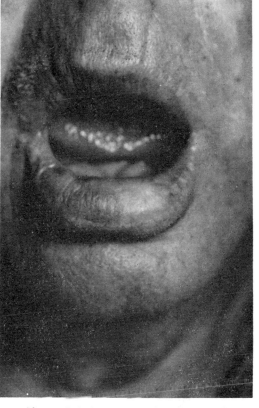

Figure 3-6. Same area after four weeks.

able with some cryosurgical instruments. The author's personal choice is a long spinal needle of appropriate diameter, e.g. #17, which can fit onto any unit equipped with a Luer-Lok. If vapors cloud the area the patient can be asked to inhale through the nose and exhale through the mouth. Still, treatment may need to be halted temporarily if this does not work.

Lesions on the tongue can be treated. However scarring has occurred if frozen too solidly. Usually thirty to forty-five seconds thaw time is adequate for most lesions and risk of resultant scarring at these figures should be minimal.

Keratoses, Seborrheic

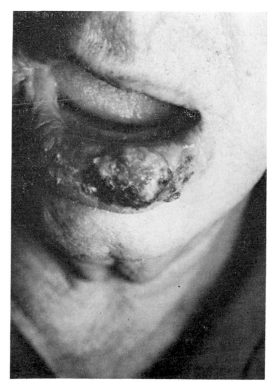

Figure 3-5. Same area after one week.

Many seborrheic keratoses are amenable

to cryosurgical techniques. These may be used alone or in combination.

Cryosurgery is a natural choice of selection as a primary method of therapy. These lesions are superficial and as such do not have to be treated deeply for eradication. Accordingly superficial freezing lends itself to little resultant scarring. With cryosurgery also, many keratoses can be treated at a single sitting and control of bleeding is usually no problem. Spray techniques are used almost exclusively. Morphology dictates whether spray is used alone or in combination with other procedures.

Flat lesions can be spray-frozen very quickly. The entire tumor is frozen solidly with a small amount of normal rim. Thaw time of thirty to forty-five seconds usually suffice. Many keratoses, depending on size, can be frozen at the same session especially on the trunk. Using this method has its drawbacks. Some lesions recur and must be re-treated. If the patient is told in advance he seldom minds, when this limitation is weighed against the obvious advantages of cosmetic elegance, speed of eradication and relative lack of complications.

Although raised tumors may be treated in the manner described, total eradication is frequently not achieved. A more successful alternative consists of spraying the lesion until lightly frozen. A curette is used for removal. The base may then be frozen again with thaw time around thirty seconds. Monsel's solution or 100 percent TCA can be employed to control bleeding of the base. Otherwise Oxycel®, Gelfoam® or similar chemical hemostatic sponges may be applied and covered with a Band-aid®. Healing is routinely uneventful. Cosmetic results in these cases are usually excellent.

Care should be taken not to freeze too hard. It is difficult to use a curette if the keratosis is frozen solidly. If this happens

the operator must wait until the lesion is partially thawed before continuing. Also, too much freezing can result in scarring or hypopigmentation out of proportion to the tumor being treated. Some amount of time is required to gain clinical experience in this judgement.

Lentigines (Senile)

Treatment for removal of senile lentigines can be a frustrating condition for the dermatologist. Poor results can be the rule rather than the exception. However, cryosurgery may be used in many cases with a moderate degree of success (Plates 19 and 20). Either the spray or probe technique is employed.

If a probe is used a flat-head type slightly smaller than the lesion should be selected. It should then be frozen lightly just to the outside of the color. For most small lentigines such as those on the hand this takes around five to ten seconds for each.

With several of the newer portable cryosurgical instruments the spray can be controlled fine enough to permit its use in treating small lesions. The spray technique is faster and might be considered providing the qualification of controlling the lateral spread of freeze is met. A small #18 gauge needle, or similar, is used. The macule is frozen completely including a small rim of normal skin. Freezing times are usually slightly faster than with probes.

Using either of these techniques results in a small blister which subsequently lifts off the lentigo in the healing process; or each may produce a small yellowish crust which gradually resolves, taking the pigmented macule with it.

These methods do not always work completely, but even when not eradicating all the lesions frequently helps to lighten them. With cryosurgery the chance of producing adequate results without complications is high enough to justify its use. It is therefore the author's treatment of choice for the condition.

Verrucae

As with most other forms of therapy, cryosurgery cannot be hailed as a panacea for verrucae. It is difficult to state precisely how effective cryosurgical techniques are for these lesions. The reason is the same as for evaluations of other techniques: warts are unpredictable. Further elaboration of this theme is unnecessary. It is assumed that the reader, having experience with warts, knows exactly the dilemma.

Digitate warts usually respond well to freezing. The entire stalk, base and a small surrounding rim of normal tissue is frozen solidly. A spray tip is used. Usually fifteen to twenty seconds is sufficient freezing time, depending upon which instrument is used. Thaw time is not necessary, but special attention should be paid to the base to make certain it is solidly frozen.

Periungual verrucae respond quite erratically to freezing (Figures 3-7 and 3-8). On attempting to assess treatment failures the author has found two common occurrences in these cases. First, and probably most im-

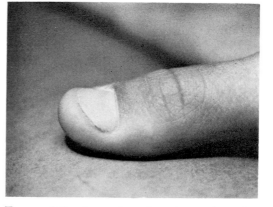

Figure 3-8. Approximately six weeks after spray-freezing.

portant, pain has prompted discontinuance of the freezing procedure prematurely. Second, the nail was not trimmed sufficiently to treat the entire lesion. Attention to these details has notably increased recent success rates.

The cotton-tip applicator or small cryosurgical unit can be used. If not using the dip-stick, a small-diameter spray tip, for example #18, should be selected. Intermittent freezing coupled with the former usually will provide adequate control of lateral spread of freeze.

After a solid freeze no thaw time is necessary. Care should be taken not to treat too much at one time; edema can cause severe pain around the periungual area. In most cases pain also occurs with thawing in this region. It is a throbbing type which some patients describe as nauseating. This can also occur around the temples and occasionally on the forehead.

The dip-stick cotton applicator has been used for years on lesions of verruca vulgaris of glabrous skin. Despite the development of several portable small cryosurgical units[13, 23] it will continue to be an effective way to use liquid nitrogen for treatment. If one wishes to use instrumentation for

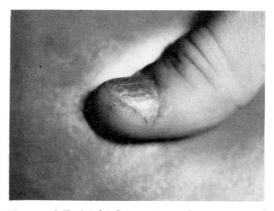

Figure 3-7. Multiple periungual verrucae of thumb.

this purpose a spray technique should be selected similar to that described for peri-ungual verrucae. Cryoprobes freeze too slowly. They are not recommended in most cases.

Limiting devices are presently being evaluated to control the lateral spread of freeze in the treatment of both benign and malignant lesions. However, for common warts on glabrous skin, these are not needed if a dip-stick is used. Similarly they are not required with instrumentation, provided a small gauge spray tip and intermittent freezing are employed. Failing to do so can create this problem, as it is sometimes difficult to spray-freeze to the deep margins of many lesions without also freezing too much surrounding normal skin.

A solid spray-freeze, when successful, usually presents a quite acceptable cosmetic final result. Hypertrophic scars, sometimes evident in wart treatment sites using E D and C, are seldom seen with cryosurgery. More frequent are hemorrhagic blisters (usually on the extremities) and hypopigmentation. The blisters are transient. The pigmentary problems may not be. Indeed, although curative, freezing can produce hypopigmentation which may last for many months. It can be somewhat disconcerting to produce a cure for a wart only to find the smooth treatment site replaced by a disturbing and cosmetically inelegant white spot. Careful attention to the depth and duration of freezing can reduce this complication.

Verruca planae can be eliminated with both spray and probe methods. If many lesions are involved, the spray is much faster, provided lateral spread of freeze can be controlled. A few seconds usually suffices to freeze most lesions. Care should be taken not to freeze too deeply or hypopigmentation might occur. Probes can be used but may be too slow if more than a few lesions are to be treated. A one or two millimeter flat-head probe is best suited. These techniques roughly approximate the results with light electrodessication. An alternative, and perhaps better, method follows the pattern which will be mentioned for molluscum lesions: lightly freeze the area with fluorethyl. This makes the lesions stand out from the surrounding normal skin. They can then be curetted.

Recurrence rate is high when using cryosurgical techniques for verrucae on the palmar or plantar surfaces. Treatment usually does not suffice for primary eradication, recurrences have been over fifty percent, and attendant pain often precludes subsequent procedures. To elaborate, it is difficult to freeze deep enough or hard enough (without exquisite pain) to eradicate a substantial percentage of palmar or plantar verrucae with multiple procedures. This is particularly true with spray-freezing. A probe might offer better results, but the dip-stick is probably best of all. Recurrences seem inordinately high. These can be reduced by combined methods. Pain, sometimes approaching the intolerable, almost always accompanies these procedures. An initial pain during the procedure is followed by a deeper, more prolonged discomfort. Some patients will not approve repeat sessions.

Condyloma acuminata can respond relatively well to freezing. Podophyllin still remains the treatment of choice. However, freezing can be used on podophyllin-resistant cases with sometimes surprisingly good results. Multiple discrete lesions respond better than do plaques. Spray-freezing should be used. Each lesion or small group is frozen entirely. A small amount of normal rim should be included. Light freezing procedures might be of benefit in or around the mucosal surfaces of the vagina and anus where untoward reactions to podophyllin might be feared.

Conditions Variously Responsive to Cryosurgery

Angiomas

Small angiomas may be benefitted by fairly solid freezing. If a spray tip is used, care should be taken to select a size which limits the lateral spread of freeze. This can also be accomplished by using a probe. De Morgan's spots may be eliminated. Rendu-Osler-Weber disease can respond to a point-tip cryoprobe. Because of the vascularity a hard freeze is necessary; but adequate depth and thus completeness may not be obtained. Larger angiomas, therefore, may not respond well.

Carbuncles

Cryosurgery can be of help in carbuncles which are chronic and do not respond well to conventional forms of therapy. As adjunctive therapy to antibiotics and incision and drainage, it can provide an extra means of attack. It can be considered as an alternative where one might use electrodessication and curettage.

The spray is used after incising and draining the wound. The entire lesion can be frozen externally, but best results are obtained by spraying into the cavity and freezing the walls solidly. To avoid splattering, complete evacuation of the cavity should be performed if possible before directing the spray therein. If the unit being used has adjustable spray pressure, it should accordingly be low. Thaw time is not necessary, but freezing time may be longer than anticipated due to vascularity.

Chondrodermatitis

It is difficult to assess the degree to which cryosurgical techniques are effective in chondrodermatitis. With other forms of therapy, these lesions can be recurrent and present long-term management problems. This is no less the case for cryosurgery. Small lesions can respond quite well.

Larger lesions may require repeated freezing. One disturbing complication deserves mention. Some lesions seem to be made more inflammatory after freezing. This does not happen often, but when it does occur, it can be quite disturbing. This possible complication should be weighed against the excellent cosmetic results achieved and the relative simplicity of the procedure as compared to more traditional forms of surgery. The author's technique is to inject intralesional triamcinolone into the lesion every two weeks for two or three injections. In some cases this is enough to cure or control the tumor. If more work is needed, the nodule is then frozen solidly until white with a spray tip with a thaw time of around forty-five seconds. Repeat procedures may be performed after four to eight weeks with a slightly longer thaw time. If imflammation results after freezing, triamcinolone is again used. This will usually "cool down" this complication.

Granuloma Pyogenicum

These lesions, like many angiomatous tumors, do not respond consistently to cryosurgery. Small lesions are sprayed until frozen solid. The rim, or cup, should also be included. A probe may be needed for larger lesions in order to obtain greater depth/lateral ratio. Thaw times cannot be used accurately in these lesions; one frozen supposedly hard will thaw with unanticipated rapidity. Small lesions appear to respond best. Also of some prognostic significance is the size of the base; the more narrow the base, the better the results using cryo techniques (Plates 21 and 22).

Hidradenitis

Cryosurgery for hidradenitis can be spoken of only as adjunctive therapy. This does not mean that for certain lesions this modality does not offer temporary and sometimes dramatic control. Indeed, this

TABLE 3-I

BENIGN AND PREMALIGNANT CONDITIONS AMENABLE TO CRYOSURGERY

Disease	Cryosurgery Can Be Used as: Therapy of Choice (C) Alternate Therapy (AT) Adjunctive or Combined Therapy (CT) Experimental but Promising (E)	Technique: Spray (S) Probe (P) Dipstick (D)	Procedure: Freeze Time (FT) Thaw Time (TT) Solid Freeze (SF) Light Freeze (LF)	Remarks
Adenoma sebaceum (Seb. hyperplasia)	C	P	FT 5-10 sec	Improvement but not necessarily eradication
Angioma	AT	S	SF	May need harder than anticipated freeze due to vascularity
Carbuncle	CT	S	LF or SF	Evacuate contents if spraying into cavity
Chondrodermatitis	AT or CT	S	SF	Caution: some are made more inflammatory
Chromoblastomycosis	E	S	TT 4 min or more	More cases needed
Dermatofibroma	C	S or P	TT 1 min or more	Repeat treatments may be necessary
Granuloma pyogenicum	AT	S	FT Judge by normal rim SF	May need harder than anticipated freeze due to vascularity
Granuloma-swimming pool	E	S	SF	More cases needed
Hidradenitis	CT	S	LF or SF	Evacuate contents if spraying into cavity
Keloid	AT or CT	S	SF	May combine with intralesional steroids
Keratoacanthoma	AT or CT	S	SF	Harder freeze and removal of core may enhance results
Keratosis, actinic	C	S	TT 20-30 sec	Ideal for cryosurgery; high cure rate
Keratosis, leukoplakia	C	S or P	FT 1 min (lip)	Spray for lip. S or P for mouth
Keratosis, seborrheic	C or CT	S	Freeze outside border LF	Combine with curettage for raised lesions
Lentigo	C	S or P	LF	Improvement but not necessarily eradication
Molluscum contagiosum	CT	S	LF	Combine with curettage for best results
Mucocele	E	S or P	SF	More cases needed
Nevus, epithelial	E	S	SF	Improvement; more cases needed
Nevus, junction	E	P	SF 1-1.5 mm beyond border	More cases and follow up needed
Verruca	AT	S, P or D	Various	Plantar, palmar types respond least. Technique & response vary with type

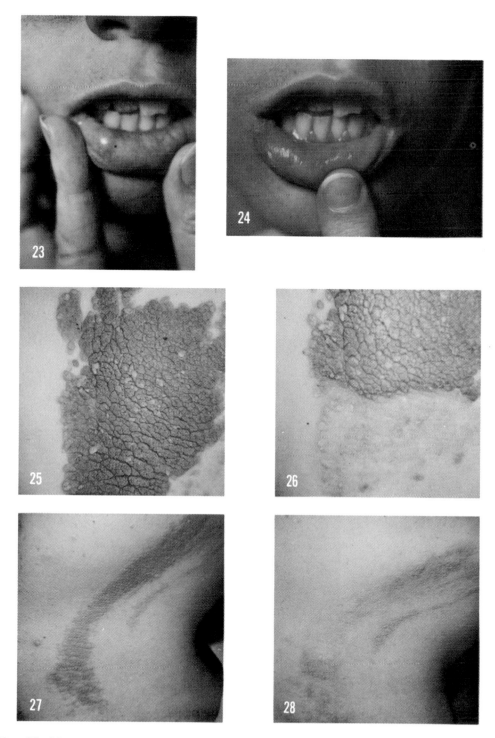

Plate 23. Mucocele right lower lip.

Plate 24. Same area after two treatments.

Plate 25. Large epithelial nevus. (Courtesy Dr. S. Zacarian)

Plate 26. Same area 3 months after lower half spray-frozen. (Courtesy Dr. S. Zacarian)

Plate 27. Epithelial nevus neck. (Courtesy Dr. G. Graham)

Plate 28. Same area approximately six weeks after spray technique used. Although complete removal has not been accomplished, much improvement is noted. (Courtesy Dr. G. Graham)

may be the case and can be a welcome therapeutic addition when treating this frustrating disease. However, cryosurgical techniques in this condition are tactical rather than strategic weapons. They are aimed at treating specific lesions and thus have limited value.

Two techniques can be used. The first is similar to treating carbuncles. The lesion is opened and drained. A spray is then inserted into the cavity and the walls and base are frozen solidly. The same admonition regarding splattering of liquid contents as in carbuncles is again given.

A simpler and less messy alternate technique is to freeze the lesion in toto without prior preparation. This may be a superior method for smaller lesions. Once the nodule is frozen solidly using either method, thaw time is not needed.

Keloids

Cryosurgery is not necessarily recommended as a primary therapy for keloids for several reasons. The first is that results using intralesional steroids certainly justifies their consideration in the same type lesions which cryosurgery seems to benefit, namely the young and/or the small. In addition no one seems to have worked with enough of them in various sizes and ages to offer definite guidelines for cryosurgical treatment. For this reason, keloids might well be argued for inclusion in the next rather than the present section.

The author has worked mainly with small keloids. Results on larger keloids have been generally unsatisfactory. Lesions 1 cm or smaller can be frozen using a spray tip with a thaw time around one minute. Larger lesions are injected with intralesional steroids once or twice with an interval of two weeks, then frozen. These injections may also be used at the time of and following treatment.

Zacarian[4] has also treated primarily small keloids 2 to 3 cm and smaller. He freezes them in their entirety. He reports variable results.

Torre[24] cites an alternative for old keloids which are unresponsive to intralesional steroids. He suggests the technique of shelling out 9/10 of the lesions surgically, then freezing the resultant cavity and borders with liquid nitrogen spray.

Keratoacanthoma (KA)

Variable response can also be expected when treating keratoacanthomas with cryosurgery. The keratotic plug in many lesions is difficult to freeze. For lesions under 1 cm, a spray-freeze of the entire lesion with a surrounding normal rim may be performed. For lesions larger than this the tumor should first be shelled out. The bleeding can be stopped with 100% TCA or Monsel's solution. Next the base should be frozen solidly using a spray tip. A local anesthetic should be used if this method is chosen.

Multiple KAs can be well suited to this modality. Recurrences as in other forms of therapy occur often enough to justify not recommending cryosurgery as the prime treatment of choice in most cases. Recurrences can be kept to a minimum by producing a solid freeze with total thaw times similar to those used for some malignancies, e.g. 2½ to 3½ minutes. Multiple freeze-thaw cycles can be used.

Molluscum Contagiosum

Freezing molluscum lesions can be helpful. However best results are obtained when used in combination with other procedures (Figures 3-9 and 3-10).

Using a cotton-tipped applicator or instrument system can be quite slow. The major drawback, though, in using cryosurgery solely is that complete eradication is

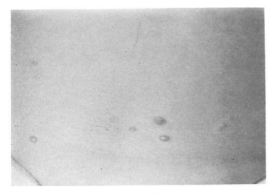

Figure 3-9. Multiple molluscum contagiosum lower abdomen.

often not achieved. In order to remedy this, freezing time must be much longer in relation to the depth of lesions. This can result in scarring which is neither aesthetic nor necessary.

There is, however, a simple technique which occasions high cure-rate and pleasing cosmetic results. This consists of lightly freezing the lesions with a spray until the papule turns white except for the central core which stands out like a small crater. The whole lesion is then plucked off with a small curette. Usually only a few seconds are needed for each papule when done in this manner. A freon such as

fluorethyl can be substituted for liquid nitrogen or nitrous oxide. It works quite well except that lateral spread of freeze cannot be well controlled. The lesions usually heal without scarring when treated in this way.

Conditions Undeterminedly Responsive to Cryosurgery

Chromoblastomycosis

The author treated a patient with chromoblastomycosis of the lip with apparent cure to date (Figures 3-11 and 3-12). This will soon be the basis of a full report.[25] The lesion extended from the left upper lip to just under the nose. After histological examination revealed chromoblastomycosis, culture methods showed *Phialophora*

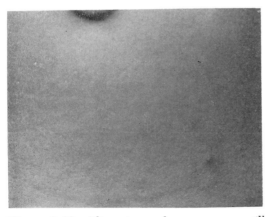

Figure 3-10. After six weeks same area still shows residual lesions. Curettage after light freezing resulted in cure.

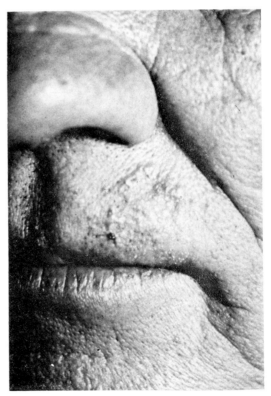

Figure 3-11. Chromoblastomycosis left upper lip and adjacent intranasal area.

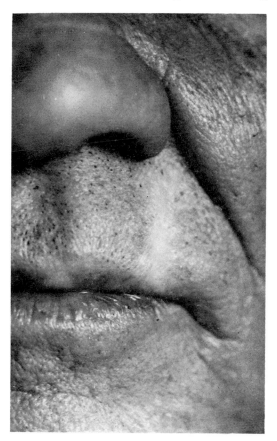

Figure 3-12. Same area approximately one year postoperative. Although cured, hypopigmentation precludes acceptable cosmetic result produced from extensive deep freezing.

pedrosoi to be the causative organism. Medical therapy was deemed contraindicated because of liver and past kidney disease. Cryosurgery was then considered.

A liquid nitrogen spray technique was used. Total thaw time was approximately four minutes. Two small areas near the border of the lesion were refrozen three months later. After one year no recurrences have been noted. Cosmetic results were not as good as the author would have liked due to depigmentation of the central lesion area. In retrospect the freezing time was probably too long. However, to the au-

thor's knowledge this was the first case treated by cryosurgery and therefore there were no precedents to follow. Knowing that certain fungal organisms can be difficult to eradicate, it was thought best to treat the lesion hard the first time around.

Granuloma, Swimming Pool

Swimming pool granuloma is often a difficult tumor to treat. They are notoriously recurrent, particularly when of larger size. Cryosurgery has been reported curative in at least some instances by Atkinson and Daniels.[26] The technique employed consisted of removal of the lesion followed by freezing the base solidly with liquid nitrogen spray. Cosmetic results were reported as excellent. *Leishmania tropica* was commented on in this same report. Therapy using solid CO_2 resulted in apparently curative response.

Mucocele

Cryosurgery may soon be advocated more strongly in the treatment of these lesions. Spiller and Spiller[21] have reported four cases on the lip which responded well with no recurrences to date. Cryoprobes were used. The author has treated several and results are in agreement (Plates 23 and 24). Both spray and cryoprobe techniques were used, but probes appear to be the better choice.

Nevi (Epithelial)

Both Graham[27] and Zacarian[27] report partial success in the treatment of several epithelial nevi (Plates 25, 26, 27 and 28). Cure was not necessarily the objective in these cases but significant improvement in appearance was obtained. Spray techniques were used. Several were treated by successive sessions, only portions being frozen at each visit.

Nevi (Junction)

Most nevi respond poorly or erratically to cryosurgery. Details of response to freezing have been reported by Lindo and Daniels.[28] Flat junctional nevi have also been subjected to clinical study by Torre,[20] and initial results were promising. He has found that many lesions disappear when using cryosurgery. Some require re-treatment. His technique is to select a probe approximately the same size as the nevus. He then freezes the lesion solidly and includes about 1 to 1.5 mm outside the border of color.

Comment

It would be inappropriate and less than candid were this chapter to close leaving an impression in the reader's mind that cryosurgery is a treatment panacea. Accordingly, certain misconceptions should be laid to rest along with other therapeutic myths. There are two major legends in this regard. The first is that cryosurgical procedures leave no scars. It should be obvious that this is a medical absurdity. Where confusion possibly occurs is that these procedures can, indeed, be well controlled as to the depth of freezing required. Thus, many lesions are not overtreated, leading to excellent cosmetic results. These results merely reflect good technique using a controllable treatment method. Even so, this is a far cry from "no scar." The second fiction is that cryosurgical methods are so simple and safe that little if any training is necessary to begin using them. As reported elsewhere[29] this naive belief is far from valid. Cryosurgical techniques are relatively simple, at least for benign lesions. It is also true that they are relatively safe. But in order to use this modality successfully, the same rules apply which govern any potential treatment program. A level of knowledge which permits an adequate understanding of the diagnosis and pathophysiology of the conditions to be treated must be a prerequisite. This is then combined with an accumulated degree of skill in dermatocryosurgical procedures which allows selection of those methods necessary to carry out the treatment plan. These skills must be acquired. Fortunately this can be done, although at some effort. There are no short-cuts.

REFERENCES

1. Lubritz, R. R.: Cryosurgery for benign and malignant skin lesions: treatment with a new instrument. *South Med J*, Accepted for publication.
2. ———: Cryosurgery of benign lesions. *Cutis, 16*:426-432 (Sept.) 1975.
3. Torre, D.: Cryosurgery of premalignant and malignant skin lesions. *Cutis, 8:* 123 (Aug.) 1971.
4. Zacarian, S.: *Cryosurgery of Tumors of the Skin and Oral Cavity,* Springfield, Thomas, 1973.
5. Nix, T. W., Jr.: Liquid Nitrogen Neuropathy. *Arch Derm,* 92:185-188 (Aug.) 1965.
6. Gage, A. A.: Deep Cryosurgery. In Epstein, E. (Ed.): *Skin Surgery.* Springfield, Thomas, 1970.
7. Greer, K. E., and Bishop, G. F.: Pyogenic granuloma as a complication of cryosurgery. (letter to the ed.) *Arch Derm,* 111:1536-1537 (Nov.)
8. *Dermatological Cryosurgery: A Coming of Age.* (Round table audio tape discussion) Distributed by Lederle laboratories. (Oct.) 1974.
9. Torre, D.: Alternate cryogens for cryosurgery. *J Derm Surg,* 1:56-58 (June) 1975.
10. ———: Freezing with freons. *Cutis, 16:* 437-445 (Sept.) 1975
11. ———: *Bits and Pieces* (Lecture). Presented at Second Annual Dermatocryosurgical Seminar (Rudolph Ellender Med Found), New Orleans, La. Oct. 4-5, 1975.
12. Torre, D. and Torre, S.: Gadgets and gimmicks. *Cutis, 12*:93, 1973.

13. Lubritz, R. R., and Johns, F.: A new simplified cryosurgical instrument: the Foster Froster. *J Derm Surg, 1:*59-62 (June) 1975.

14. Torre, D.: Cutaneous cryosurgery. *Journal Cryosurgery, 1:*202-209 (Oct.) 1968.

15. ———: Cradle of cryosurgery. *NY State J Med, 67:*465-467, 1967.

16. ———: Cryosurgery in dermatology. *Physicians' Panorama, 6:*4-8, 1968.

17. Cahan, W. G.: Five years of cryosurgical experience. In Rand, R. W., Rinfret, A. P., Von Leden, H. (Eds.): *Cryosurgery.* Springfield, Thomas, 1968.

18. Zacarian, S. A. and Adham, M. I.: Cryotherapy of cutaneous malignancy. *Cryobiliogy, 2:*212-218, 1966.

19. Zacarian, S. A.: *Cryosurgery of Skin Cancer.* Springfield, Thomas, 1969.

20. Torre, D.: Dermatological cryosurgery: a progress report. *Cutis, 11:*782, 1973.

21. Spiller, W. F. and Spiller, R. F.: Cryosurgery in dermatologic office practice. *South Med J, 68:*157-160 (Feb.) 1975.

22. Grimmett, R. H.: Liquid nitrogen therapy, histological observation. *Arch Derm, 83:*563, 1961.

23. Tromovitch, T. A.: An intermediate cryosurgical unit: the TT 32. *Cutis, 16:*502-503 (Sept.) 1975.

24. Torre, D.: Cryosurgery in Dermatology. In Von Leyden, H. and Cahan, W. (Eds.): *Cryogenics in Surgery.* Flushing, NY, Med Exam, 1971.

25. Lubritz, R. R.: Cryosurgery for chromoblastomycosis: case report. In preparation for publication.

26. Atkinson, S. C. and Daniels, F., Jr.: Swimming pool granuloma: treatment with cryosurgery. *Cutis, 11:*818, 1973.

27. Seminar In Depth: *Cryosurgery.* Presented at Amer Acad Derm, San Francisco, Calif, Dec. 10, 1975.

28. Lindo, S. D. and Daniels, F., Jr.: Cryosurgery of junction nevi. *Cutis, 16:*492-496 (Sept.) 1975

29. Lubritz, R. R.: Dermatocryosurgery: status in general medicine. (Editorial) *Med Digest, 21:*21-22 (Nov.) 1975.

CHAPTER FOUR

Cryosurgery in Treatment of Acne and Specific Cutaneous Neoplasia

GLORIA F. GRAHAM, M.D.*

HISTORY AND BACKGROUND

CRYOSURGERY USING LIQUID nitrogen or nitrous oxide spray or probe applications offers the physician an effective means of managing both acne and acne scarring. Minimal complications have been encountered and discomfort from the procedure has not been a problem. The simplicity and excellent cosmetic results of cryosurgery gives the dermatologist a valuable technique in dealing with the physical disfigurement and psychological trauma of acne and its scarring.

Liquid nitrogen applied with a cotton swab was first used by Allington[1] for the treatment of skin diseases including acne. More recently, Graham[2] reported on liquid nitrogen spray in the treatment of the inflammatory lesions of acne and acne scarring; and Kligman,[3] using liquid nitrogen on cotton swab, and Leyden,[4] using cryoprobes utilizing carbon dioxide or nitrous oxide, reported on the effectiveness of treating acne conglobata. Torre[5] has reported on freezing milia with a large-sized probe and acne scars with freons.[6] Pierce[7] and Zacarian[8] found cryotherapy to be effective therapy for keloids; and Shalita[9] and Goette[10] confirmed the usefulness of

freezing in the treatment of cystic acne lesions. Epstein[11] too found cryorolling to be useful in the treatment of acne scarring.

The author's experience with cryotherapeutic management of acne now extends over five years and exceeds four hundred cases. In 1970, utilizing the Kryospray, several patients with acne scarring were treated with twenty seconds of freezing with liquid nitrogen. The resultant blistering, crusting and peeling was followed by an improvement in scarring that approached that of dermabrasion and surpassed results obtainable with dry ice slush. The liquid nitrogen spray was later used to treat acne cysts, papules and pustules, gradually replacing the previous routine of application of dry ice slush, liquid nitrogen swab or ultraviolet light. This experience allowed an assessment of the clinical benefits and limitations of managing acne and acne scarring with cryosurgery as an adjunctive procedure. The overall effectiveness, efficiency, and enthusiastic patient acceptance have made cryosurgery a preferred treatment for acne and acne scarring, especially for nodulocystic acne and superficial to medium depth scars (Plates 29-48).

Technique

Equipment

Numerous types of equipment are available for the controlled application of liq-

* Dr. Gloria Graham gratefully acknowledges with thanks the advice, encouragement and assistance of Dr. Clayton Wheeler, Dr. Daniel Lowe, Dr. Jerry Klingler, Ms. Ruth deBliek, Mrs. Helen Simpson and Mrs. Martha Barnes.

uid nitrogen or nitrous oxide in spray and probe form. The author's experience has centered on several commercially available units. Two hand-held units, the Kryospray and the Zacarian C-21 are easy to use but require refilling with liquid nitrogen several times each day. More recent portable units such as the Foster Froster and the Cry-Ac are capable of liquid nitrogen applications for six to eight hours without refilling. A floor model, the CE-8 Cryoderm, with both spray and probe capabilities, is large enough to function for several weeks without refilling and is the unit used primarily in the author's practice. Although nitrous oxide is not an appropriate cryogen for use in treating malignancies, it is adequate for freezing acne and other benign skin lesions. The Dynatech Dermadyne is used with a six-pound cylinder of readily available nitrous oxide which will last for two weeks during moderate use. (See Chapter two of this volume for additional information concerning the equipment.)

Probes and Spray Tips

For both spray and probe units, metal probes and tips are available. A stainless steel acne tip is available commercially and is adequate if care is used not to rest it against the skin, allowing the metal to act as a probe producing an area of freezing greater than anticipated. A plastic tip* has been found particularly advantageous in treating acne scarring since it can touch the skin if necessary without acting as a probe. Further, with the CE-8 Cryoderm floor model unit, since the cryogen Dewar is separated from the spray or probe applicator tip by a long delivery tube, the freezing time may need to be slightly longer than

---

* Acne spray tip developed by Robert Williams, Smithfield, North Carolina.

with hand-held units. Once the tube is cooled, freezing is rapid. The amount of refrigerant being emitted may vary with the tip size, amount of refrigerant in container and even atmospheric pressure.

Procedure

Patients are seated for the cryosurgical procedures and plastic drapes are worn to prevent accidental drippage of liquid nitrogen onto the chest. Goggles are placed over the eyes (Plate 33). For treatment of only a few acne lesions on the face this is not necessary. The operator's hand is sufficient for protecting the eyes from the spray.

Treatment

Treatment of Inflammatory Lesions of Acne

Cryotherapy in the form of liquid nitrogen or nitrous oxide sprays is used as an adjunct to the routine acne regimen.† Patients are seen every two to six weeks until their acne is controlled.

The cryospray has proved more advantageous than the cryoprobe for inflammatory lesions, although the probe is useful in confining treatment to small lesions, milia, and deep cysts. Generally the cryo-

---

† Cryotherapy is used in conjunction with standard acne therapy: removal of comedones, a variety of cleansing agents, a well-balanced diet, adequate rest, antibiotics where indicated and avoidance of tension and stress. Benzoyl perioxide sulfur and sodium sulfacetamide topical medications were being used at the time this study was started and more recently retinoic acid as well as topical agents containing a combination of benzoyl peroxide with polyoxyethylene lauryl ether or sulfur have been available. These more effective agents have lessened the need for cryotherapy since cysts, papules and pustules are cleared more rapidly by them than previous topical treatments and comedones have been lessened by retinoic acid as well as by the use of the Buf-Puf®, a polyester sponge.

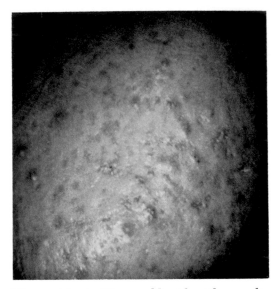

Figure 4-1. A 13-year-old girl with papular pustular acne was treated with two to five seconds of freezing with liquid nitrogen spray on individual lesions prior to initiation of any other therapy.

spray is quicker to use, does not require cleaning of the tip and allows for prompt visual appreciation of the extent of freezing while the solid cryoprobe largely obscures the treatment site.

Freezing time varies from two to five seconds for pustules, papules, nodules, and cysts up to 1 cm and five to fifteen seconds for larger cysts and nodules. The spray nozzle is held 3 to 5 cm from the lesion and is moved rapidly from one lesion to another. Comedones do not respond to freezing.

Some stinging or burning of treatment sites is noted for a few minutes following the procedure. Contrary to some reports[9] pain has not been a significant problem with liquid nitrogen and may even be less than with other cryogens because of its potential for more rapid analgesia. Occasionally an urticarial wheal will be seen at the site, persisting for several hours. Often erythema will be noted and on the following day vesiculation followed by crust-

ing is noted after freezing some cysts. Usually only erythema followed by gentle desquamation complete in four to five days is noted.

In a few patients atrophic and hypertrophic scars have been observed following freezing of acne cysts on the back and chest. These sequelae had been observed prior to freezing in these patients and it is difficult to say whether the procedure caused increased scarring or not. The cysts have been more efficiently controlled with cryosurgery than with incision and drainage or with intralesional steroids and the recurrence rate appears to be decreased after each freezing treatment.

Results: Inflammatory Lesions and Cysts (Plate 29-32; 45-48)

Residual erythema and crusting may be seen for a few days following freezing, rarely persisting over several weeks. Even with shorter freezing times vesiculation may develop in twelve to twenty-four hours, especially in fair-skinned patients, but this is not a frequent occurrence. Freezing generally results in the involution

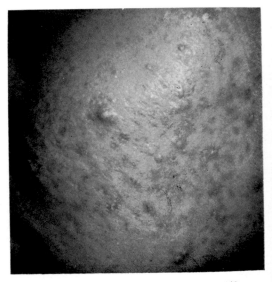

Figure 4-2. Two days later there was a 50 percent decrease in number of countable lesions.

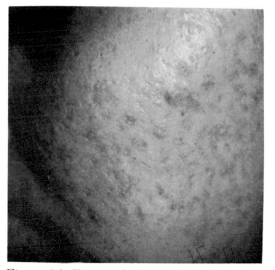

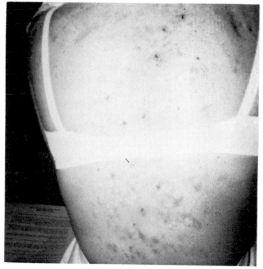

Figure 4-3. Two weeks later only a few active lesions remain and patient was then started on topical therapy for use at home.

Figure 4-5. A fourteen-year-old girl with cystic acne of the back as well as the face developed anemia while on tetracycline. Her hematologist requested that antibiotics be withheld until the anemia was corrected and patient was referred for cryosurgery. Twelve acne cysts treated initially.

of most papules, pustules, and cysts within two to four days (Figures 4-1 through 4-6). Larger cysts which require a freezing treatment of five to fifteen seconds do not resolve as rapidly as with intralesional steroids; however, it is the impression[12, 13]

that the recurrence rate is definitely less. The speed and ease of cryotherapy, the avoidance not only of injections but also of more involved surgical procedures makes cryosurgery a preferred therapy for both patient and physician.

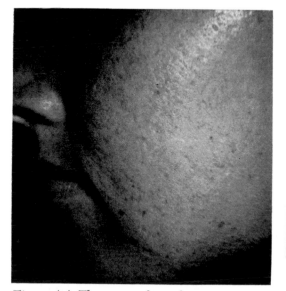

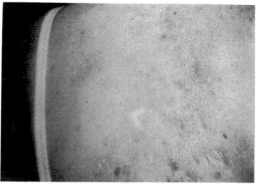

Figure 4-6. Two months later after four treatments with liquid nitrogen spray her acne is controlled and no further treatments have been required. Her only other treatment is Panoxyl Gel.®

Figure 4-4. Three years later there was no significant sequela from acne and Retin A cream had been used for control over the past year.

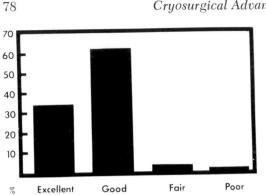

Figure 4-7. Evaluation of response in over 150 patients treated with the cryospray.

Subjective evaluation in over 150 patients[13-15] showed good to excellent results in 95 percent of the cases (Figure 4-7). Several patients required continued use of intralesional steroids in firm nodular cysts. For cysts on the back and chest a decreased recurrence rate has made cryosurgery the primary treatment even for patients with acne conglobata. The percentage reduction in number of countable inflammatory acne

lesions was determined in thirty-eight patients (Figure 4-8). After two weeks there was a 50 percent reduction in countable lesions. After six weeks there was a 67 percent reduction and after twelve weeks a 97 percent reduction in countable lesions. Individual inflammatory lesions subsided in an average of two to three days in 76 percent of 100 patients, three to four days in 21 percent, and four to five in 3 percent. An evaluation of the results relative to acne grade[13-15] using the system of Pillsbury, Shelley and Kligman[16] (Table 4-I) showed excellent results in sixteen of forty-eight (33%) grade II acne patients and good results in thirty-one of forty-eight (65%). Excellent results were noted in twenty-seven of seventy-six (35%) grade III acne patients and good results in forty-six of seventy-six (61%). In grade IV acne patients excellent results were noted in six of twenty-six (23%), and good results in seventeen of twenty-six (65%).

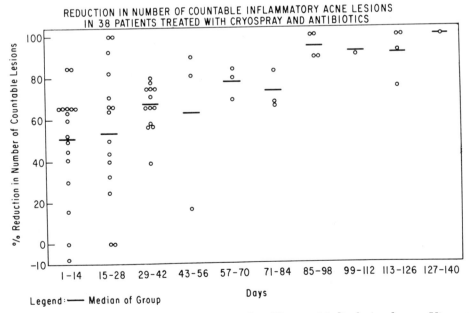

Figure 4-8. Reduction in the number of acne lesions treated cryosurgically in thirty-eight patients. Reproduced with the permission of the Vienna Medical Academy, Vienna, Austria, International Congress of Cryosurgery, Vienna, Austria, 1972.

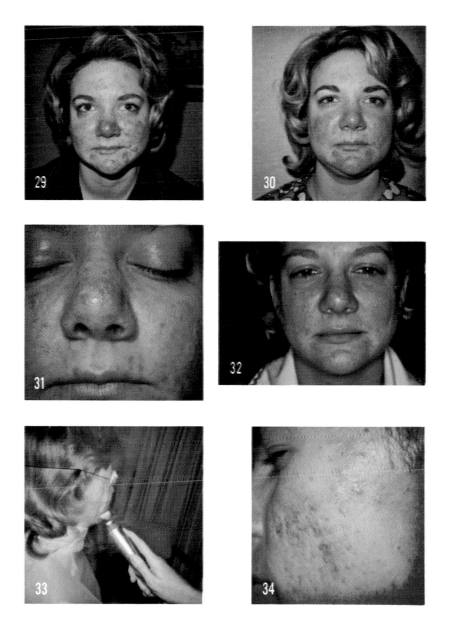

Plate 29. A twenty-five-year-old woman with severe acne rosacea since age 18 had failed to respond to multiple antibiotics, hormonal therapy, vaccines, X-ray therapy, systemic steroids and many forms of topical therapy. On her first visit she had multiple cysts, papules and pustules in addition to intense erythema and telangiectasia of the nose, chin and cheeks. Liquid nitrogen spray was used for two to five seconds on all of the active lesions. Prednisone was reduced from 40 mgm a day to 5 mgm every other day over the following three weeks.

Plate 30. Three weeks later the patient showed marked clearing of inflammatory lesions. Erythema and telangiectasia remained. Additional freezing to these areas was performed.

Plate 31. Liquid nitrogen spray used every three weeks brought about significant improvement with essentially no activity two months later. Systemic steroids were discontinued.

Plate 32. The patient required only occasional freezing over the past 28 months and minimal antibiotics for control of acne which remained essentially quiescent. Dermabrasion produced additional improvement in scarring and especially in telangiectasia.

Plate 33. Plastic tip for treating acne attached to handle of CE-8 Cryoderm manufactured by Frigitronics is used to freeze areas sectioned off for treatment of acne scarring. Patient wears goggles and a raincoat which is snug around the neck to prevent dripping of liquid nitrogen on the chest or neck.

Plate 34. This fourteen-year-old male patient with superficial acne scarring of the cheeks was treated with fifteen seconds of freezing using liquid nitrogen spray.

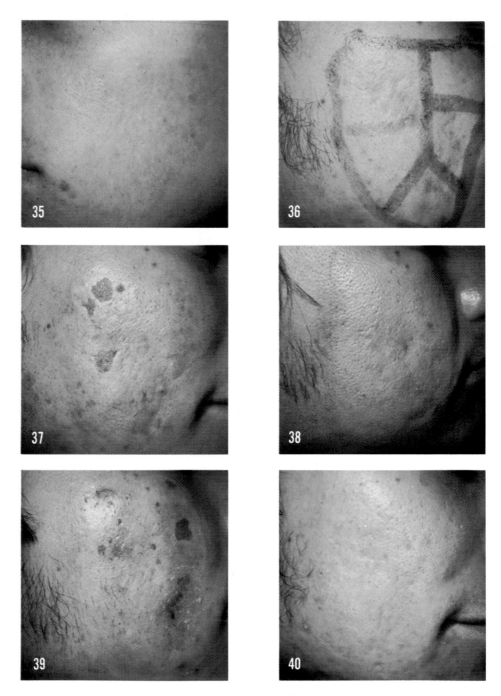

Plate 35. Several months later the patient showed significant improvement in scarring. From G. F. Graham, Cryosurgical treatment of acne, *Cutis, 16*:509-513, 1975. Courtesy of Yorke Medical Journals, Dun Donnelley Publishing Corp.

Plate 36. A nineteen-year-old male patient with moderate number of irregular shaped acne scars following severe cystic acne of the cheeks. Gentian violet used to outline areas for freezing with fifteen seconds of liquid nitrogen spray.

Plate 37. One week later a few areas of superficial eschar remained in an otherwise erythematous zone.

Plate 38. Two months later significant improvement in scarring observed. A second freeze was carried out at that time.

Plate 39. Six days later erythema and superficial crusting noted.

Plate 40. Three months later no pigment alteration observed despite sun exposure.

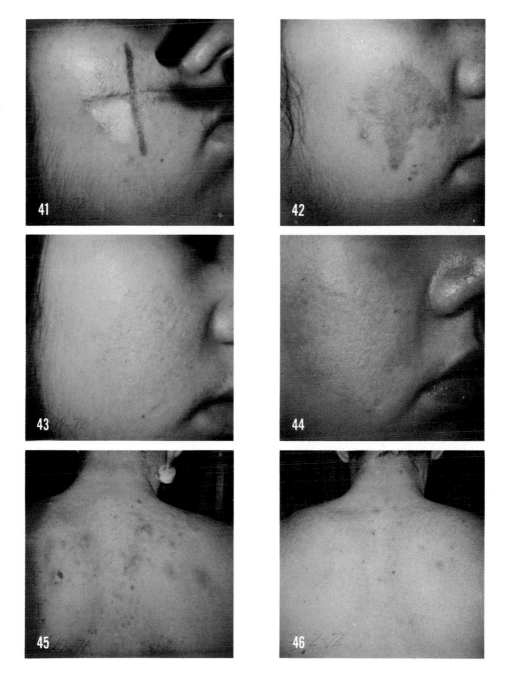

Plate 41. A seventeen-year-old female patient with moderately deep circinate acne scars on only one cheek was treated with nitrous oxide spray for twenty seconds in the outlined areas.

Plate 42. Five days later a superficial brown crust was observed.

Plate 43. One month later the patient showed moderate improvement in scarring.

Plate 44. Three years later dermabrasion of this area produced additional improvement.

Plate 45. Eighteen-year-old male paitent with cystic acne of the back. This patient had previously had a severe flare of acne due to proteus infection with high fever, requiring hospitalization and intravenous antibiotics, primarily ampicillin for control. The patient required continued ampicillin for control of the proteus infection and despite this cystic lesions developed on the back. These were controlled with liquid nitrogen spray weekly. From G. F. Graham, Cryocurgical treatment of acne, *Cutis, 16*:509-513, 1975. Courtesy of Yorke Medical Journals, Dun Donnelley Publishing Corp.

Plate 46. Five months later activity was essentially quiescent and the patient required only occasional freezing for control. From G. F. Graham, Cryosurgical treatment of acne, *Cutis, 16*:509-513, 1975. Courtesy of Yorke Medical Journals, Dun Donnelley Publishing Corp.

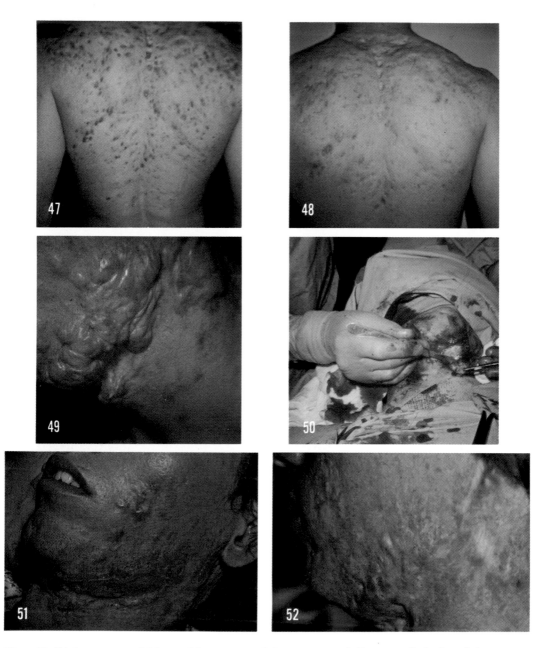

Plate 47. Eighteen-year-old boy with acne conglobata was partially controlled after eight months of cryosurgery and tetracycline.

Plate 48. Thirteen months later he remained controlled and subsequently had very minimal activity.

Plate 49. This nineteen-year-old boy was referred for cryosurgery of extensive keloids on the face, chest and back as a sequela of acne.

Plate 50. Under general anesthesia the keloids on both sides of the face and neck were removed by surgical excision and the base treated with intralesional steroids and cryosurgery for one minute.

Plate 51. Three weeks later some recurrence of keloid was noted, but freezing and intralesional steroids were continued every two to three weeks for five months, each side being treated approximately once every four to six weeks.

Plate 52. Significant improvement was noted after five months of therapy.

TABLE 4-I

EVALUATION OF RESPONSE IN ACNE
PATIENTS°

	Patients	Excellent	Good	Fair	Poor
Grade II	48	16	31	2	0
Grade III	76	27	46	3	0
Grade IV	26	6	17	2	1
Totals	150	49	94	7	1

° Reproduced with the permission of the Vienna Medical Academy, Vienna, Austria, International Congress of Cryosurgery, Vienna, Austria, 1972.

Treatment: Acne Scarring

Unless the patient is unusually anxious no preoperative medication is necessary. With a skin marker, the face is divided into approximately six rectangles 2 by 4 cm on each cheek (Plate 33). Liquid nitrogen spray is applied via a plastic tip with a horizontal opening 2 cm in width, allowing for uniform application of the refrigerant. The spray tip is moved downward with a shaving motion several times through each rectangle for a total of ten to twenty seconds, but usually not over fifteen seconds. The freezing time should be shorter when treating the skin under the eyes, over the mandible and on the neck since excessive freezing in these areas could result in hypopigmentation or atrophy.

The patient will experience moderate stinging and burning and may require a brief rest period of a minute or so after several areas have been treated. This also allows time for dissemination of vapor which may obstruct vision if it clouds the treatment field.

In the case of acne scarring, not more than one to three treatments are generally used. The second is administered if some improvement is noted with the first or if the first treatment failed to produce sufficient peeling. This may happen, especially in males with thicker skin types which may require longer freezing—fifteen to twenty seconds rather than the usual ten to fifteen seconds.

Although some discomfort may persist for several hours after freezing, postoperative medication is rarely required. The patient is instructed not to sleep on the face since edema fluid may accumulate more rapidly. Topical medications are withheld, but a mild emollient, such as Aloe Vera Gel® may be applied. Every effort to avoid premature removal of the crust is made since this might allow secondary infection to occur. The patient is advised to avoid sun exposure for at least six weeks. Sunscreens may be used when sun exposure is unavoidable.

Longer freeze times of twenty to forty seconds, and occasionally up to sixty or ninety seconds are required to treat hypertrophic scars and keloidal acne with either spray or probe. In combination with intralesional steroids, keloids resulting from acne require thirty to sixty seconds of freezing (Plates 49-52).

Side Effects

As with any other therapy, complications may arise from events such as an idiosyncratic reaction, a secondary infection or premature removal of the crust. Although significant complications have been rare, the physician is urged to be both experienced in the modality, and—before freezing extensive areas on patients not previously subjected to freezing—to consider the use of a test site to rule out an idiosyncratic response to the refrigerant.

Edema of the face, especially the periorbital areas, may be seen following the fifteen-second freeze. A patient treated by another dermatologist[15] developed marked periorbital edema several hours following a ten to fifteen second freeze. An emergency room physician suspected angioedema and administered intravenous steroids and adrenalin. The patient developed an area of delayed healing with an eschar removed surgically several weeks later. It is possible that treatment with intravenous steroids and adrenalin, in addition to premature removal of the eschar, contributed to scarring in the treatment site. A patient should be informed that periorbital edema may develop when freezing around the eyes and that this is not cause for alarm.

Hyperpigmentation has been noted in only five patients following the ten to fifteen second freeze. In three patients this increased pigmentation faded in two to six months. Two brunette patients required the application of Eldopaque Forte® to assist in lightening of the pigment. Hypopigmentation of a transitory type is often seen following freezing but has not been permanent in the author's experience. After sun exposure patients resume normal pigmentation. Hypopigmentation in several Negro patients had been transient with repigmentation occurring within few months, however, caution should always be exercised when treating dark or black-skinned individuals. Although permanent pigmentary changes have not been observed following freezing for fifteen to twenty seconds, freezing beyond this limit or multiple repeated freezings in the same location could prove detrimental to the melanocyte and lead to aberration of normal pigmentation.

Results: Acne Scarring
(Plates 34-44)

The skin is erythematous and occasionally urticarial after a ten to fifteen second freeze. The patient may experience a burning or stinging sensation for up to several hours following the freeze. Redness, vesiculation, edema and occasionally bullae may be present the following day. After a few days a superficial crust forms and is followed by desquamation which is generally complete in five to seven days. Erythema may persist for up to one month and occasionally longer.

Over 200 patients have been treated for acne scarring with a ten to fifteen second freeze. Patients with mild to moderate circinate scars especially on the cheeks respond best to freezing. Irregular deep scars, pits and atrophic areas show less response due to their depth and configuration. A transitory improvement of atrophic areas may result from edema during the first month. Patients should be informed of this since they may be disappointed as the edema subsides. Patient appraisal of the results has generally been good. Several patients were sufficiently improved to forego their desire for dermabrasion. The freeze may be repeated two or three times with at least a one month rest period between freezes. Additional improvement has rarely been seen after the third or fourth freeze.

Cryosurgery and Dermabrasion

Cryosurgery and dermabrasion are not necessarily mutually exclusive techniques. The ten to fifteen second freeze several weeks prior may serve as a prelude to dermabrasion in order to allow for abrasion to be carried out on cyst-free skin. Dermabrasion, using a wire brush, has resulted in additional improvement in a number of the patients treated initially with freezing. Since permanent pigmentary alteration could develop with repeated freezing, dermabrasion should be considered for those patients who do not show significant improvement after at least two to three freezing treatments and especially for patients with deeper, irregular scars. In dermabraded patients pigmentary changes have been more apparent than with patients treated exclusively with cryosurgery. Cryosurgery preceding dermabrasion, however, does not appear to increase the tendencies for pigment alteration (Plates 41 44).

General Precautions in Freezing

Cryotherapy appears to be an effective, safe procedure yielding excellent cosmetic results. Cryosurgeons should, however, give particular attention to the individual with a fair skin type or to the patient using retinoic acid since their skin may require less freezing. In certain facial regions, especially under the eyes, on the neck, the temples, and on the angles of the mandible, the epidermal thickness may allow for a reduction of freezing time. The use of a test site has not been routine in the author's practice up to this point, but in an effort to rule out the possibility of an idiosyncratic response or cold urticaria, this could prove useful. Although the response in a test site would not necessarily mirror the final results of the completed treatment, it might exclude the possible rare patient who could have an idiosyncratic response.

History of intolerance to cold such as cold urticaria and cryofibrinogenemia. Patients with auto-immune diseases such as: Lupus Erythematosis and ulcerative colitis, cryosurgery should be used with caution. The possible resulting necrotic tissue in this group of patients might unduly delay wound healing.

Central to the cryosurgeon's experience is a visual and tactile appreciation of the degree of freezing necessary in treating a particular lesion or disorder. If during treatment the physician recognizes that freezing has progressed further than is necessary, the site may be thawed rapidly by massage with the fingertips.

Although we have not seen a case of secondary infection following a freeze for acne the physician should be alert to signs which may indicate its presence such as purulent discharge, increased temperature, or cervical lymphadenopathy. If infection should develop, and this is exceedingly rare in cryosurgery, an appropriate systemic antibiotic is indicated. Antibiotic ointments soften the crusts and make premature removal more likely. Cleansing the skin with Betadine Skin Cleanser® or other antiseptic cleansers has not appeared to delay healing and could prove useful. Herpes simplex infection following freezing has not been reported but is a possibility. Freezing of extensive areas should be delayed if herpes simplex infection is observed at the time of a procedure. Instruct patients to avoid contact with persons with herpes simplex infections, smallpox vaccinations, or a bacterial infection such as impetigo or furuncles. Any such infection could prove detrimental to the excellent cosmetic result expected with cryosurgery.

As with any treatment modality, an understanding of possible pitfalls is important. The major concern in acne cryotherapy is to protect the melanocyte as much as possible from permanent damage, particularly in black-skinned and brunette patients, as well as avoiding rare atrophic changes or idiosyncratic reactions to cold.

Theory of Cryosurgery

The resolution of the acne cyst is not necessarily due to cell necrosis, since only superficial epidermal necrosis is incurred with a limited freezing. Leyden[4, 12] found in histopathologic sections of an acne nodule taken forty-eight hours after freezing with a carbon dioxide cryoprobe that there were superficial crusting with edema and liquifaction of the abscess in the dermis. A normal epidermis and dense collagen in the dermis appeared seventy-two hours after freezing. Leyden also found that during the fifteen to thirty-five second freeze the temperature drop at the 1 mm level was $23°C$ and at a depth of 6 mm the drop was around $8°C$, not sufficient for dermal

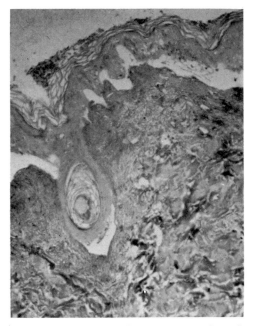

Figure 4-9. Histopathologic section of epidermis showing epidermal-dermal separation following freezing with liquid nitrogen. The separation produced extends around the follicle. Reproduced with the permission of Dr. Farrington Daniels, Jr.

necrosis. Leyden suggests freezing may result in liberation of enzymes which aid in clearing the abscess rapidly or in the increase of blood flow through the cyst. In his studies, a frozen nodule was cleared of injected fluorescein dye and had subsided in six to seven days while an untreated nodule continued to fluoresce at twelve days. This experiment confirms what has been observed clinically—the treated nodule subsides in half the time of an untreated nodule. More importantly, the recurrence rate is lessened.

A reduction of scarring following freezing with the spray is related to the greater depth of freezing possible with liquid nitrogen spray. Unlike fluroethyl spray, dry ice slush, and liquid nitrogen on cotton which can only freeze to the 2 mm level, liquid nitrogen in spray form can incur epidermal separation of even the follicle

wall from its dermal bed (Figure 4-9). The basement membrane remains intact and there is rapid regrowth of the epidermis following a freeze. The fibroblast is highly resistant to freezing, and Daniels[17] found that the preservation of the normal substrate is a factor in rapid re-epithelization. Zacarian[18] has shown that, in contrast with the liquid nitrogen swab, the deeper freezing possible with copper disc freezing, as with liquid nitrogen spray, degenerates skin appendages, sebaceous glands, and the hair matrix in the skin. These findings support the perspective that cryogenic probes and sprays using liquid nitrogen are more advantageous than are more superficial forms of freezing in attacking the deeper dermal lesions of acne such as cysts and scars.

Conclusion

Freezing sprays and probes in the treatment of acne have been in use for over six years. This method offers the dermatologist a fast and effective way of treating the inflammatory lesions of acne and acne scarring, especially mild to moderate depth scars. Cryosurgery may be used in conjunction with all other forms of acne therapy and may be used as a prelude to dermabrasion.

CRYOSURGERY OF BENIGN AND PREMALIGNANT LESIONS

The scope of cryosurgery is wide and its use in many benign and premalignant conditions is encouraging. Actinic and seborrheic keratoses, lentigos, pyogenic granulomas, and many other conditions have been treated often with good or even excellent response. Table 4-II lists many of the conditions the author has treated with their results. Several disorders are shown to illustrate the versatility of cryosurgery with pigmented, vascular, keratotic, dermal and epidermal lesions (Figure 4-10 through 4-19).

TABLE 4-II

CRYOSURGERY OF SELECTED BENIGN AND PREMALIGNANT LESIONS

Type	Results* Unaffected	Improved	Resolved
Actinic keratoses		most	many
Adenoma sebaceum	few	many	some
Chondrodermatitis	2	2	10
Comedonal nevus		4	
Dermatofibroma	few	most	few
Elastosis perforans		multiple lesions in one patient	
Ephelides		most	many
Epidermal nevus		5	
Fordyce condition		1	
Glomus tumor		1	
Granuloma annulare	1	5	5
Granuloma faciale†		1	
Hemangioma		4	
Herpes Simplex	several	several	
Insect bite granuloma		4	2
Keloids		20	
Lentigos		most	many
Lentigo maligna			2
Leukoplakia	2	13	10
Lichen sclerosus et atrophicus		1	1
Lymphangioma circumscripta			1
Lymphatoid papulosis			4 lesions in 2 patients
Molluscum contagiosum		most	many
Mucocele	3	4	2
Nevi—junctional		@ 30	
compound		@ 20	1
intradermal		@ 50	
(persistent pigmentation at base after biopsy only)			
Oral florid papillomatosis		2	
Porokeratosis	few	most	many
Port-wine stain	8	4	
Prurigo nodularis	few	many	some
Pseudopyogenic granuloma			1
Psoriasis (localized plaques)	2	8	
Pyogenic granuloma		1	8
Sebaceous cysts	few	many	some
Seborrheic keratoses		most	many
Senile angiomas	few	most	many
Syringomas	few	most	some
Spider angioma	few	most	some
Telangiectasia	some	some	some
Trichoepithelioma		5	3
Verrucae	few	most	many
White sponge nevus (mouth)	1	1	
Xanthelasma	5	5	3

* Numbers represent approximations only
† Patient of Dr. Roger Stewart

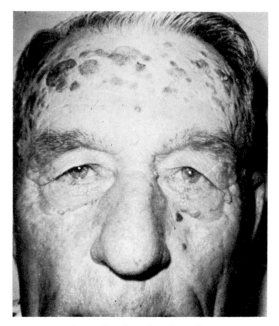

Figure 4-10. Multiple seborrheic keratoses are noted in a sixty-eight-year-old man.

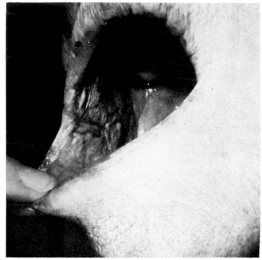

Figure 4-12. Diffuse leukoplakia in a seventy-year-old woman who had been a life-long snuff dipper.

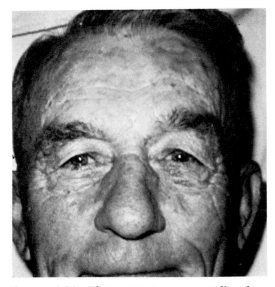

Figure 4-11. This patient is essentially clear after being treated with a combination of cryosurgery and curettage.

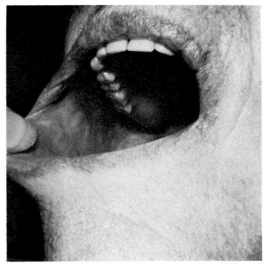

Figure 4-13. Leukoplakia is resolved after freezing with ten to fifteen seconds with liquid nitrogen spray. Patient had developed one area of epidermoid carcinoma on the gingiva prior to freezing.

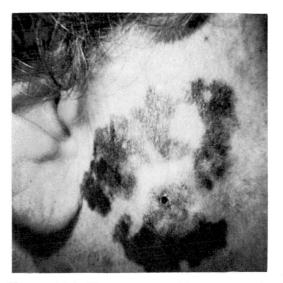

Figure 4-14. This sixty-year-old woman with a 4 cm lentigo maligna had refused surgical treatment of this site. Biopsy confirmed the clinical impression.

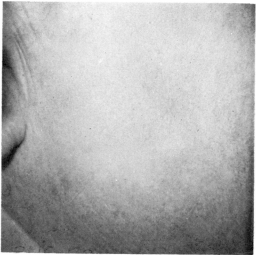

Figure 4-16. One year later some hypopigmentation is present but no evidence of the lentigo. There has been no recurrence in six years.

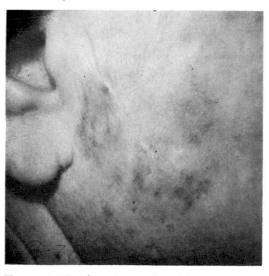

Figure 4-15. After six months of freezing areas approximately 1 to 2 cm every few weeks the area was cleared except for spots of pigment which on biopsy were found to be in the melanophages in the superficial dermis. It was the pathologist's opinion that the pigment previously in the cells prior to freezing became incontinent and was phagocytized by macrophages in the dermis. This cleared in several months.

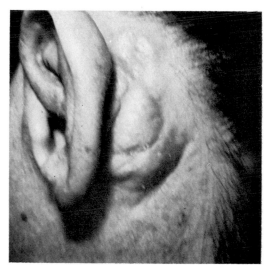

Figure 4-17. A forty-two-year-old patient with pseudopyogenic granuloma of Wilson Jones involving the external ear and ear canal. Tumor had been resistant to radiation therapy, intralesional steroids and desiccation and curettage. Pruritus had been her chief complaint.

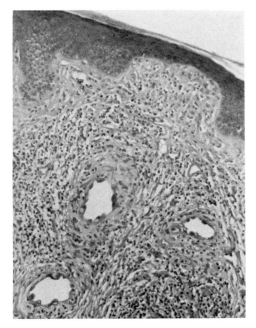

Figure 4-18. Histopathologic section through the lesion of pseudopyogenic granuloma shows thick-walled blood vessels with hypertrophic endothelium and a perivascular dense infiltrate primarily composed of lymphocytes and a few eosinophils. Courtesy of Dr. Herbert Z. Lund.

STATISTICAL EVALUATION IN THE TREATMENT OF SKIN CANCERS BY CRYOSURGERY

Cryosurgery has become a primary treatment for skin cancers in the author's dermatology practice in North Carolina. The patient population* is perhaps unique in the degree of actinic skin damage. It is not

---

* This patient population puts cryosurgery to the ultimate test. Most of these patients are of Scotch-Irish descent with fair skin and blue eyes. Many are farmers, fishermen, gardeners, and golfers, with a lifetime of exposure to the southern sun. Many of the farmers are engaged in tobacco farming and have been exposed to arsenic based pesticides in the past. Thus, many of these patients now presenting skin cancers have a long history of involvement with two major environmental carcinogens.

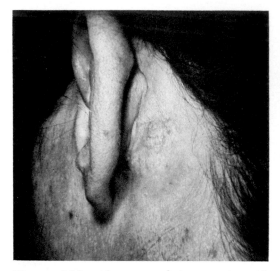

Figure 4-19. After several treatments with cryosurgery using a freeze time of one and one-half to two minutes the lesion resolved. An extension of tumor in the ear canal was treated with a probe developed for this purpose. The patient has been free of symptoms for over a year.

uncommon for patients to present multiple skin cancers. The three cryotherapeutic approaches used in this study have all provided results rivalling those of other methods. Only Mohs' chemosurgery yields better cure rates overall.[19]

Introduction

In the mid-nineteen-sixties the successful cryosurgical work of Torre[20] and Zacarian[21] with skin cancers encouraged the au-

TABLE 4-III

Tumor Type	Frequency	Percent
Basal cell epithelioma	591	69.5
Squamous cell carcinoma	186	21.9
Bowen's disease	11	1.3
Superficial BCE	23	2.7
Morphea type BCE	23	2.7
Keratoacanthoma	14	1.6
Other	2	0.2
	850	100

TABLE 4-IV

Description of Tumor Area	Frequency	Percent
Ear	55	6.5
Nose	189	22.2
Eyelids	12	1.4
Nasolabial fold	26	3.1
Other on face	340	40.0
Trunk	75	8.8
Upper extremities	56	6.6
Lower extremities	11	1.3
Lip	14	1.6
Scalp	11	1.3
Neck	38	4.5
Other	23	2.7
	850	100

thor to explore the potential of cryosurgery. Beginning in 1969 treatment of skin cancers with liquid nitrogen was initiated using the Kryospray, a hand-held unit manufactured by Brymill. An earlier report[22] describes this initial experience.

This present study details the cryosurgical treatment of 850 skin cancers in 424 patients and has been evaluated with the assistance of a computer data bank. The majority of the cancers treated were basal cell epitheliomas (637) including superficial and morphea (sclerosing) types. In addition 186 squamous cell carcinomas have been treated. Lesions of Bowen's disease and keratoacanthoma account for the remaining tumors in the study (Table 4-III). Of the total tumors, 719 (84.6%) were new tumors; 123 (14.5%) were recurrent and 8 (0.9%) were persistent following

previous treatment. The frequency of tumors at various locations is included in Table 4-IV. Table 4-V provides categorization of tumors by size.

Technique

Liquid nitrogen is the only cryogenic agent capable of freezing malignant lesions to the degree and depth necessary for cancer cell destruction. Instrumentation in the author's practice centers on the spray or probe application of liquid nitrogen. The CE-8 Cryoderm, a floor model unit manufactured by Frigitronics, together with a recent hand-held unit, the Cry-Ac, manufactured by Brymill, are the two basic instruments presently being used. Since regulation of both the length and depth of freezing is central to the cryosurgical process, a temperature monitoring device with thermocouple needle and pyrometer is an important component of the liquid nitrogen system. Such a monitoring system manufactured by Brymill has proven very satisfactory.

Freezing is carried out for one to two minutes as noted in Table 4-VI and then the lesions are allowed to thaw. A single application of freezing and the resulting thawing is referred to as a single freeze-thaw cycle. A repeat of the above process is referred to as a double freeze-thaw cycle. Of the cryosurgical methods employed, 414 (48.7%) were treated with a single

TABLE 4-V

Tumor Size	Frequency	Percent
Data not available	5	0.6
0.0-0.5 cm	262	30.8
0.6-1.2 cm	385	45.3
1.3-2.4 cm	148	17.4
2.5- and up cm	50	5.9
	850	100

TABLE 4-VI

Freeze Time	Frequency	Percent
Data not available	3	0.4
0-60 seconds	385	45.3
61-90 seconds	239	28.1
91-120 seconds	97	11.4
121-up seconds	125	14.7
	1	0.1
	850	100

TABLE 4-VII

Thaw Time—Thermocouple	Frequency	Percent
Thermocouple not employed ..	355	41.8
0-60 seconds	124	14.6
61-90 seconds	128	15.1
91-120 seconds	97	11.4
121-up seconds	146	17.2
	850	100

freeze, 172 (20.2%) with a double freeze, and 263 (30.9%) were treated with curettage and cryosurgery.

Both the freezing of a lesion to −20°C and the thawing which occurs at the base of a lesion from −20°C to 0°C is monitored with a thermocouple needle in place and is recorded respectively as freeze time (FT) and as thermocouple thaw time (TTT) (Table 4-VII). In over 60 percent of cases in the study, the microthermocouple needle and pyrometer were used in monitoring the freeze time to −20°C or in some cases −30°C and the thaw time from −20°C back to 0°C. The thermocouple needle should be autoclaved prior to each use. The clinical thaw time (CTT—the time from cessation of freezing until the tumor has visually thawed) is recorded on all patients and does not require thermal monitoring, only visual appreciation of the surface thawing (Table 4-VIII). Since it is a retrospective event, CTT cannot be used as an exclusive indicator of the length of freezing required. Thermocouple monitoring, measuring the peripheral spread of

TABLE 4-VIII

Clinical Thaw Time	Frequency	Percent
Data not available	157	18.5
0-60 seconds	75	8.8
61-90 seconds	154	18.1
91-120 seconds	104	12.2
121-up seconds	360	42.4
	850	100

freezing as used by Torre,[23] or fixing the site to underlying cartilage must be used to determine freezing time.

Tumor characteristics such as type, size, possible lateral extension, and depth are principal considerations for assigning cryosurgical methods. The thaw time also becomes significant since it may determine whether a second freeze-thaw cycle is required.

1. Single Freeze-Thaw Cycle

A single freeze-thaw cryosurgical application is used to treat superficial basal cell epitheliomas as well as many other basal cell epitheliomas, Bowen's disease, or squamous cell carcinomas if the thermocouple thaw time is at least sixty seconds and/or the clinical thaw time is at least ninety seconds.

2. Double Freeze-Thaw Cycle

Cryosurgery utilizing a double freeze-thaw cycle is used for more difficult tumors, either because of location, size, or

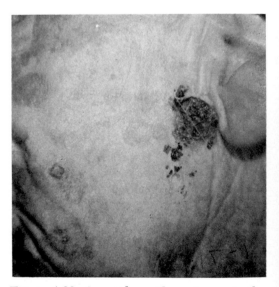

Figure 4-20. An epidermoid carcinoma in the preauricular area arising from actinic damaged skin.

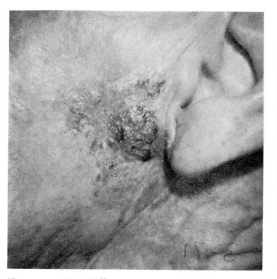

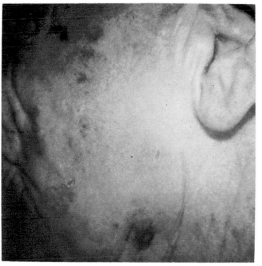

Figure 4-21. Following use of 5-fluorouracil the actinically damaged skin of the surrounding area and a portion of the tumor was eradicated.

Figure 4-23. The patient remains tumor free five years following treatment.

recurrence. In addition, if the thaw time following the initial single freeze application is less than sixty seconds (TTT) or ninety seconds (CTT) a second freeze-thaw cycle is utilized. The second cycle im-

mediately follows the first upon completion of thawing.

3. Curettage and Cryosurgery

Thorough curettage followed by cryosurgery is often used, especially in treatment of nodular lesions. This allows better definition of depth and lateral extension of tumors. A single freeze-thaw cycle following curettage is sufficient for many tumors, especially if the TTT and CTT are in the range of sixty to ninety seconds respectively. If the thaw time has been insufficient a second freeze is used. When extension of tumor into subcutaneous fat is discovered, total excision of the area with grafting is necessary, or Mohs' chemosurgery should be considered.

Results

The cure rates presented in the following statistics include those treatment sites which were followed for a minimum of three months. As of August 1975, 850 tumors had been treated with cryosurgery. Of this total, follow-up time has been up

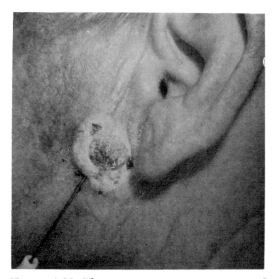

Figure 4-22. The remaining tumor was treated cryosurgically using thermocouple monitoring.

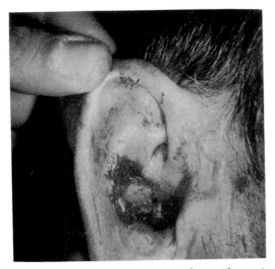

Figure 4-24. An extensive epidermoid carcinoma recurrent following cryosurgery and curettage and electrodesiccation. The site is shown following more extensive curettage extending into the ear canal. A biopsy of underlying cartilage failed to reveal invasion.

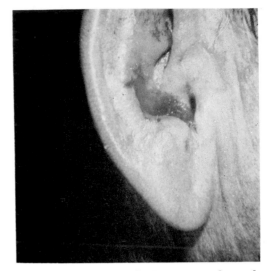

Figure 4-26. Edema fluid was noted in the area the following day. The patient was instructed to keep cotton in the ear canal to prevent the fluid draining into the canal.

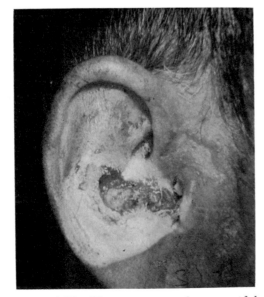

Figure 4-25. The area was frozen widely using, in addition to curettage, a double freeze-thaw cycle.

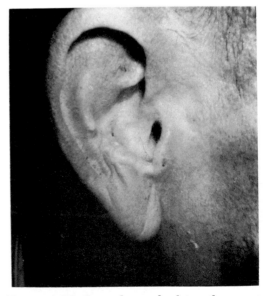

Figure 4-27. Several months later there was no evidence of tumor remaining. The patient has been tumor free for over five years.

to six months in 26.2 percent; seven to twelve months in 12.2 percent; thirteen to twenty-four months in 23.8 percent; twenty-five to forty-eight months in 17.9 percent and forty-nine months or more in 13.9 percent. Follow-up time was not available in 6 percent. The subsequent statistics will deal with the 739 tumors for which sufficient follow-up data is available.

New Basal Cell Epitheliomas

The data on basal cell epitheliomas would seem to indicate that the single freeze-thaw cycle is equivalent to a double freeze-thaw approach—both achieving a cure rate of approximately 97 percent. A reasonable case can be made, using this data, for a single freeze-thaw cycle for smaller and more superficial basal cell epitheliomas and a double freeze-thaw approach for more difficult lesions. The use of the single freeze-thaw cycle in the treatment of certain tumors was prompted because of rather striking hypopigmentation developing in several patients treated by

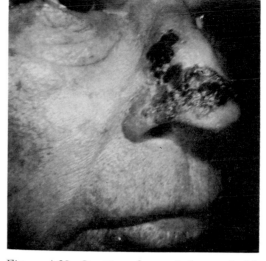

Figure 4-29. Crusting observed the week following a double freeze-thaw cycle.

the double freeze-thaw cycle. The highest cure rate for all new basal cell eiptheliomas was achieved with curettage followed by cryosurgery, a rate of 98.4 percent. Superficial basal cell epithelioma and morphea type basal cell epithelioma further demonstrates a very high success rate

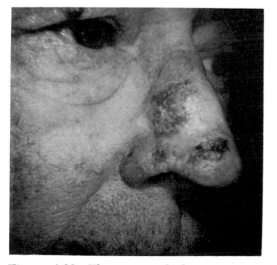

Figure 4-28. This patient had an extensive epidermoid carcinoma of the nose treated previously with cryosurgery. A recurrence appeared around the periphery of the initial site.

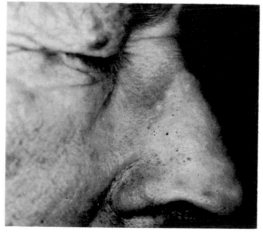

Figure 4-30. The patient is tumor free several months later. Note hypopigmentation in treatment site as well as milia and comedones which are often seen on the nose following freezing.

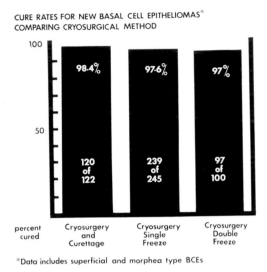

CURE RATES FOR NEW BASAL CELL EPITHELIOMAS*
COMPARING CRYOSURGICAL METHOD

percent cured	Cryosurgery and Curettage	Cryosurgery Single Freeze	Cryosurgery Double Freeze
	98.4%	97.6%	97%
	120 of 122	239 of 245	97 of 100

*Data includes superficial and morphea type BCEs

Figure 4-31. A comparison of cure rates for new basal cell epitheliomas treated by three different methods.

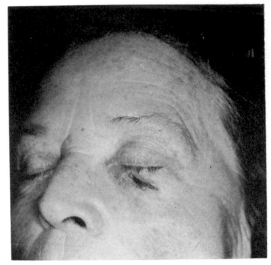

Figure 4-33. An excellent cosmetic result was obtained despite the use of curettage. Also a basal cell epithelioma under the eye was removed by curettage and treated cryosurgically.

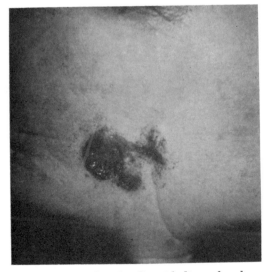

Figure 4-32. A basal cell epithelioma has been removed by curettage. Note the extension of tumor into surrounding area which did not appear to be involved. The base is treated with a one minute freeze.

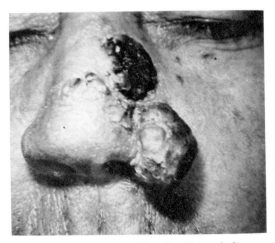

Figure 4-34. Extensive basal cell epitheliomas of the nose in an elderly patient.

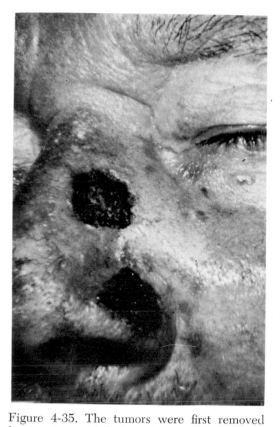

Figure 4-35. The tumors were first removed by curettage and the base frozen.

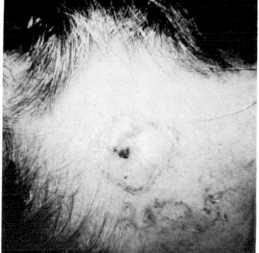

Figure 4-37. A 2 cm morphea type basal cell epithelioma on the forehead was treated with a double freeze-thaw cycle. Freeze time to –20°C was four minutes and thaw time to 0°C required 4 minutes. From *N C Med J, 32* (3): March 1971. Copyright 1971 by the North Carolina Medical Society.

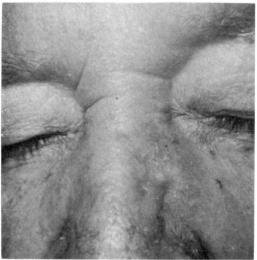

Figure 4-36. A very acceptable cosmetic result is obtained. The patient remained tumor free until his death several years later.

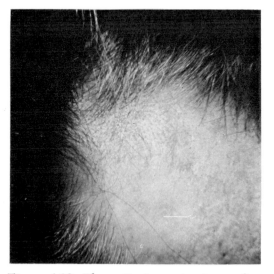

Figure 4-38. The patient remains tumor free six years later. From *N C Med J, 32* (3): March, 1971. Copyright 1971 by the North Carolina Medical Society.

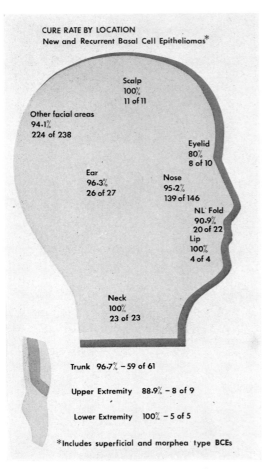

CURE RATE BY LOCATION
New and Recurrent Basal Cell Epitheliomas*

Scalp
100%
11 of 11

Other facial areas
94.1%
224 of 238

Eyelid
80%
8 of 10

Ear
96.3%
26 of 27

Nose
95.2%
139 of 146

NL Fold
90.9%
20 of 22

Lip
100%
4 of 4

Neck
100%
23 of 23

Trunk 96.7% – 59 of 61

Upper Extremity 88.9% – 8 of 9

Lower Extremity 100% – 5 of 5

*Includes superficial and morphea type BCEs

Figure 4-39. Cure rate of new and recurrent basal cell epitheliomas by location.

with all cryosurgical techniques, achieving a cure rate approaching 100 percent (43 of 44) cases.

Recurrent Basal Cell Epitheliomas

Cryosurgery proved to be effective therapy for recurrent basal cell epithelioma. Of the total of eighty-eight recurrent basal cell epitheliomas treated cryosurgically, seventy-six remained tumor free (86%). The combination of curettage plus cryosurgery was effective in 90.9 percent of the cases (10/11). A single freeze-thaw cycle was effective in 93.87 percent of cases (46/49). The double freeze-thaw approach was

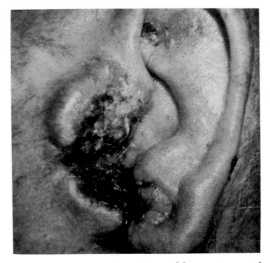

Figure 4-40. A ninety-year-old patient with extensive recurrent tumor, originally a basal cell epithelioma found at the time of surgery to have epidermoid carcinoma extending into the ear canal.

effective in only 71.4 percent (20/28), but this lower success rate is in part made artificially low by the selection of this form of therapy not only for those very exten-

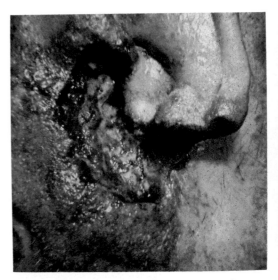

Figure 4-41. One day following general anesthesia extensive curettage and cryosurgery of this area has produced edema and serosanguineous drainage.

sive recurrences, but also as a means of palliation. These were the most difficult of the tumors treated and some of these had been recurrent in the same location more than once.

Squamous Cell Carcinomas New and Recurrent

Cryosurgery was found to be a successful treatment for squamous cell carcinomas (Figures 4-20 to 4-30). Cure rates for new squamous cell carcinomas treated in the above fashion were as follows: curettage plus cryosurgery (98.6 percent (70/ 71), single freeze-thaw cycle 96.2 percent (51/53), double freeze-thaw cycle 82.4 percent (14/17). Again, note there was a tendency to assign the more difficult squamous cell carcinomas to the category of the double freeze-thaw cycle. An acceptable cure rate for recurrent squamous cell carcinoma was achieved with results as follows: curettage followed by cryosurgery 85.7 percent (6/7); a single freeze thaw cycle 71.4 percent (5/7); and a double freeze-thaw cycle 66.7 percent (2/3).

Comparison of Results

A comparison of the cryosurgical methods and their cure rates for all new basal cell epitheliomas is shown in Figure 4-31: 98.4 percent (120/122) of new basal cell epitheliomas were cured by cryosurgery and curettage, 97.6 percent (239/245) by a single freeze-thaw cycle, and 97 percent (97 of 100) by a double freeze-thaw cycle. This includes all types of basal cell epitheliomas (Figures 4-32 to 4-38) and would indicate little statistical significance between the three methods used.

Comparison of cure rates by location of combined new and recurrent basal cell epitheliomas is shown in Figure 4-39. Of the two tumors which recurred on the eyelid, one was subsequently eradicated with cryosurgery while the other required Mohs'

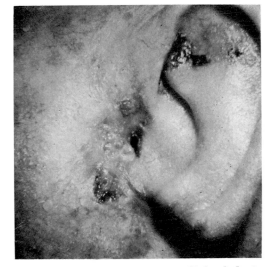

Figure 4-42. The area was well healed. Six weeks later the patient did develop recurrent disease superior to the treatment site. This was eradicated with cobalt therapy and the patient lived two years. The palliative procedures combining several techniques resulted in significant relief in this elderly patient.

chemosurgery. The cure rates were somewhat lower in the nasolabial fold (90.9%), but this area is known to yield lower cure rates for other methods as well, excepting Mohs' chemosurgery. The results achieved on the scalp have not been confirmed by others and may be due to the relatively small number of tumors in this location. Zacarian[24] and Torre[25] have both expressed concern over the use of cryosurgery in the scalp because of recurrences noted there. The author believes it is important in this location to use thermocouple monitoring and a double freeze-thaw cycle.

Certain tumors probably should not be treated with cryosurgery, for example a tumor recurrent several years following excisional surgery in which tumor boundaries have been obscured. Mohs' chemosurgical technique, in the author's opinion, is the preferred method in this type of recurrence. However, tumors recurrent after irradiation, curettage and desiccation, or cryosurgery have been treated successfully with cryosurgery.

Cosmetic Results

A subjective evaluation of cosmetic results following cryosurgery, dependent on the degree of atrophy, hypopigmentation or hypertrophic scarring, was made on many of the tumors treated. The results were considered excellent in 68 cases (8%), good in 680 cases (80%), and fair in 21 cases (2.5%). Since hypopigmentation is the most common and unwanted side effect, it is fortunate that most patients who develop skin cancers are fair-skinned individuals where this does not become a significant problem.

Complications

Serious complications stemming from cryosurgery are unusual although a degree of morbidity, including edema, vesiculation, and weeping (Figure 4-40 to 4-42), followed by crusting for two to three weeks are to be expected. Periorbital edema following treatment of tumors around the eyes and a severe vascular type headache following freezing of tumors on temple or scalp are to be expected and the patient should be so warned. For the beginning cryosurgeon, a thermocouple needle and pyrometer should be used to monitor freeze and thaw times. The physician should be alert to any sign of secondary infection in the treatment site and premature or accidental removal of the eschar should be guarded against, since such removal may enhance the possibility of infection and scarring. The use of appropriate systemic antibiotics, as well as antibiotic powder or spray rather than creams or ointments, seems preferable in handling such a complication. Pigmentary changes, scarring, and idiosyncratic effect are dis-

cussed earlier in the chapter in the section on acne.

Conclusion

The gratifying response of skin carcinomas to cryosurgery is well supported by this data. The good cosmetic results, ease of therapy, and overall cure rates competitive with other treatment methods establishes cryosurgery as a major technique in skin cancer therapy.

REFERENCES

1. Allington, H. D.: Liquid nitrogen in the treatment of skin diseases. *Calif Med,* *12*:153-155, 1950.
2. Graham, G. F.: Liquid nitrogen spray found useful in treating acne. *JAMA,* *215*:1901-1904, 1971.
3. Kligman, A. M.: Tropical acne. Paper read before the Academy of Dermatology Meeting in Chicago, December, 1970.
4. Leyden, J. J.: Cryoprobes in the treatment of acne conglobata. Paper read before Society for Cryosurgery, Miami, Florida, March, 1971.
5. Torre, D. P.: Cryosurgery in dermatology. In Von Leyden, H., and Cahan, W. G. (Eds.): *Cryogenics in Surgery.* Flushing, NY, Med Exam, 1971.
6. Torre, D. P.: Freezing with freons. *Cutis,* *16*:437-445, 1975.
7. Pierce, H. W.: One-time combination cryotherapy may flatten small keloids. *Dermatology in practice,* *6* (5):4-5, 1973.
8. Zacarian, S. A.: Cryosurgery of Tumors of the Skin and Oral Cavity, Springfield, Thomas, 1973, pp. 121-122.
9. Shalita, A. R.: Surgical procedures for the treatment of acne vulgaris. *J of Dermatologic Surgery,* *1*:46-48, 1975.
10. Goette, D. K.: Liquid nitrogen in the treatment of acne vulgaris, a comparative study. *South Med J,* *66*:1131-1132, 1973.
11. Epstein, E. H.: Cryorolling for acne and acne scarring. Paper read before the Academy of Dermatology Meeting in San Francisco, Calif., December, 1975.

12. Leyden, J. J., Mills, O. H., Kligman, A. M.: Cryoprobe treatment of acne conglobata. *Brit J Derm*, 90:335-341, 1974.

13. Graham, G. F.: Liquid nitrogen and nitrous oxide sprays in the treatment of acne vulgaris. Proceedings, Latest Developments in Cryosurgery, International Congress of Cryosurgery. Vienna, June, 1972, pp. 351-358.

14. Graham, G. F.: Cryosurgical treatment of acne. *Cutis, 16:*509-513, 1975.

15. Graham, G. F.: Cryosurgery in the treatment of acne. In Epstein, E.: *Skin Surgery*, 4th ed. Springfield, Thomas, 1976.

16. Pillsbury, D. M., Shelley, W. B., and Kligman, A. M.: *Dermatology*. Philadelphia, W. B. Saunders, 1956, pp. 810-811.

17. Daniels, F., Jr.: Some of the cryobiology behind cryosurgery. *Cutis, 16:*421-424, 1975.

18. Zacarian, S. A.: *Cryosurgery of Skin Cancer and Cryogenic Techniques in Dermatology*. Springfield, Thomas, 1969, p. 60.

19. Mohs, F. E.: Chemosurgery for basal cell carcinoma. *JAMA, 210:*1759-1761, 1969.

20. Torre, D.: New York: Cradle of Cryosurgery, *NY State J Med, 67:*465-667, 1967.

21. Zacarian, S. A. and Adham, M. I.: Cryotherapy of cutaneous malignancy. *Cryobiology, 2:*212-218, 1966.

22. Graham, G. F.: Cryosurgery of Skin Tumors. *NC Med J, 32:*81-87, 1971.

23. Torre, D.: Cryosurgery in dermatology. In Von Leden, H. and Cahan, W. G. (Eds.): *Cryogenics in Surgery*. Flushing, NY, Med Exam. 1971, pp. 500-529.

24. Zacarian, S. A.: Cryosurgery of skin cancer—in proper perspective. *J of Derm Surgery, 1:*33-38, 1975.

25. Torre, D.: Personal communication, October 1975.

CHAPTER FIVE

Cryosurgery for Cancer of the Skin

SETRAG A. ZACARIAN, M.D., F.A.C.P.

I. CANCER OF THE SKIN— A GENERAL REVIEW

S KIN CANCER is by far the most common malignant tumor of man. No less than 250,000 patients are treated annually in the United States, many of whom have multiple skin cancers at the time of their initial examination by their physician. The number of patients with premalignant tumors of the skin each year is in excess of 5,000,000.[1] Cutaneous malignant tumors account for approximately 25 percent of all malignant disease in the United States and some 2 to 2½ percent of all cancer deaths, approximately 5000 per year.[2] A large proportion of mortality from skin malignancy is attributed to melanomas. The early recognition of skin cancer is extremely important and of equal significance is the proper selection of the most effective modality. One must consider the histology, anatomical site and the age of the patient. An added consideration is whether one is confronted with a primary or a recurrent tumor.

There are two interacting influences in the development of skin cancer, namely *genetic* and *sunlight*. The highest incidence of skin cancers are found in patients with light pigmentation, with a relative infrequency in the deeply pigmented races. In Australia for example, the incidence of cutaneous carcinoma constitutes approximately 60 percent of all malignancies seen on the continent, the highest in the world. This is due to the influence of British descent in the populace who are exposed to prolonged high-intensity sunlight.[3] The critical and detrimental wave lengths of ultraviolet light appear to be within the range between 290 mn to 332 mn.[4] The evidence of actinic damage upon the integument and its pathogenesis leading to skin cancer have been well established.[5-8]

We must not overlook other inciting factors and carcinogens which produce skin cancers, such as ionizing radiation,[9-11] ingestion of arsenicals,[12-16] trauma,[17-19] neglected ulcers of the skin,[20-21] and post vaccinia scars.[22-24]

The most common skin cancer encountered in man is the *basal cell epithelioma* (rodent carcinoma), followed with *squamous cell carcinoma* (prickle cell or epidermoid carcinoma). Less frequently noted are *basosquamous* cell carcinoma and *Bowen's disease* (carcinoma in situ). This group of four malignant tumors of the skin constitutes approximately 96 percent of all skin cancers observed in man. Less frequently noted neoplasms are melanomas, cutaneous tumors associated with basal cell nevus syndrome, erythroplasia of Queyrat, extramammary Paget's disease, and intraepidermal epithelioma of Jadassohn, the rare adenocarcinoma and metastatic carcinomas to the integument from internal visceral malignancies.

It is not unusual for a patient with skin cancer to present multiple tumors at his initial examination. In a series of 5,840 patients who had a combined total of 14,383 skin cancers, excluding melanomas, Mac-Donald[26] observed that approximately 40 percent of the patients presented multiple lesions at their first examination. She further observed that twelve of every one hundred patients treated for primary lesions returned within twelve months with a second carcinoma. In a more recent study, Spoore[27] observed that approximately a third of his patients returned within a year for the treatment of additional primary skin cancers. In stressing the importance of long-term follow-up for patients treated for basal cell carcinomas, Ernst Epstein[28] noted some 20 percent of his patients previously treated for skin cancers during a one year period had developed new cutaneous cancers and some 75 percent of the patients examined were unaware or did not suspect the presence of another skin cancer when examined.

Approximately two-thirds of all cutaneous carcinomas are observed between the fifth and seventh decade of life. In a series of 488 patients with skin cancer, Schrek and Gates[29] observed that the median age for the time of onset for basal cell carcinomas was 52.3 and for epidermoid carcinomas, 66.2; only 1.5 percent of skin cancers seem to appear under thirty years of age.[30]

It is important to appreciate the histological characteristics of a given skin cancer to properly assess the best therapeutic approach. Basal cell carcinomas may be multicentric, nodular, ulcerative, syringoid, adenoid and sclerosing. Some of these are more invasive to underlying subcutaneous tissue, as with the ulcerative type, while others like the sclerosing are more radioresistant as well as resistant to freezing. The reader is referred to the classic monograph written by Lund.[31]

The size and the anatomic site of the tumor will very often dictate the choice of modality to effectively eradicate the neoplasm. Fortunately most skin cancers are not very large. In a twelve year study of collected cases of both basal cell epitheliomas and epidermoid carcinomas, Macomber[32] recorded the size of the tumors. He observed that two-thirds of the neoplasms were 1.0 cm in size or smaller. In a series of 634 basal cell epitheliomas in 375 patients, Griffith and McKinney[33] found 38 percent measured under 0.5 cm and 38.2 percent between 0.6 cm to 1.0 cm; i.e. 76.2 percent were 1.0 cm or less in size. They noted 17.5 percent of the tumors were between 1.1 and 2.0 cm; 4.5 percent measured 2.1 to 3.0 cm and only 1.8 percent of the lesions were over 3.0 cm.

It is an acknowledged fact that most cutaneous carcinomas are observed on sun-exposed portions of the body. In a large series of 836 cases of basal cell epitheliomas, Owen[34] noted 92.5 percent were found on the head and neck. As much as 50 percent of skin cancers are observed on the nose and cheeks.[35] Cancers situated on the arms and legs constitute a small percentage, and when noted, very often (10:1) favor an epidermoid carcinoma over a basal cell epithelioma.[36] Less than 2 percent of cancers of the integument are situated upon the scalp. Frequently cutaneous neoplasms in this area may prove to be sarcomas or even melanomas. Conley[37] in a series of 150 patients with malignant tumors of the scalp found fifty-eight were malignant melanomas, fifty-seven were basal cell epitheliomas, twenty-six were squamous cell carcinomas and nine were sarcomas.

Malignant tumors of the skin in critical areas, such as the eyelids, nose and ears will be discussed in detail further along in this chapter.

Metastasis from basal cell epitheliomas are extremely uncommon. In a series of

9,050 basal cell epitheliomas, Cotran[38] found only six to demonstrate metastasis, an incidence of 0.09 percent. There have been approximately seventy-six cases of metastasis from basal cell carcinoma reported in the literature since 1894.[39] Be aware, however, that once these tumors metastasize, mortality rate is high, within the range of 50 percent.[39, 40] The lungs[41, 42] and bones[43-45] appear to be favored sites. Although metastasis is rare in these tumors, there is no room for complacency for their vigorous treatment. Some basal cell epitheliomas are extremely aggressive in behaviour and involve underlying bone. When they approximate and extend into mucous membranes or facial orifices, these tumors will become treacherously invasive.[46]

Epidermoid carcinomas on the other hand have a higher incidence of metastasis. Clinicians, however, differ in their reported data. In a five year study of 340 skin cancers, eighty of which were epidermoid carcinomas, Rueckert[47] observed seven which metastasized. Metastatic capacity of epidermoid carcinomas is very often dependent upon the size of the tumor. In a study of 507 epidermoid carcinomas, Warren and Hoerr[48] noted the neoplasms under 1.0 cm showed a metastasis of 3 percent, while those between 1.5 to 2.5 cm showed a propensity to metastasize in the vicinity of 12 percent. On the other hand, Ackerman and del Regato[49] have reported only 5 percent incidence of metastasis of epidermoid carcinomas of the face and neck. Lower figures from 2 to 3.5 percent metastasis of epidermoid carcinomas have been reported by other investigators.[50-52] Despite the divergence of opinions regarding the incidence of metastasis of epidermoid carcinomas, all authorities agree that neoplasia which arise from preexisting precanceroses or trauma manifest a greater potential to metastasize.[53-55]

The management of skin cancers will vary among physicians, and the choice of his therapeutic regimen will depend upon his specific skill and his judgment as to the specific site of the tumor, its histology, size, an in particular whether the tumor is primary or recurrent. The existing modalities are well known: surgical excision, irradiation, curettage and electrodesiccation, Mohs' chemosurgery, topical chemotherapy, 5-FU, and cryosurgery.

It is not the intent nor the purpose of this monograph to review each and every technique, but to discuss briefly the overall cure rate of the long-established modalities, to fully comprehend and evaluate the cryosurgical approach to skin malignancy, and to properly assess its effectiveness. It is extremely difficult to compare cure rates among various modalities, for much is dependent upon the skill of the cancer therapist, the selectivity and location of the neoplasia, and other factors already cited above.

An interesting paper was recently published by Crissey.[56] He cites the composite of five-year cure rates of 14,114 carcinomas of the skin drawn from thirteen published studies. The comparative modalities employed were cold knife surgery, curettage and electrodesiccation, radiation therapy and Mohs' chemosurgery. He noted the cure rate from chemosurgery was 99.1 percent followed with cold-knife surgery which was 95.5 percent. Radiation therapy yielded a 94.7 percent cure rate while curettage and electrodesiccation offered a 92.6 percent cure rate. We are all aware of many published reports citing varied statistical cure rates for the modalities cited above, some of which may be considerably higher. However, after a thorough review of the literature, the author finds Crissey's overall view a fair assessment. Cure rates for carcinoma of the scalp, nose, and eyelid do not generally demonstrate the high cure rates as in other cutaneous sites. This will be discussed in further detail later in this chapter.

A word or two regarding the pattern of recurrence of skin cancers is in order. In an interesting study of 1,196 surgically excised basal cell carcinomas, Gooding and his associates,[57] followed for five years the recurrence rate of sixty-six lesions (5.5%) which were reported by the pathologist as inadequately excised, i.e. tumor showing at the excised margins. They found only twenty-three of the sixty-six basal cell carcinomas (34.8%) recurred at the end of five years. In a similar study by Pascal et al.,[58] they noted that in 42 of 361 patients who underwent a primary excision for a basal cell carcinoma, the pathologist reported inadequate excision of their tumors in 11.5 percent. These patients were followed for ten years and the recurrence rate was 30 percent. Does this mean that we should not reexcise or re-treat neoplasms reported by the pathologist as inadequately excised? Not necessarily, although both authors felt a watchful observation was mandatory. Pascal advised a conscientious postoperative follow-up would be the procedure of choice in such instances where further surgery, particularly on the face, "might result in cosmetic or functional embarrassment."

As to the peak incidence of recurrences following treatment of cancer of the skin, there is a firm agreement among clinical investigators. Grover[59] cites the following incidence in 118 patients with a combined total of 138 basal cell carcinomas. The observed recurrences within the first year was 46.4 percent; second year, 23.7 percent; the third year, 13.5 percent; fourth year 10.1 percent; fifth year 3.9 percent; sixth year 1.4 percent; and seventh year 1.0 percent. It is quite clear that at the end of the third year, most recurrences will have manifested themselves, i.e. 83.6 percent, while at the end of the fifth year 97.6 percent. The author's own statistical follow-up with cryosurgery closely correlates with Grover's studies. Lauritzen and his associates[60] noted in their series of 2,900 basal cell carcinomas followed for a ten year period, that 76 percent of the recurrences were within the first three years. This data along with our knowledge that a high percentage of patients with skin cancers develop new tumors, makes it mandatory that we follow our patients with cutaneous carcinoma for no less than five years.

A final remark regarding the depth of invasion of the average skin cancer is pertinent, not only in surgical excision, irradiation, and curettege and electrodesiccation, but also in cryosurgery. There is much paucity in the literature in this area and much more is needed. Ebbehoj,[61] interested in the depth of ionizing radiation within the skin from grenz rays in patients with skin cancer, obtained a biopsy of each lesion prior to treatment and measured the depth of invasion of the neoplasm from the surface epithelium. He observed that in 208 skin cancers, 50 percent of the tumors did not exceed 2 mm from the cutaneous surface, and 82.5 percent of the cancers did not exceed 5 mm in depth. Some 11.5 percent of the malignant tumors exceeded 5 mm and the majority of them were epidermoid carcinomas. In a much smaller series, Newell[62] in 1968 observed that 96.0 percent of 67 basal cell carcinomas carefully biopsied and measured did not extend beyond 3 mm from the integumentary surface. In the author's own series of 123 consecutive patients with basal cell carcinomas, biopsy specimens were submitted to Dr. Theodore Brand, pathologist in Springfield. We observed that 96.0 percent of these tumors did not extend beyond 3 mm from the epithelial surface. Only 3.2 percent of the tumors invaded to the depth of 4 to 5 mm from the surface of the skin and a mere 0.8 percent invaded beyond 5 mm depth.

The depth of invasion of a given skin cancer is but one consideration. An equally important consideration is the unknown and unpredictable lateral extension of its pseudopods and tiny nests of tumor cells beyond surgical excision, curettage, irradiation, and even cryosurgery. Clinicians often ask what constitutes an adequate margin of normal skin, 0.5 cm or 1.0 cm? Much of this decision rests upon the site of involvement of the tumor. Cancers located on the ala nasi and nasolabial fold may extend far beyond the nominal margins which we would ordinarily consider adequate for other sites. Basosquamous cell carcinomas, in particular, may extend far beyond the anticipated nominal margins and also have a higher propensity to metastasize than basal cell epitheliomas.[63] Ernst Epstein,[64] in a series of 200 surgically excised cell carcinomas, found 2 mm margin of normal appearing tissue proved quite satisfactory, rendering a cure rate of 98 percent followed for over two years. This is a provocative study and worthy of deliberation, but the author would like to see a five year follow-up on his observations. The author believes most clinicians would favor at least 0.5 cm margin of normal skin beyond the tumor margin whenever possible.

II. CLINICAL APPLICATION OF CRYOSURGERY IN SKIN CANCERS

A. Instrumentation

Contemporary cryosurgery began fifteen years ago by its founder, Irving S. Cooper.[65] His influence and meticulous work captured the imagination of many clinical investigators in all surgical specialties, in-

cluding dermatologists. Early pioneers in this new surgical technology learned much from the cryobiologists and worked closely with engineers. As a consequence, we now have a clearer understanding of cryonecrosis and have available a number of cryogenic instruments suitable for one's own specific needs. Throughout this book, the various instruments currently in use are fully discussed.

For the past six years, the author has consistently used a self-pressurizing hand-held cryogenic unit, the C-21 (Figure 5-1). This vessel holds 250 cc of liquid nitrogen and will allow the free flow of this refrigerant in an acceptable liquid-vapor state for over five continuous minutes. The amount of flow can be controlled by interchangeable plastic needles varying in gauge from number 18 to 22. The unique feature of this unit is that one can instantly stop the flow of the cryogen and start again by a simple metal rod attached to the cap held in one's hand. This instrument has also two escape valves should the pressure of the refrigerant rise too rapidly. If one does not wish to use an open spray, the unit is equipped with various sized closed discs (Figure 5-2). For the most part, the

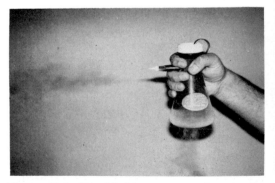

Figure 5-1. Hand-held cryosurgical unit, the C-21, for the treatment of benign and malignant tumors of the skin. The amount of spray of liquid nitrogen can be controlled with interchangeable plastic needles. Courtesy of Frigitronics Inc., Shelton, Ct.

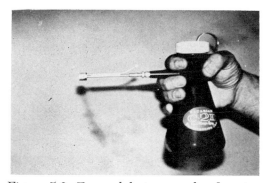

Figure 5-2. For oral lesions, a closed system may be used by attaching a disc to the apperture of the unit. Courtesy of Frigitronics Inc., Shelton, Ct.

author uses the open spray of liquid nitrogen. An exception would be for keloids or an angioma where he wishes to use pressure or compression upon the given tissue.

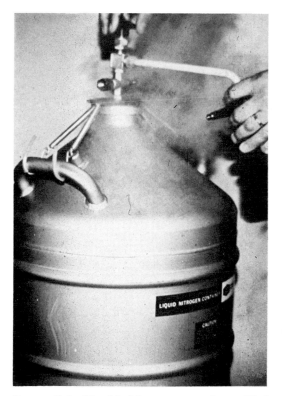

Figure 5-3. Hand-held unit must be refilled from time to time with liquid nitrogen from a larger reservoir of the refrigerant.

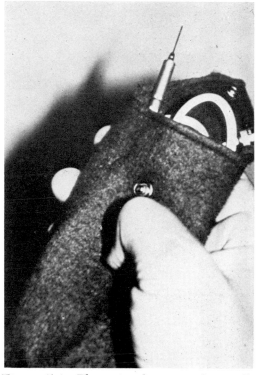

Figure 5-4. The microthermocouple needle along with its attached insulated tubing is placed in a paper or cloth receptacle.

A single disadvantage, as with some other hand-held units, is that the cryogen empties within the vessel and must be refilled from a large Dewar container (Figure 5-3). This disadvantage is compensated by the fact that it is mobile and the unit can be used at a hospital, a clinic, or a nursing home. In a group practice with an extra unit, inexpensively purchased, one doctor can use the instrument while an associate does not have to wait for its use, as with a large floor model. At a single filling, a doctor can freeze multiple skin cancers and, while waiting for the thawing period of the tumors to end, can readily refill the vessel. On humid days and with repetitive use of this unit, moisture will on occasion trap itself and the free flow of liquid nitrogen will temporarily stop. Fortunate-

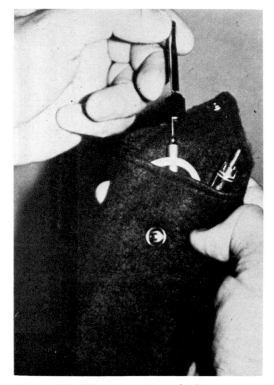

Figure 5-5. The protective shield is placed over the microthermocouple needle.

ly, with the improvement of the ball-valve system, this does not occur too often. This unit does not drip liquid air droplets from its outer shell when in use because of its plastic construction.

In order to measure the advancing ice front within and below the tumor during a freezing experience, the need for micro-thermocouple needles is essential (Figure 5-4). These are tiny 22 gauge needles, 15 mm or ¾ inch long, with a sensitive constantan tip which will sense the temperature. With each use, the needle can be cleaned and covered with its protective shield, placed in a cloth or paper container, and autoclaved (Figure 5-5). The monitored temperature is registered upon the pyrometer capable of recording two channels within the turn of the knob (Figure 5-6). Try to get into the practice of *testing out the thermocouple needle* before using it. Dipping the tip in ice water and in liquid nitrogen will quickly establish its integrity.

In the first chapter the author discussed the evolvement of the cryolesion and also the development of a small clinically applicable template or jig. For the clinician who first begins to freeze malignant tumors of the skin, the author recommends that the template be used very often. In a short time one develops the sense of duration of freeze through ballottement

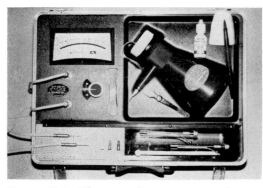

Figure 5-6. The complete cryosurgical unit, the delivery system, microthermocouple needles in place and pyrometer. Courtesy of Frigitronics Inc., Shelton, Ct.

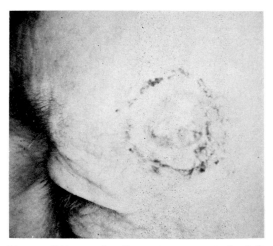

Figure 5-7. Basal cell epithelioma of the left temple just above the left eyebrow, prior to freezing.

and duration of thaw period in relation to the varied morphological shapes and size of the neoplasia. With experience he will become adept and selective in the application of the template in tumor sites such as the cheeks, anterior to the ears, the neck, and nasolabial areas. For malignant tumors situated upon the scalp, forehead, temples, and upper bridge of the nose, as well as the paranasal areas, one can continue freezing until the ice front has extended to the underlying periosteum and the overlying skin becomes immobile (Figures 5-7 to 5-10). Rarely will a cancer of the skin extend down to the periosteum and freezing to this depth will give the needed assurance to the clinician of the adequacy and extent of the ice front.

B. Cryosurgical Technique

The management of skin cancers by means of cryosurgery as an effective and useful modality has been well established[66-93] in the past fifteen years. The patient in Figure 5-11 presented a 0.8 cm ulcerated biopsy-proven basal cell carcinoma of the nasolabial area. A safe margin of normal skin approximately 0.5 cm beyond

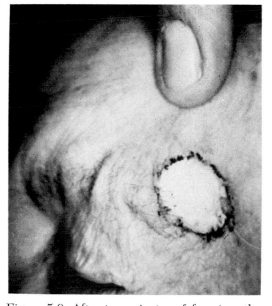

Figure 5-9. After two minutes of freezing, the ice front had reached down to the periosteum and the overlying skin is immobile. The freezing was terminated, allowed to completely thaw, and a second freeze was instituted.

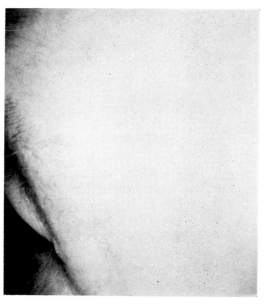

Figure 5-10. Six weeks following cryosurgery, there was complete healing and elimination of the epithelioma. This patient has been followed for over five years now without a recurrence.

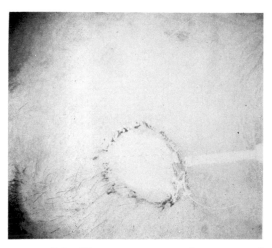

Figure 5-8. The same tumor during initial freezing.

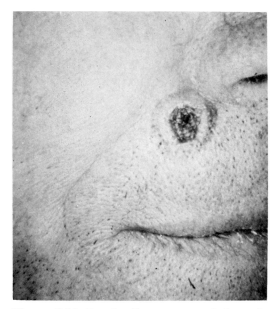

Figure 5-11. Basal cell carcinoma of the right nasolabial fold. Five mm beyond the visible margin of the tumor has been outlined with a skin marker.

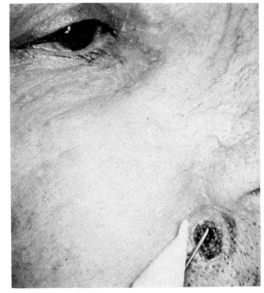

Figure 5-12. A side view of the thermocouple needle as it is passed through the 5 mm track of the template.

the visible margins of tumor was outlined with a skin marker. The microthermocouple needle is passed through the 5 mm depth tract of the template, demonstrating the eventual position of the tip of the needle to be in the midcenter of the tumor (Figure 5-12). The cancer site is locally anaesthetized to allow the insertion of the thermocouple needle through the template into the skin at the free margin of the growth. The needle penetrates below the neoplasm at 5 mm depth, the tip resting midcenter below the lesion (Figure 5-13). The hub of the needle is fastened firmly to the skin with tape to prevent mobility and to maintain the desired position of the needle and template. Direct spray of liquid nitrogen is delivered to the center of the lesion and applied on an *intermittent* basis until *two criteria* have been fulfilled: Continue freezing until the monitored temperature is recorded to a mini-

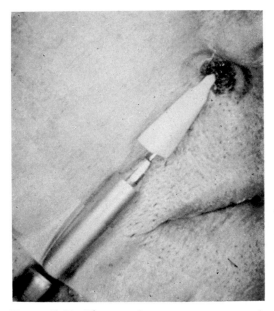

Figure 5-13. The template is in position with its tip resting upon the midcenter of the tumor. The thermocouple needle has been passed through the template and it is buried 5 mm below the midcenter of the surface tumor.

mum of $-25°$ to $-30°C$, and extend the freezing up to and even beyond the marked safe area of normal skin beyond the visible margins of the tumor (Figure 5-14).

Once these two criteria have been met, stop freezing, allow the tumor and adjacent skin to thaw *completely* and freeze once again. This is referred to as a double freeze-thaw cycle. In such areas as the nasolabial fold, ala nasi, eyelid, and in particular the medial canthus, the author has recently subjected tumors to a *triple* freeze-thaw cycle to enhance a greater degree of cryonecrosis and to achieve a higher cure rate.

The importance of intermittent spray of liquid nitrogen needs to be stressed. The author has observed that with a continuous spray of liquid nitrogen there is a rapid peripheral spread of the ice front

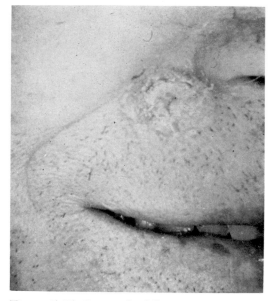

Figure 5-15. Six weeks following cryosurgery, there was present a pseudoepitheliomatous hyperplasia at the site of freezing.

at the expense of in-depth freeze below the tumor mass. With continuous freezing, you will also experience a roll-off of the refrigerant. The initial freeze time will be the longest and with each subsequent sequential freezing, the time required to reach the desired temperature will be shortened. The reason for this is explained on the basis that the tiny microvessels are still under semi-vasoconstriction and will offer less resistance to the subsequent development and extension of the ice front. Also once cells and tissue are frozen, their subsequent conductivity is increased. Freezing time will also be somewhat shortened when local anesthetic is used, in particular, when it contains epinephrine.

The thaw period which is undoubtedly more lethal to normal than malignant tissue, is totally out of the control of the clinician. If the freeze time takes one and a half minutes, anticipate the thaw period to be in the vicinity of two and one-half

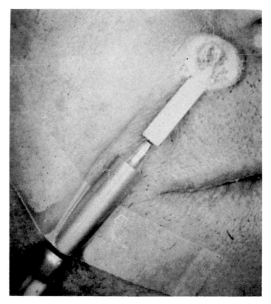

Figure 5-14. At the end of two minutes of intermittent freeze, the temperature of the cryolesion produced at 5 mm depth was recorded at $-25°C$ and the surface spread of the ice front had extended laterally to the safe margin of normal skin.

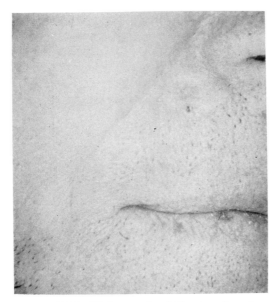

Figure 5-16. Eight weeks following freezing, there was present some hyperpigmentation. This patient has been followed for three years without a recurrence.

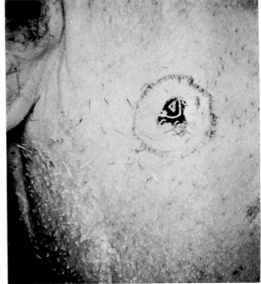

Figure 5-17. A small but ulcerated 0.6 cm biopsy-proven basal cell carcinoma of the right cheek. From Zacarian, *Comprehensive Therapy*, Harvard, Book Associates International, Inc., Aug. 1975. Reprinted by permission.

to three minutes, which is one and a half to two times the length of the freezing time. The author considers the *termination of the thaw period to be when both the tumor and adjacent normal skin have resumed its original color,* then will consider a second freeze or a third, if so desired.

Six weeks following cryosurgery (Figure 5-15) the patient presents an epitheliomatous hyperplasia at the site of treatment, referred to as pseudorecidive. This has been reported following irradiation of skin cancer[94, 95] and will infrequently develop following cryosurgery. One should be aware of it, however, lest one mistakes it for inadequate freezing or an early recurrence of the tumor. Eight weeks following treatment (Figure 5-16) one still observes a minimum degree of residual hyperplasia which soon spontaneously disappeared.

Cancers of the cheek, particularly an-

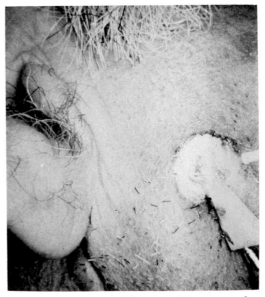

Figure 5-18. After infiltration of local anesthesia, the template was positioned and thermocouple needle was positioned through the 5 mm track and freezing commenced. From Zacarian, *Comprehensive Therapy*, Harvard, Book Associates International, Inc., Aug. 1975. Reprinted by permission.

terior to the ears, can be elusive in appearance and deceiving in depth. The extension of the skin and its appendages in this area is quite deep, as much as 2.5 mm in thickness, compared to the skin overlying the eyelid where it is only 0.5 mm.[96] The patient in Figure 5-17 presented a two-year history of a slowly growing and recently bleeding basal cell epithelioma of the right cheek. The tumor itself did not measure over 0.6 cm in size but a wide safe margin of 0.8 cm distal to the visible margin of the ulcerated lesion was delineated. Careful examination of his recurrences has alerted the author to the fact that failures have been for the most part at the margins and therefore, he freezes as wide a margin of normal skin as possible. The microthermocouple needle was passed through the 5 mm tract of the plastic jig

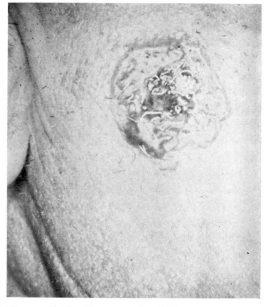

Figure 5-20. Two weeks following cryosurgery, the tumor site shows a hemorrhagic scab. From Zacarian, *Comprehensive Therapy*, Harvard, Book Associates International, Inc., Aug. 1975. Reprinted by permission.

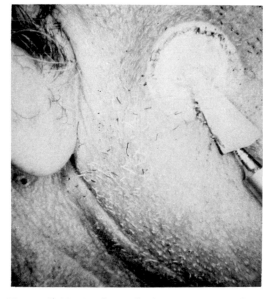

Figure 5-19. At the end of two minutes of intermittent spray of liquid nitrogen, the temperature at 5 mm depth was −35°C and the lateral spread had extended beyond the safe delineated margins of normal skin. From Zacarian, *Comprehensive Therapy*, Harvard, Book Associates International, Inc., Aug. 1975. Reprinted by permission.

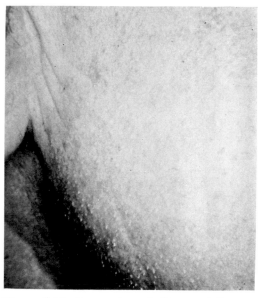

Figure 5-21. Two and one-half years following freezing, there is no recurrence of the BCE with almost perfect skin without depigmentation. From Zacarian, *Comprehensive Therapy*, Harvard, Book Associates International, Inc., Aug. 1975. Reprinted by permission.

and commenced freezing (Figure 5-18). The tumor mass was subjected to intermittent freezing until the depth temperature was monitored at −35°C, and the ice front extended peripherally far beyond the delineated ink marker (Figure 5-19). The freeze time was two minutes; the thaw period was three and one-half minutes. Should the temperature extend to −40° or −50°C, do not be concerned. These lower temperatures will in no way disturb your freezing experience. This carcinoma was subjected to a double freeze-thaw cycle. Two weeks following cryosurgery, the tumor site and adjacent skin showed the classic hemorrhagic eschar (Figure 5-20). Healing time was four weeks. Two and one-half years following cryosurgery (Figure 5-21), there is very little evidence of scarring, no recurrence of the tumor, and the cosmetic end result is superb.

The above descriptive clinical cases clearly outline the important essentials for cryosurgery of malignant tumors of the skin, which are summarized below.

The Essential Parameters for Effective Cryosurgery of Malignant Tumors of the Skin

1. *Delivery System* must be versatile with controlled delivery of liquid nitrogen as a direct spray or closed disc. Intermittent spray is extremely important.
2. *Freezing Time* will vary from one to several minutes, dependent upon the size of the tumor. When monitored, the temperature achieved below the neoplasm should record −25° to −30°C.
3. *Temperature Monitoring* is important for tumors situated upon the cheeks, nasolabial areas, ala nasi and just anterior to the ears.
4. *Freeze-thaw Cycles* of a minimum of

two is recommended and in critical areas, three times is desirable. A complete thaw is recommended before refreezing.
5. *Extend Freezing* to 5 mm beyond the visible margin of the tumor.
6. *Thaw-Time* will vary from one-and-a-half to two times the duration of the freeze period.

C. Critical Areas of Skin Cancers Amenable to Cryosurgery

In the author's experience in the management of skin cancers subjected to cryosurgery, neoplasia of the nose, ears and eyelids have constituted 38 percent of malignant tumors encountered and indeed present a challenge to all cancer therapists (Table 5-I).

Freezing tumors upon these anatomical sites demands serious consideration of not only the size of the tumor, but also its histology and in particular, whether it is a primary or a recurrent lesion. The author has established a firm rule in this regard. If the neoplasm is a recurrent one, he refers the patient to Mohs' chemosurgery or to a plastic surgeon for a more definitive approach. Only in cases of marked debilitation in the patient will the author perform cryosurgery and only as a palliative measure. He would also hesitate to freeze large epidermoid carcinomas of the nose because of its invasiveness and predilec-

TABLE 5-I

CRITICAL AREAS OF SKIN CANCERS

Nose
    25% of all skin cancers
 Ears
     8% of all skin cancers
 Eyelids
     5% of all skin cancers
    38% of all skin cancers occur in critical
      areas of the face.

tion to early metastases. For the most part, he does not hesitate to perform cryosurgery on primary cutaneous carcinomas at these critical sites.

1. Cancer of the Nose

In a large series of 590 patients who had a combined total of 817 basal cell carcinomas of the skin, Taylor and Barisoni[97] found 26 percent of the tumors were situated on the nose and an additional 20 percent in the periorbital region. In the 82 recurrences observed, 13.2 percent were recorded on the nose and 15.8 percent in the periorbital area. Of the 817 lesions, 280 had received one or more previous treatments including surgery or irradiation prior to referral to the authors.

An excellent paper recently published by Conley[98] clearly discusses the seriousness of cancer of the nose. In a series of 456 cases of cancer of the skin of the nose, 87 percent were basal cell epitheliomas occurring predominantly on the ala, tip and root. Squamous cell carcinomas constituted

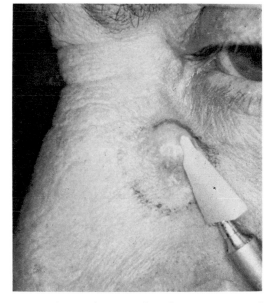

Figure 5-23. The template being positioned in place prior to freezing.

10.7 percent and were more common on the lateral borders and columella. Metastases developed in 0.25 percent of basal cell epitheliomas and *18.5 percent of the squamous cell carcinomas.* He also found that 51 percent of the cases had been previously treated inadequately and had developed recurrences. A little over a half of the recurrences were from previous irradiation and the remaining from previous surgery, electrodesiccation and curettage. After definitive treatment of 456 cases, predominantly by means of surgery, Conley had a recurrence of only 9 percent, which is remarkable when one considers the large number of difficult and previously recurrent tumors he had to treat.

An ideal cancer of the nose to treat cryosurgically is shown in Figure 5-22. This is a primary, biopsy-proven, nodular basal cell epithelioma, 1.2 cm in size, on the upper lateral margin of the nose. After marking a safe margin beyond the borders of the tumor (Figure 5-23), the template

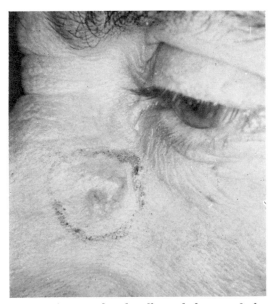

Figure 5-22. A basal cell epithelioma of the left side of the nose measuring 1.2 cm in size.

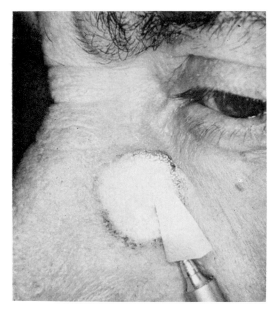

Figure 5-24. At the end of two and one-half minutes of intermittent spray of liquid nitrogen, the initial thaw time was four minutes.

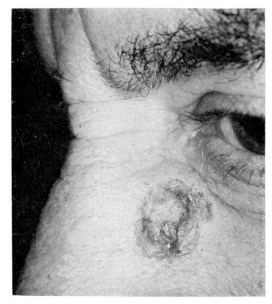

Figure 5-25. Two weeks following cryosurgery, an adherent scab was present.

is positioned in place and the thermocouple needle is passed through the 5 mm track and fastened. The freezing is carried on with the direct spray of liquid nitrogen with three significant end points. One, the freezing must extend to the normal skin edges as previously marked (Figure 5-24). Second, the tumor is frozen until the microthermocouple monitors the temperature 5 mm below the lesion to a minimum of −25° to −30°C. As an added assurance of depth of freeze, your third end point at this site is to continue to freeze until the periosteum of the nose has been reached and the overlying skin becomes immobile. Once the tumor has thawed, a second freeze was delivered. Two weeks following cryosurgery, one notes the expected hemorrhagic eschar (Figure 5-25). Final healing was accomplished in four weeks and a six months follow-up shows a slight degree of depig-

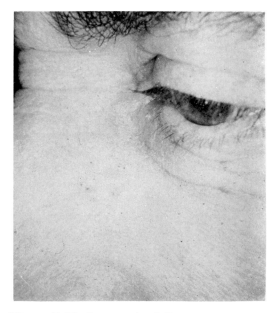

Figure 5-26. Six months follow-up show tiny islands of hyperpigmentation at the previous tumor site. In three years postcryosurgery, no recurrence has been observed.

mentation (Figure 5-26).

Frequently patients present multiple cancers at the initial examination. This situation often proves ideal for cryosurgery. The patient in Figure 5-27 revealed two tumors of the nose, quite apart and distinct and histologically confirmed to be basal cell carcinomas. After freezing the lesion on the lobule of nose, while waiting for it to thaw, the second and larger lesion was subjected to cryosurgery (Figure 5-28). When both tumors had fully thawed, they were frozen again.

A more difficult cancer of the nose is one which has had previous treatment. The patient in Figure 5-29 presents multiple sites of ulcerated basal cell carcinoma along the tip and side of the nose including the ala. They appear distinct, but clinically the author was certain they were all interconnected. This woman had a basal cell epithelioma of the lobule of the nose some twelve years earlier which had been surgically ex-

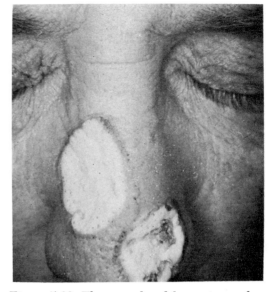

Figure 5-28. The second and larger tumor has been frozen, while the first is undergoing thawing.

cised. Three years later with evidence of recurrence, she had been given a full course of irradiation. Two years following this, when further recurrences were noted, she had repeated curettage and electrodesiccation until the author first saw her three years ago with the involvement as shown in Figure 5-29.

He frankly told her that her epithelioma was not amenable to cryosurgery and a definitive approach would be Mohs' chemosurgery or plastic surgery with reconstruction. She told the author that she had been suggested the latter and had refused. In fact she wanted no further surgery in any form. He informed her that freezing would simply prove palliative and tried earnestly to persuade her but to no avail. The implications were explained to the patient. The tumor sites were then subjected to a triple freeze-thaw cryosurgical procedure (Figure 5-30). Please observe from the previous figure that the cancer had al-

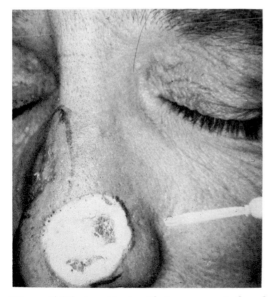

Figure 5-27. A patient with two separate basal cell epitheliomas of the nose. The one on the lobule is being frozen.

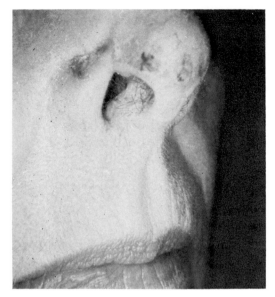

Figure 5-29. Multiple foci of recurrent basal cell epitheliomas of the nose from previous surgery and irradiation.

ready produced scarring and constriction of the nares and atrophy at the tip of the nose. Six months follow-up showed no clinical evidence of her cancer (Figure 5-

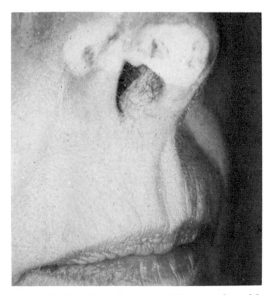

Figure 5-30. After the second freeze of visible tumor sites.

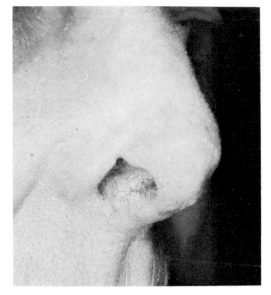

Figure 5-31. Six months following cryosurgery, there was no clinical evidence of any recurrent sites. Since this writing, she developed some ulcerated recurrences and the author sent her for definitive surgery and reconstruction of the nose.

31). One year following freezing, she presented small 0.2 to 0.3 cm pockets of clinical recurrences. These areas were frozen again. It has been over two years and a careful watch is being maintained. Recurrent cancers carry a very low cure rate, whatever modality is used. Estimates of recurrence in a previously treated skin cancer varies from 15 to 50 percent.[32, 99–101]

The above patient was not an ideal case for cryosurgery but it does serve to point out two distinctive features of freezing as a technique. First, it is a palliative measure and the second more important reason is that cryosurgery is safe upon previously irradiated skin or tumor sites without the fear of possible delayed or poor wound healing.

Approximately one of every four carcinomas of the skin of the nose in the author's series were situated at the ala nasi,

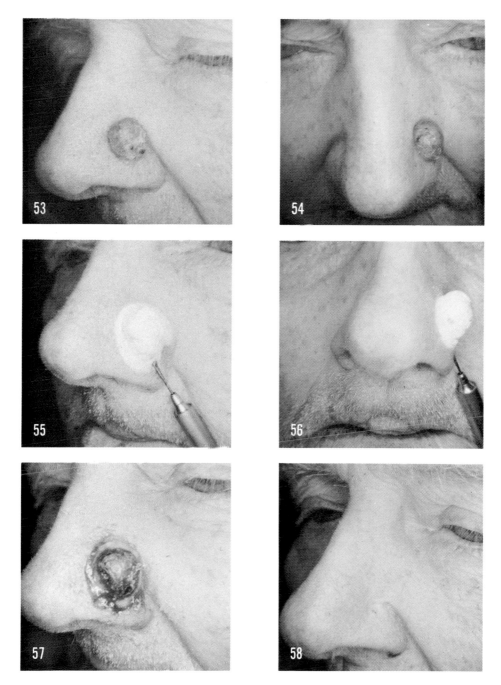

Plate 53. Basal cell carcinoma left ala nasi, 1.3 cm in size.

Plate 54. Anterior view of the nodular tumor; note how raised it is.

Plate 55. Three minutes of freezing; monitored temperature below the tumor was -40°C.

Plate 56. Anterior view of frozen tumor mass.

Plate 57. Seven days postcryosurgery; note the hemorrhagic crust.

Plate 58. One year following freezing, there is superb cosmetic end result. Three year follow-up, no recurrence.

a critical and difficult area to affect a permanent cure. The patient in Plate 53 is a 79-year-old male patient with a two-year history of a tumor at the ala nasi, measuring 1.3 cm in diameter. The biopsy showed an adenoid basal cell carcinoma. An anterior view of the patient demonstrates a raised nodular component to the tumor extending 0.5 cm above the cutaneous surface of the nose (Plate 54). After imbedding the tip of the microthermocouple needle at the base of the tumor into the underlying cartilage, the lesion was frozen for a period of three minutes, at which time the registered temperature was recorded at $-40°C$ (Plate 55). Note the wide margin frozen beyond the visible margin of the tumor.

The anterior view of the patient reveals the amount of tumor mass which was frozen and how deeply the microthermocouple needle is imbedded within the skin of the nose (Plate 56). A simple clinical evaluation of the depth of freeze is to observe the ice front extended onto the posterior aspect of the nares. In this patient both the thermocouple needle and clinical visualization of the ice front through the cartilage was employed to assure a thorough and energetic freeze. Seven days following cryosurgery, there is evident a serous exudate from the frozen site (Plate 57). Except for a daily change of dressing and cleansing of the wound site with soap and water or hydrogen peroxide, no further care is needed for tumors subjected to cryosurgery. It is on rare occasion that the author has encountered secondary infection and cancers of the face generally heal within four weeks following freezing. As with this patient, healing was complete within the specified time. One year following cryosurgery, the cosmetic end result is superb with no underlying disturbance of the cartilage of the nares (Plate 58) except for a minimal area of depigmentation.

A distinct and superior advantage of cryosurgery for skin cancers overlying cartilage is that chondronecrosis or perforation of the nose or ear is nearly absent—the author has not encountered a case in over twelve years of experience. At the expense of being redundant, but for the purpose of emphasis, cancers of the nose are to be highly regarded and respected. The author would defer cryosurgery for the larger lesions, i.e. over 2.0 cm, and in particular epidermoid carcinomas or recurrent cancers of the nose, unless palliative. From their vast experience in treatment of skin cancers by means of chemosurgery, Mohs and Lathrop[102] point out the selective affinity of these neoplasms, particularly the nasal area to specific tissues and structures. They enumerate as follows: (1) dermis, (2) facial planes, (3) periosteum, (4) perichondrium, (5) embryologic planes, (6) nerve sheaths, (7) lymphatic vessels, and (8) blood vessels. These concepts are more formidable with epidermoid carcinomas.

2. Cancer of the Ear

The ear is not a common site for malignant tumors. In the author's series, it represented approximately 8 percent of skin cancers encountered. Not infrequently they are epidermoid carcinomas or basosquamous cell carcinomas and therefore must be more vigorously treated to affect a cure. Because of underlying cartilage, the radiotherapist is not too anxious to employ irradiation. The average surgeon or plastic surgeon, because of his disciplined training, is often prone to radical surgery, i.e. partial ablation or extirpation or extensive reconstructive surgery. This is not to criticize but to point out that cryosur-

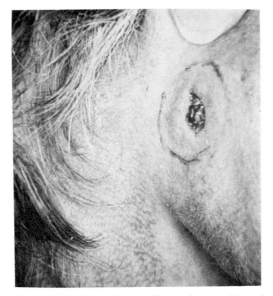

Figure 5-32. A patient with an ulcerated basal cell epithelioma behind the right ear.

gery has a definite place in the management of cancer of the ear.

The patient in Figure 5-32 presented an ulcerated 1.0 cm lesion on the posterior as-

pect of his ear of three years' duration. The microscopic examination of the tumor revealed a basal cell carcinoma. After a careful demarcation of a safe zone, 0.5 cm outside the visible margins of the neoplasm, it was subjected to two and one-half minutes of freezing. The cryosurgery was pursued to the safe zone of normal skin (Figure 5-33) and freezing was delivered until the ice front extended to the anterior aspect of the uninvolved ear and cutaneous surface (Figure 5-34). The thaw period was three and one-half minutes. A second freeze was executed. Two weeks following cryosurgery, the wound site was clean and showed no secondary infection (Figure 5-35). The patient was without symptoms and presented no evidence of chondronecrosis. Four weeks following cryosurgery, there is no clinical evidence of the carcinoma (Figure 5-36) nor perforation of the cartilage of the ear. There is no need to measure the ice front with cancers of the ear. Do not hesitate to

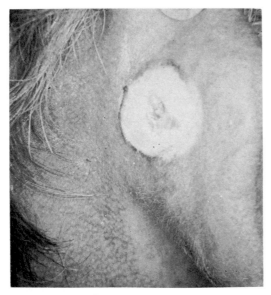

Figure 5-33. After two and one-half minutes of freezing with liquid nitrogen spray. Note the lateral extent of the ice front to at least 5 mm beyond the ulcerated tumor.

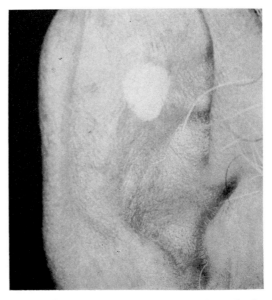

Figure 5-34. Freezing was carried through the cartilage to the uninvolved anterior cutaneous surface of the ear.

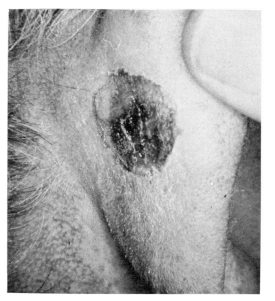

Figure 5-35. Two weeks following freezing, there was some exudation from the wound site.

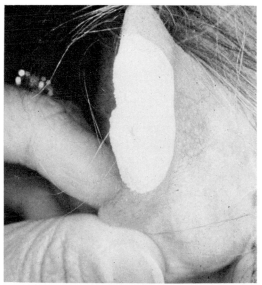

Figure 5-37. An extensive ulcerated and nodular epidermoid carcinoma of the ear, eroded into the cartilage itself. The tumor size was 2.5 cm.

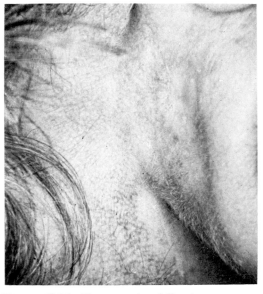

Figure 5-36. Four weeks following cryosurgery, the epithelioma was eradicated without perforation or evidence of chondronecrosis. No evidence of recurrence four years following treatment.

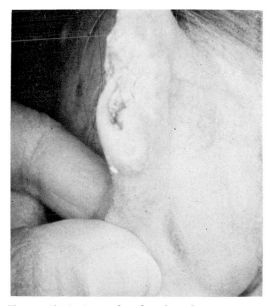

Figure 5-38. Immediately after three minutes of freezing time. The initial thaw period was five minutes. A second freeze was initiated after complete thawing.

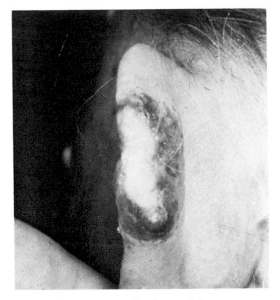

Figure 5-39. Forty-eight hours following cryosurgery, there was still intact a hemorrhagic bullus. Note the wide margin of freeze beyond the visible borders of the tumor.

surgery, the malignant tumor was no longer clinically evident (Figure 5-40). There was some loss and integrity of the integument of the ear; however, this was not due to cryosurgery. The carcinoma had already eroded deep within the skin and underlying cartilage. The cosmetic end result was far more satisfying to her than a wedge resection of the ear.

A more extensive and erosive neoplasm of the ear was a biopsy-proven basal cell carcinoma in the posterior aspect of the ear in a forty-two-year-old male (Plate 59). This tumor measured 2.5 by 3.0 cm in size invading the underlying cartilage. He was sent to a plastic surgeon by his personal physician who advised total ablation of the ear. Quite alarmed over this verdict, he sought the advice of a radiotherapist who declined to treat him because of the extent of the tumor and the degree of in-

freeze through the cartilage for thoroughness to eradicate the given carcinoma.

A more extensive tumor of the ear was observed in an elderly female patient who had neglected to obtain medical attention. This tumor measured over 2.5 cm and was definitely ulcerated with elevated margins to the cutaneous surface with clear evidence of extension to the underlying cartilage (Figure 5-37).

The biopsy proved to be an epidermoid carcinoma. She was advised to have a wedge excision by her surgeon and she refused. She was referred to me for consideration of cryosurgery as an alternative procedure. The tumor site was thoroughly frozen for three minutes and subjected to a second freeze-thaw (Figure 5-38). The initial thaw period was five minutes. Within forty-eight hours the tumor site and adjacent skin manifested considerable edema and hemorrhagic bullous reaction (Figure 5-39). Four weeks following cryo-

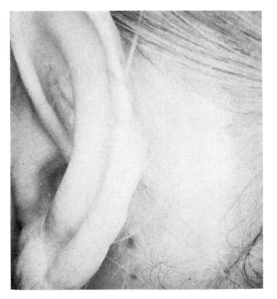

Figure 5-40. Four weeks following cryosurgery, there was minimal evidence of granulation tissue. The loss of some integrity of the margin of the ear was due to the underlying neoplasm. A four-year follow-up showed no recurrence.

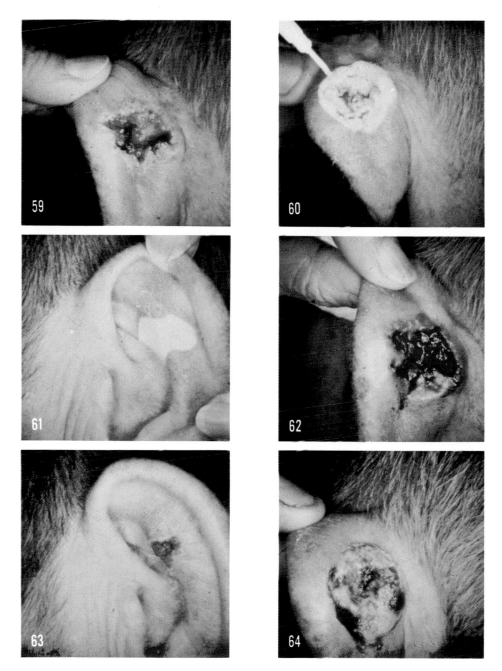

Plate 59.* An extensive ulcerated basal cell carcinoma of the ear, extending into the cartilage.
Plate 60.* After four minutes of freezing.
Plate 61.* Freezing extended through the ear onto the anterior uninvolved aspect.
Plate 62.* Two weeks following cryosurgery with marked exudation of wound site.
Plate 63.* The anterior aspect of the ear shows a superficial crust.
Plate 64. Eight weeks following cryosurgery. There is still active granulation tissue.

*From S. A. Zacarian, Cryosurgery of skin cancer: Fundamentals of technique and application, *Cutis, 16*:449-460, 1975. Courtesy of Yorke Medical Journals, Dun Donnelley Publishing Corp.

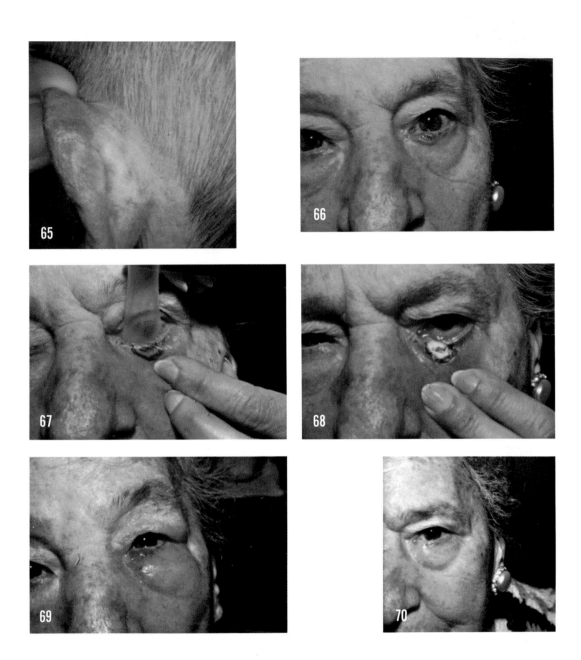

Plate 65. Three years following cryosurgery, excellent end result without perforation of the cartilage.

Plate 66. Ulcerated nodular basal cell carcinoma of the free margin of left lower eyelid.

Plate 67. Placement of the plastic eyelid retractor.

Plate 68. The frozen tumor mass after sixty seconds. A triple freeze-thaw cycle was executed and freezing carried into the tarsus.

Plate 69. Twenty-four hours following cryosurgery; note the marked periorbital edema.

Plate 70. Four weeks following freezing, complete healing without ectropion or eversion of the lid. No visible recurrence after eighteen months of follow-up.

volvement of the underlying cartilage, and referred him to the author for possible consideration of cryosurgery as an alternative procedure. The carcinoma was subjected to four minutes of intermittent spray of liquid nitrogen (Plate 60). Freezing was continued until the anterior uninvolved site of the ear, including the cutaneous surface, demonstrated the visible extension of the ice front (Plate 61). This tumor was subjected to a double freeze-thaw cycle, each time carrying the ice front through the cartilage to the anterior aspect of the ear. The initial thaw period lasted seven minutes. No local anesthesia was used and the patient tolerated the procedure quite well. Two weeks following cryosurgery, there is present a moderate degree of edema with extensive exudation of serous fluid (Plate 62). The patient was essentially without symptoms; other than the exudate he offered no complaints suggesting a chondritis. The anterior uninvolved area of the ear developed an eschar with minimal edema (Plate 63). Eight weeks following freezing, the wound site was still undergoing healing with an extensive development of granulation tissue (Plate 64). The final healing and full epithelialization did not occur until ten weeks following cryosurgery. This was not unusual considering the degree and intensity of freezing. Three years following cryosurgery, there was no clinical evidence of the earlier carcinoma nor perforation of the cartilage of the ear (Plate 65).

3. Cancer of the Eyelids

a. General Remarks

Malignant tumors of the eyelids constitute approximately 5 percent of all skin cancers.[103, 104] This small percentage however, presents a real challenge to the dermatologist, ophthalmologist, plastic surgeon, and the radiotherapist. In this critical area several considerations come to mind, such as: (1) to obtain as high cure rate as possible, (2) to obtain an acceptable and functioning cosmetic end result, and (3) to avoid permanent damage, particularly to the lacrimal duct apparatus with resulting epiphora.

The outer mantle of the lids is the continuum of the integument to the free margin of the lids. Whereas the overall thickness of the skin of the face averages 2.5 mm, the integument of the eyelids measures merely 0.6 mm. The firmness of the lid is due to the tarsal plate and elements of muscle fibers. The overall thickness of the lids measures 2.0 mm, being somewhat thicker in the orbital segment.

Cancers of the eyelids carry an extremely high rate of mortality (11%)[105] as compared to other integumentary sites. The danger is not only from metastasis; even more treacherous is the inherent ability of the tumor to directly extend into the orbit and cranial vault. Involvement of the bulbar conjunctiva is an ominous sign of early extension into the orbit with the eventual potential of global destruction. In all fixed lesions of the lids, particularly the medial canthi, X-ray film of the sinuses (ethmoid) and orbit is mandatory to rule out possible invasion of underlying bone. As early as 1938, Birge[106] stressed the importance of early recognition and treatment of malignant neoplasia of the lids, particularly the basal cell carcinomas. The lower lids are common sites for the development of cancer. The upper eyelids are protected from the sun by the overlying brow. It is also interesting to note that the medial canthus constitutes almost one quarter of all tumors observed on the lower lid.

Before discussing the management of eyelid carcinomas by means of cryosurgery, a brief review of the literature of other

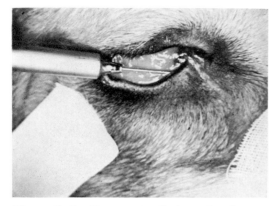

Figure 5-41. Placement of the microthermocouple needle within the lacrimal duct of a dog. From *Cutis, 16:* Sept. 1975. Courtesy of the Yorke Medical Journals, Dun Donnelley Publishing Corp.

therapeutic modalities is germane. With the exception of Cole's[107] series of 293 carcinomas of the eyelids surgically excised, where he found only one recurrence and that of Domonkos,[108] with a recurrence rate of 2 percent, most other authors place the recurrence rate in the range between 8 to 12 percent. Rakofsky[109] in a series of 95 basal cell carcinomas surgically excised found a recurrence rate of 12 percent. He also noted that 50 percent of the specimens submitted showed inadequate excision. In the inadequately excised carcinomas, he found 23.4 percent recurrence. In another series of 273 eyelid cancers surgically excised by Payne and his associates,[110] the reported recurrence rate was 12 percent. They also observed complications in 18 percent of the patients. Epiphora was cited as the most common. In forty surgically excised cancers of the eyelids carefully examined histologically, Einangler[111] found twenty to be inadequate and carcinoma extended beyond the margins of the submitted surgical specimen. Abraham and his associates,[112] in a review of 116 cases of medial canthus carcinomas treated by X ray and surgical excision, found an overall recurrence of 8 percent.

Complications following therapy averaged 9.1 percent, half of which were to the lacrimal duct, resulting in epiphora. Frozen section control of cancer of the lids undoubtedly yields the highest cure rates.[113, 114]

The first substantial series of lid cancers treated with cryosurgery were by this author in 1969.[89] Since then there have been other clinical investigators, particularly ophthalmologists.[115, 116] Human and animal eyelid tumors, benign and malignant also have been reported. There is at the present time positive preliminary laboratory and clinical evidence to support that freezing neoplasia of the eyelids is effective and cosmetically acceptable with minimal functional loss and preservation of the lacrimal apparatus.

Tumors of the medial canthus are in critical sites and their eradication is as important as the preservation and integrity of the lacrimal duct and puncta.

b. The Effects of Freezing on Canine Eyelids

To determine the effects of freezing temperatures upon the lacrimal duct, Dr.

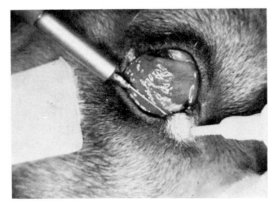

Figure 5-42. Freezing the medial canthus of the canine lower lid. Monitored temperature within the lacrimal duct was −25° to −30°C. From *Cutis, 16:* Sept. 1975. Courtesy of Yorke Medical Journals, Dun Donnelley Publishing Corp.

Stoyak and the author passed a microthermocouple needle into the lacrimal duct of the right eyelid of a dog (Figure 5-41). The medial canthus was frozen along with the puncta (Figure 5-42), and the temperature within the duct was monitored at −25° to −30°C. After thawing, a second freeze was instituted (Figure 5-43). On the opposing eyelid, the punctum itself was subjected to a double freeze-thaw cycle (Figure 5-44). Dr. Stoyak followed the course of the freezings and, after eight weeks, the lacrimal ducts remained patent with no eversion or damage to the lids or the tarsal plates. A more precise and extensive study of the effects of freezing temperatures with liquid nitrogen on the puncta and lacrimal canaliculi[120] upon the rabbit was investigated by Bullock. He not only monitored temperatures during freezing at the punctum, but also the canaliculi with post-freezing histological examination to observe patency. He noted the canaliculus remained open to −10°C. At −30°C, 67 percent of the canaliculi were still patent; at −50°C only 50 percent remained open. The puncta remained patent and functional in all observed rabbits at temperatures car-

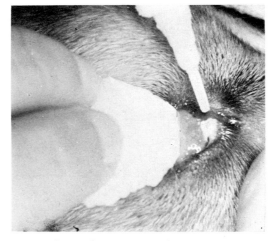

Figure 5-44. The punctum of the opposite eyelid was subjected to a double freeze-thaw cycle.

ried to −50°C. At −70°C, 67 percent of the puncta were still patent. The results following cryosurgery were observed eight weeks after the freezing experiments. These animal studies corroborate the clinical observations in man by both dermatologists and ophthalmologists in freezing tumors of the medial canthus. Subzero temperatures are not as damaging to the can-

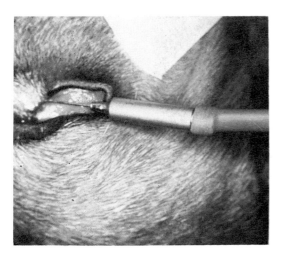

Figure 5-43. After thawing a second freeze was executed.

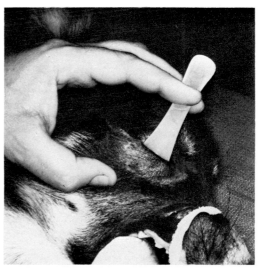

Figure 5-45. Placement of the Jegher plastic eyelid retractor behind the right lower lid.

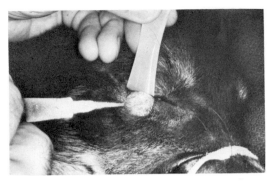

Figure 5-46. After ninety seconds of intermittent spray of liquid nitrogen to the right lower lid.

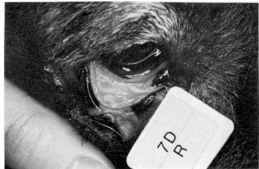

Figure 5-49. Seven days following freezing, the bulbar conjunctiva was clean without perforation of the tarsal plate.

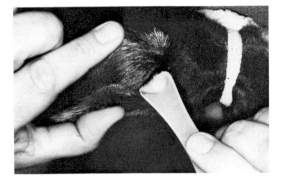

Figure 5-47. At the same time as in Figure 5-46, the ice front has extended through the tarsal plate on to the bulbar conjunctiva.

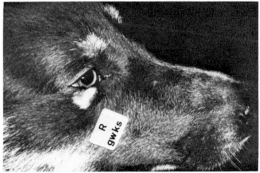

Figure 5-50. Eight weeks following cryosurgery, the right lower lid was intact without eversion or perforation. The hypopigmentation and loss of some lid hair was expected.

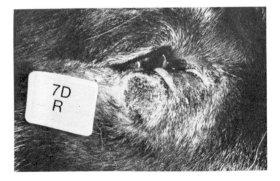

Figure 5-48. Seven days following cryosurgery, there was considerable edema of the right lower lid as expected.

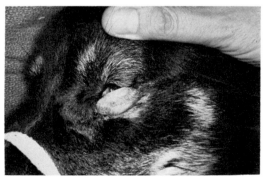

Figure 5-51. A more extensive freeze of the entire left lower lid was undertaken.

aliculi and puncta as irradiation, and their functional integrity is far more preserved from cryosurgery.

One of the concerns the author has had in freezing eyelid tumors has been the tolerance of the tarsus to freezing, in particular, when the freezing is extended throughout. Cartilage can be frozen through the nose and ear without the sequelae of chondronecrosis. Freezing through the tarsal plate has been reported in a nominal number of cases, although the need for it does not present itself very often. To evaluate its response to freezing, once again the author returned to canine studies with Dr. Stoyak.

Under anesthesia, after shaving the fur of both lids, a plastic retractor was placed in the right eyelid of a dog (Figure 5-45). The thickness of the entire lower lid of the dog was measured at 3 mm. Freezing was undertaken with liquid nitrogen for ninety seconds, at which time a substantial portion of the right lower lid appeared totally frozen (Figure 5-46). The plastic retractor became adherent to the bulbar conjunctiva and upon eversion and careful inspection, one observes that the freezing has extended right through the tarsus (Figure 5-47). After thawing, the lid was subjected to a second freeze-thaw cycle. Seven days following cryosurgery, the lid showed a moderate degree of edema (Figure 5-48). Careful examination of the bulbar conjunctiva during the same period showed minimal inflammatory response (Figure 5-49). Diligent observation of the animal throughout eight weeks following cryosurgery demonstrated an intact tarsus without perforation or eversion of the lid margin. There is however loss of pigment and hair at the frozen site of the lid (Figure 5-50).

A more vigorous freezing of the entire left lower lid was executed (Figure 5-51),

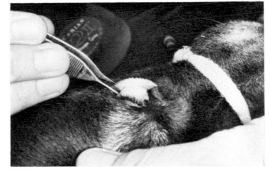

Figure 5-52. After 120 seconds of freeze time, one observes the depth of freezing through the left lower lid to the conjunctiva.

with extension of the ice front to the anterior surface of the bulbar conjunctiva (Figure 5-52). Eight weeks following cryosurgery the animal had functional lid without perforation of the tarsus. This study was repeated with a second animal with similar results. The evidence thus far from clinical experience and experimental studies on the dog seems to support that the tarsus, like cartilage, is quite resistant to freezing temperatures and its integrity and function is maintained.

c. Cryosurgery of Eyelid Cancers

A frequent site for malignant tumors seems to be at the upper paranasal areas which very often extend to the lower lid (Figure 5-53). This tumor, measuring 1.5 cm, was a basal cell carcinoma of two years duration. The microthermocouple needle was passed through the 5 mm track to demonstrate its position when properly stationed below the tumor (Figure 5-54). After infiltration of local anesthesia, the template was perpendicularly placed with its tip resting approximately upon the midcenter of the tumor and the microthermocouple needle was passed through the 5 mm track (Figure 5-55). The tip of the microthermocouple needle was then 5 mm

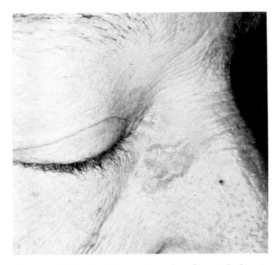

Figure 5-53. A 1.5 cm basal cell epithelioma of the right paranasal area, extending to the right lower lid. From *Cutis, 16:* Sept. 1975. Courtesy of Yorke Medical Journals, Dun Donnelley Publishing Corp.

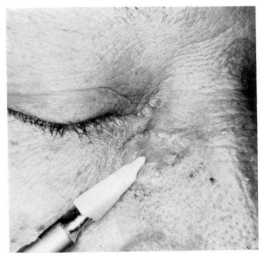

Figure 5-55. The template in position with the thermocouple inserted and its tip resting 5 mm below the cutaneous surface of the tumor. From *Cutis, 16:* Sept. 1975. Courtesy of Yorke Medical Journals, Dun Donnelley Publishing Corp.

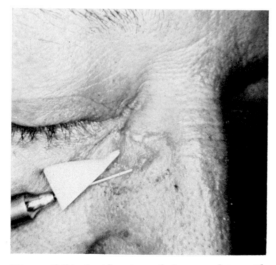

Figure 5-54. A side view of the template with the thermocouple needle passed through the 5 mm track. From *Cutis, 16:* Sept. 1975. Courtesy of Yorke Medical Journals, Dun Donnelley Publishing Corp.

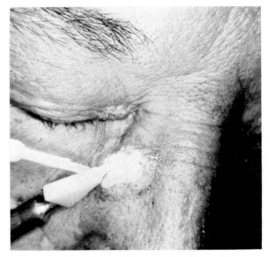

Figure 5-56. During the initial phase of intermittent spray of liquid nitrogen directed to the center of the tumor. From *Cutis, 16:* Sept. 1975. Courtesy of Yorke Medical Journals, Dun Donnelley Publishing Corp.

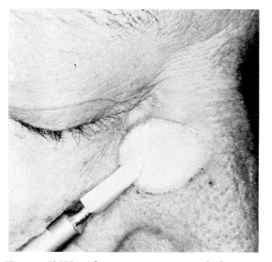

Figure 5-57. After two minutes of freezing time. From *Cutis, 16:* Sept. 1975. Courtesy of Yorke Medical Journals, Dun Donnelley Publishing Corp.

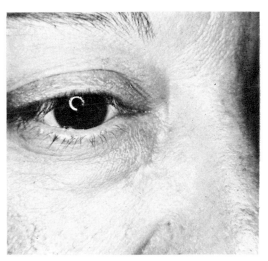

Figure 5-59. Four weeks following cryosurgery, there is no clinical evidence of the tumor, now followed for three and one-half years. From *Cutis, 16:* Sept. 1975. Courtesy of Yorke Medical Journals, Dun Donnelley Publishing Corp.

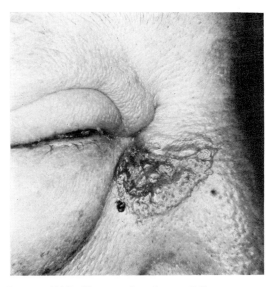

Figure 5-58. Twenty-four hours following surgery, there is a marked degree of periorbital edema with serous exudation of the frozen tumor site. From *Cutis, 16:* Sept. 1975. Courtesy of Yorke Medical Journals, Dun Donnelley Publishing Corp.

below the midcenter of the growth. Freezing was begun with an intermittent spray of liquid nitrogen (Figure 5-56). Cryosurgery was pursued until two important parameters had been fulfilled: (1) Freezing was extended to 5 mm of safe margin of skin beyond the visible borders of the tumor, as outlined with a skin marker (Figure 5-57) and (2) The temperature at 5 mm depth below the tumor was monitored at $-25°$ to $-30°$C. This was achieved in this patient within two minutes of freezing. The initial thaw period was three and a half minutes. A second freeze was directed to the carcinoma after the initial thaw was completed. The second freeze time was one and a half minutes and the second thaw period was three minutes. Twenty-four hours following cryosurgery, the expected marked degree of periorbital edema was observed (Figure 5-58). This swelling may last for several days and, if the pa-

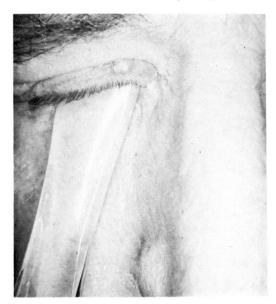

Figure 5-60. A small nodular basal cell carcinoma of the right upper eyelid.

tient is properly advised, will not be unduly concerned. The author has made a point to see patients the following day if their tumors are situated near the eyes.

Four weeks following cryosurgery, there is no evidence of the previous carcinoma (Figure 5-59), and the residual hyperpigmentation will resolve within a few months.

Carcinoma of the upper eyelid is quite uncommon as compared to the lower lid. The patient in Figure 5-60 presented a small 0.6 cm nodular basal cell carcinoma of the upper eyelid; the Jagher plastic retractor is inserted behind the upper lid after one drop of Pontacaine® was instilled in the eye. The tumor was subjected to one minute of freezing with safe margins beyond the tumor edge (Figure 5-61). Ballottement of the frozen tumor mass was used as clinical judgment regarding the duration of freeze time. Four weeks following cryosurgery, except for slight hyperpigmentation, there is no clinical evidence of the preexisting carcinoma (Figure 5-62).

The patient in Figure 5-63 is a woman in her forties, with a biopsy-proven basal

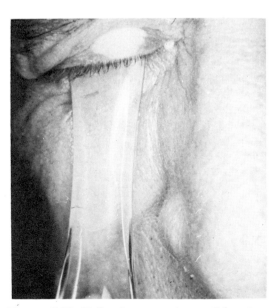

Figure 5-61. Following one minute of freezing of the above epithelioma.

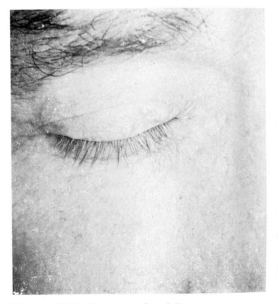

Figure 5-62. Four weeks following cryosurgery, the only residue was slight degree of hyperpigmentation.

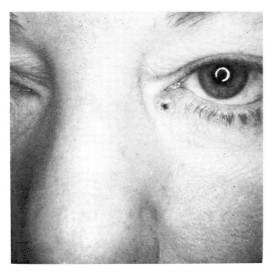

Figure 5-63. A nodular basal cell epithelioma of the left medial canthus, 3 mm below the punctum.

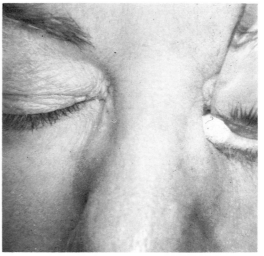

Figure 5-65. After sixty seconds of freezing, a wide margin was included extending into the punctum.

cell carcinoma of the medial canthus. She was referred by her ophthalmologist. The tumor measured 0.5 cm in size, somewhat ulcerated and nodular with its visible margin approximately 1 mm from the punctum. A drop of Pontacaine was placed in her eye and a plastic retractor was inserted

into the fornix to protect the globe from liquid nitrogen spray (Figure 5-64). Intermittent spray with liquid nitrogen was induced for a period of sixty seconds. A wide margin was frozen extending into the free margin of the medial canthus lid including the punctum (Figure 5-65). Forty-

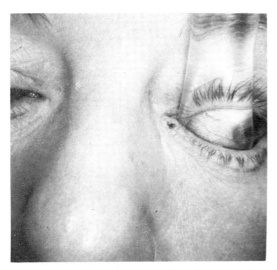

Figure 5-64. Placement of the plastic Jegher retractor on the lower lid.

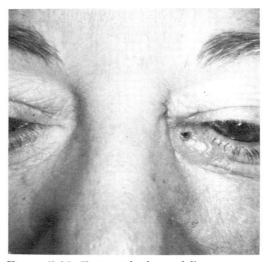

Figure 5-66. Forty-eight hours following cryosurgery, there was nominal edema at the tumor site.

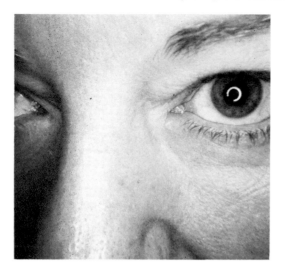

Figure 5-67. Four weeks following cryosurgery, the tumor was not evident with absence of lacrimal obstruction and also preservation of the lid margin.

eight hours following cryosurgery, there is moderate edema at the medial canthus but the patient is without subjective symptoms or discomfort (Figure 5-66). With the mechanical insertion of the plastic lid retractor and exudation of serous material from the adjacent frozen tumor, a mild noninflammatory conjunctivitis is often observed for several days following cryosurgery of tumors of the lids. To help cleanse the eye and relieve any symptoms of smarting, the daily application of Ocurins® (.85% sodium chloride) or Eye Stream® several times a day has proven beneficial. Four weeks following cryosurgery the carcinoma is clinically eradicated with no eversion of the eye margin nor obstruction of the puncta and there is an absense of epiphora (Figure 5-67).

The patient in Plate 66 presented a 0.8 cm ulcerated histologically-proven basal cell carcinoma of the left lower lid extending into the free lid margin. After carefully outlining a 0.4 cm of skin margin outside the visible tumor border of the tumor, the plastic lid retractor was placed within the fornix of the lower lid (Plate 67) after proper anesthesia with Pontocaine in the eye. The tumor was subjected to sixty seconds of intermittent freeze with liquid nitrogen. The ice front was extended clearly to the lid margin and peripherally to normal skin (Plate 68). The frozen tumor site measured over 1.3 cm. Twenty-four hours following cryosurgery, the expected periorbital edema was observed with mild noninflammatory conjunctivitis (Plate 69). Four weeks following cryosurgery, the carcinoma is totally absent without any evidence of eversion or damage to the lid or tarsal plate (Plate 70).

A more advanced basal cell carcinoma of the left paranasal area extending to the left lower eyelid and approximating the free lid margin of the medial canthus is depicted in a sixty-three-year-old patient (Plate 71). The tumor measured 2.2 cm x 2.6 cm x 0.6 cm in elevation. This tumor had been slowly growing for over twelve years and she had avoided any medical attention. She finally sought the attention of Dr. George Zippin, Schenectady, New York. A biopsy quickly affirmed his clinical suspicions of a basal cell carcinoma and he urged immediate surgical excision. The patient refused and as an alternative, he referred her to the author. Realizing the extent of the tumor and its critical anatomical site, the author recommended either Mohs' chemosurgery or surgical excision with plastic reconstruction but she refused. The advanced nature of her neoplasm, the limitation of cryosurgery, and the strong possibility of possible recurrence from freezing were fully explained. She still preferred cryosurgery. The neoplastic mass was subjected to five minutes of freezing (Plate 72). After eight minutes of thawing, the carcinoma was re-

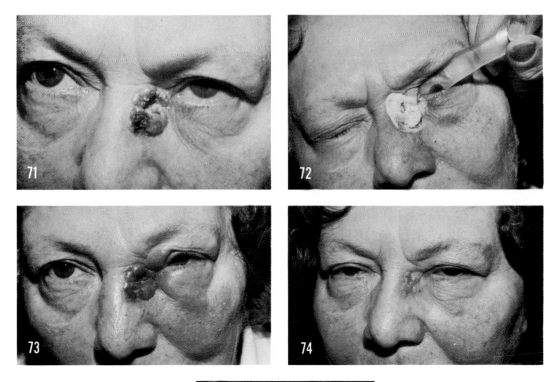

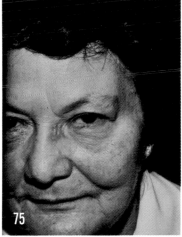

Plate 71. A large basal cell carcinoma of left paranasal area and medial canthus, measuring 2.2 x 2.6 x 0.6 cm.

Plate 72. After five minutes of freezing. This tumor was subjected to a triple freeze-thaw cycle.

Plate 73. Forty-five minutes after the third freeze. An extensive periorbital edema.

Plate 74. Five weeks following cryosurgery, there is present some epitheliomatous hyperplasia (pseudorecidive).

Plate 75. Two and one-half months after cryosurgery, there is minimal hypertrophic scarring. This was eliminated with the use of Cordran tape.

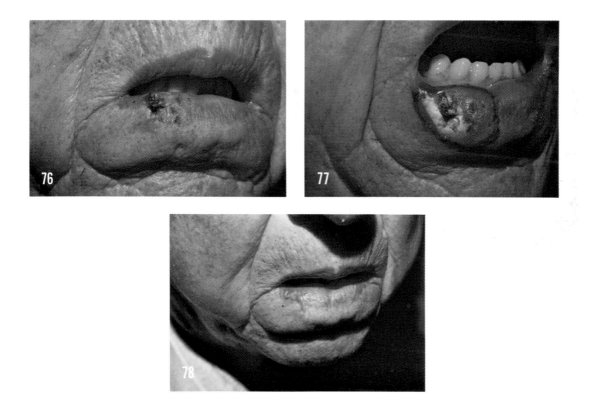

Plate 76. An epidermoid carcinoma of the lower lip.
Plate 77. During the second thaw phase. Frozen tumor was 1.5 cm in area with the initial freeze time of two and one-half minutes.
Plate 78. Four weeks following freezing, there is no clinical evidence of the carcinoma, nor after two and one-half years' follow-up.

frozen and, after thawing, was again re-frozen. Within forty-five minutes follow-ing the third freeze, she demonstrated a marked degree of periorbital edema, as an-ticipated (Plate 73). She presented a mod-erate degree of epithelomatous hyperplasia (Plate 74). Two and one-half months fol-lowing cryosurgery, there is no clinical evi-dence of the carcinoma (Plate 75). The small hypertrophic scar was treated with Cordran® tape.

The author's experience in the manage-ment of eyelid cancers in the past twelve years has been limited to one hundred pa-tients (Table 5-II). The recurrence rate of 8.0 percent is unacceptably high—over twice that of cryosurgery of skin cancer in general. Three of the recurrent carcino-mas were recurrences from either surgery or irradiation and three others subjected to freezing were palliative procedures in very old debilitated patients who could not undergo surgery. Doctors Beard and Sulli-van will discuss in more detail their own experience in cryosurgery of eyelid can-cers in chapter eight. As ophthalmologists, their assessment of this modality for tu-

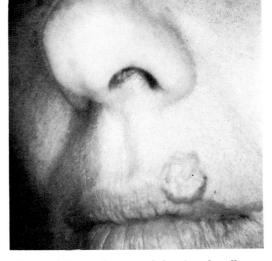

Figure 5-68. A large nodular basal cell epi-thelioma of the lip including the vermilion border. This tumor is amenable to cryosurgery but the risk of deformity in the contour of the lip is high.

mors of the lid will perhaps be more meaningful.

It is fair to say, however, that cryosur-gery offers some distinct advantages in the management of eyelid cancers and time alone and larger series by both dermatolo-gists and ophthalmologists will place this modality in its proper prospective.

d. Cancers of the Lip, Scalp and
Large Tumors

Cancers situated upon the lips can readi-ly be eradicated by means of cryosurgery. A singular exception may be tumors which are deep and infiltrating, as a sclerosing type or those extending into the vermilion border (Figure 5-68). These tumors will require extremely deep freezing and a cicatrizing scar will often develop at the vermilion border, disfiguring the normal contour of the lip.

An ideal tumor of the upper lip is shown in Figure 5-69. This patient (age 74) had a biopsy-proven basal cell carci-

TABLE 5-II

EYELID CANCERS TREATED BY MEANS
OF CRYOSURGERY

Histology
93 Basal cell carcinomas
5 Epidermoid carcinomas
2 Basosquamous cell carcinomas
100 Carcinomas in total
Location
17 Upper lid (17.0%)
83 Lower lid (83.0%)
29 of lower lid tumors situated in the medial canthus (35.0%)
Recurrences
Average follow-up of 5 years, 8 recurrences or 8.0%
3 of the 8 recurrences were recurrent to start with and 3 additional tumors were palliative procedures.

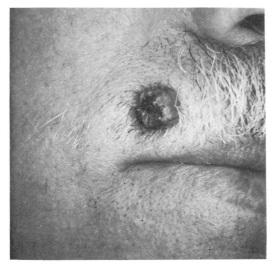

Figure 5-69. A large 1.5 cm nodular basal cell carcinoma of the upper cutaneous lip.

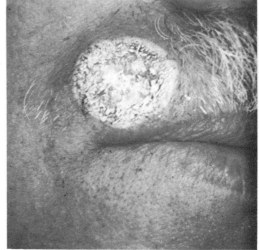

Figure 5-71. The base of the tumor after three minutes of freezing. The thaw time was five minutes.

noma, measuring 1.5 cm and presenting a nodular and ulcerated morphology 0.6 cm above the cutaneous surface of the lip. The first step was to cut away some of his mustache, 1 cm beyond the delineated margin of the cancer. This is important, for *hair will conduct the liquid nitrogen* far

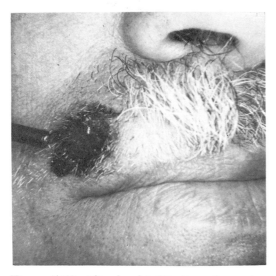

Figure 5-70. After local infiltration of anesthesia, the fungating portion of the tumor was removed with bipolar cutting current.

beyond the freezing target. The base of the tumor was then anesthetized and, to assure adequate freezing in depth, most of the surface tumor mass was removed with a bipolar cutting current (Figure 5-70). With large bulky tumors, the author often uses the cutting current to remove most of the growth and then freezes the base. Carefully extending the freeze to 5 mm beyond the surface margin of the cancer, it was frozen for three minutes (Figure 5-71). The thaw time was five minutes and a second freeze was instituted. Clinical judgment and ballottement of the frozen mass were used to insure adequate freezing.

Three days following cryosurgery (Figure 5-72), there was considerable edema and hemorrhagic exudate from the frozen site. Simple daily washing with soap and water or cleansing with hydrogen peroxide was quite adequate. Six weeks following cryosurgery, there were traces of pseudo-recidive tumor (Figure 5-73), not to be mistaken for residual unfrozen tumor or an early recurrence. Ten weeks following

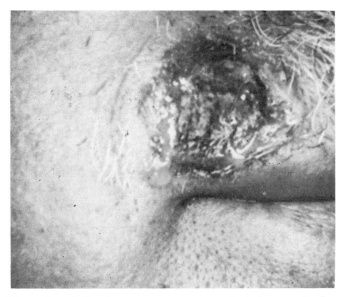

Figure 5-72. Three days following cryosurgery, a marked degree of edema and exudation was evident.

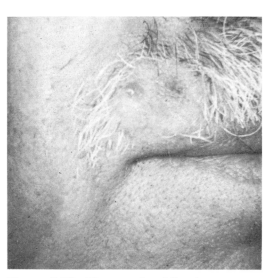

Figure 5-73. Five weeks following cryosurgery, small islands of pseudorecidive are present.

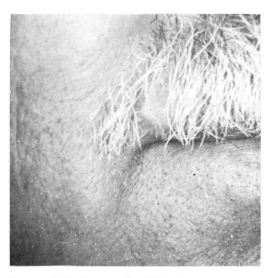

Figure 5-74. Ten weeks following cryosurgery, except for some depigmentation and loss of mustache, the neoplasm is totally eradicated. There has been no occurrence in over two years' observation.

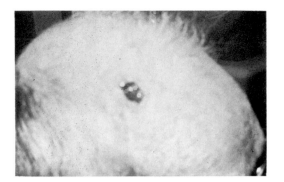

Figure 5-75. An ulcerated basal cell carcinoma of the scalp measuring 1.5 × 2.0 cm. It is not adherent to the underlying bone.

cryosurgery (Figure 5-74), there was no clinical evidence of the tumor; slight depigmentation and loss of hair was observed at the frozen site. This attests to depth of freezing deep into the hair follicles where one often finds nests of tumor extension. The surrounding hair from his mustache very nicely covers the previous site of the tumor.

The patient in Plate 76 presented a two-year history of a microscopically-proven epidermoid carcinoma of the lower lip. There were no palpable submental or submaxillary nodes. The tumor surface measured 1.5 cm. A wide safe margin beyond the visible tumor site (0.8 cm) was marked and the carcinoma was subjected to a double freeze-thaw cycle. The initial freeze time was two and one-half minutes and thaw period was four minutes; Plate 77 shows the tumor site during its second thaw phase. Complete healing was noted on the fourth week (Plate 78).

As a general rule, the author avoids freezing skin cancers upon the scalp, because recurrence has been too high and unacceptable. There are situations, however, such as the age of the patient or his poor health, when cryosurgery can be considered. The patient in Figure 5-75 is a ninety-two-year-old man with an ulcerated

tumor of his scalp of four years' duration. The microscopic examination of the biopsy of this tumor was a basal cell carcinoma. The neoplasm measured 1.5 by 2.0 cm. A safe margin of 1.0 cm was marked outside the visible margins. From observation of histological sections it is noted that tumors of the scalp extend deep, with considerable peripheral extensions—more so than with cancers elsewhere on the face. The carcinoma was subjected to a double freeze-thaw cycle (Figure 5-76). The ice front was carried down to the periosteum until the overlying skin of the scalp was totally immobile and the thaw period was seven minutes. The importance of intermittent freezing upon the center of the tumor, and not a continuous stream of liquid nitrogen, cannot be overstressed.

The patient sustained a migraine-like headache for five minutes following cryosurgery and upon its cessation, he was dismissed from the treatment room. No local analgesia was used during cryosurgery; the author has found that even with local anesthesia the transitory headache cannot be averted. A week following cryosurgery, there was present the expected hemor-

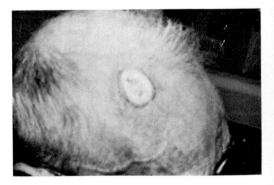

Figure 5-76. The epithelioma, after a second freeze, extended 1.0 cm beyond the visible margins of the tumor and down to the underlying periosteum. The freeze time was four minutes and the initial thaw period was seven minutes.

rhagic crust and slight oozing from the wound site (Figure 5-77). Two months following cryosurgery, there was no evidence of the carcinoma and the only residual effect was a transitory mild erythema at a small focal area of the previously larger frozen tumor site (Figure 5-78).

Large multicentric tumors of the chest and back over 10 cm are best treated with cryogenic surgery, providing freezing is executed in two separate sittings. Very often the author will freeze one half of the tumor and six or eight weeks later, with complete healing, will then freeze the other half of the tumor. The patient in Plate 79 presented a large 2.5 x 3.5 cm basal cell carcinoma of the left upper cheek. After a safe margin of 0.5 cm was outlined beyond the visible margin of the tumor and after local anesthesia of the tumor site, the modified template (Figure 1-11) was placed between the midcenter of the tumor and its edge. One thermocouple was passed through the five mm track with its tip imbedded five mm below the midcenter of the tumor. The second thermocouple needle was placed horizontally through the base of the template with its tip extending 3 mm below the skin surface at the perimeter edge of the cancer (Plate 80). Freezing was executed, directing the liquid ni-

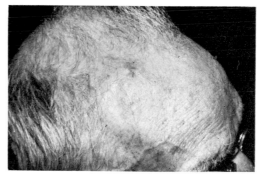

Figure 5-78. Two months following freezing, there was complete healing. Two years following cryosurgery, there is no sign of a recurrence.

trogen spray intermittently to the center of the tumor until the ice front extended peripherally. After four minutes of freezing, the measured temperature at 5 mm depth from the center of the cancer was recorded at $-35°C$ and the temperature at the margin of the tumor, 3 mm below, was monitored at $-25°C$ (Plate 81). The freezing was terminated at this point and the tumor site was allowed to thaw. The thaw period was seven minutes. A second freeze was executed. Two months following cryosurgery, except for a slight degree of erythema at the previous site of the cancer, there was complete eradication of the malignancy, with no evidence of atrophy or hypertrophic scars (Plate 82).

The measurement of the ice front at the margin of the cancer is very vital for large tumors, to insure a higher cure rate. There is indeed a place for monitoring *two focal* points in cryogenic surgery.

The use of bipolar cutting current to remove bulky tumors before freezing is an added adjunct and assurance of thorough in-depth cryonecrosis. Employing two thermocouple needles to simultaneously monitor the depth and temperature of the ice front at the center and margin of the cancer will further enhance the destruction

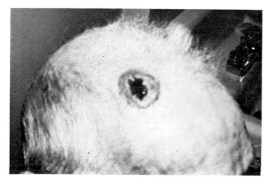

Figure 5-77. One week following cryosurgery, there was considerable edema and exudation at the tumor site.

of the carcinoma and will avoid the recurrences observed at the margins.

e. Lentigo Maligna—Hutchinson's Melanotic Freckle

Malignant melanomas occur in three distinct clinical and histological forms. They have been classified as superficial spreading, nodular melanoma and lentigo maligna melanoma.[121, 122] The present management of human melanomas, so far as cryogenics is concerned, is limited to lentigo maligna. This precancerous tumor was first recognized by Hutchinson in 1892[123] and later described by Dubreuilh[124] as a circumscribed precancerous melanosis. It is a relatively uncommon tumor of the skin appearing most often in the sixth and seventh decade of life. It must not be overlooked, however, in the younger patient, for in a series of eighty-five patients with melanotic freckle of Hutchinson, nine were observed under the age of forty.[125] Sun-exposed areas are the most common sites of involvement, in particular the malar eminences.[126]

The lesion begins as a small, light to dark brown macule, and in the course of time spreads peripherally with irregular edges. With progression of time, the neoplasm will assume a pattern of colors mottled with speckled and concentrated areas of pigment from jet black to brown to blue; in time there may develop areas of nodular outgrowth. Tumor growth is extremely slow and may take a decade or more to reach the dimensions of 1 or 2 cm. In a series of forty-eight cases studied by Clark and Mihm,[127] the average lesion occupied an area of 8.4 sq cm. These tumors have a tendency to invade deep within the dermis into the hair follicles and pilosebaceous elements. Microscopic sections will often show the proliferation and extent of atypical melanocytes within

and beyond the epidermal-dermal junction. This is an important consideration in the selection of modality to eradicate this tumor. Malignant transformation of lentigo maligna to a melanoma has been cited to occur from 30 to 50 percent of the reported cases in the literature.[125–127]

The conventional treatment for lentigo maligna is surgical excision or vigorous curettage and electrodesiccation. Mohs' chemosurgery and irradiation therapy have also been successful in the eradication of this tumor.[128] Cryosurgery for this neoplasia is relatively new and will require several years to properly assess its efficacy. The pathogenesis of cryonecrosis and the fact that melanocytes are extremely sensitive to freezing temperatures[129] as cited in the first chapter, clearly indicates that cryosurgery in sufficient depth will be curative. The largest series (eleven patients) with Hutchinson's melanotic freckle treated successfully with cryosurgery was reported by Lorenc and Wooldridge.[130]

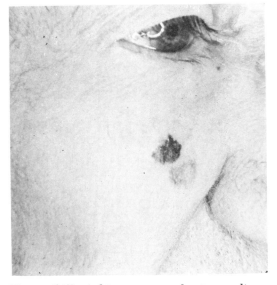

Figure 5-79. A biopsy-proven lentigo maligna approximately 1.8 cm in size. This tumor was subjected to two minutes of freeze.

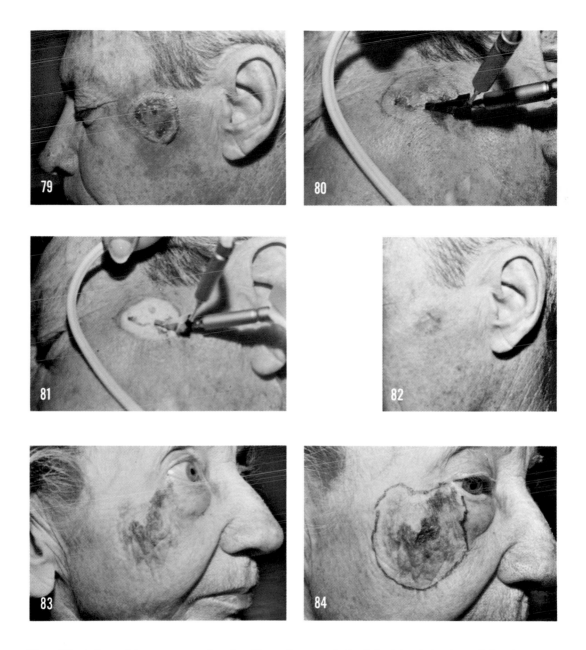

Plate 79. A large biopsy-proven basal cell carcinoma of the left side of the face, 2.5 x 3.5 cm.

Plate 80. Placement of two microthermocouples; one at midcenter 5mm below the tumor, the other at the edge of the tumor at 3 mm depth.

Plate 81. After four minutes of freezing, the monitored temperature midcenter below tumor was -35°C and at 3 mm depth at the edge of the tumor, -25°C.

Plate 82. Two months following cryosurgery, there is still present some erythema. One year follow-up shows no recurrence.

Plate 83. A large lentigo maligna of the right cheek, 4.5 x 5.5 cm.

Plate 84. A safe margin of 0.6 cm was outlined beyond the visible margin of the tumor.

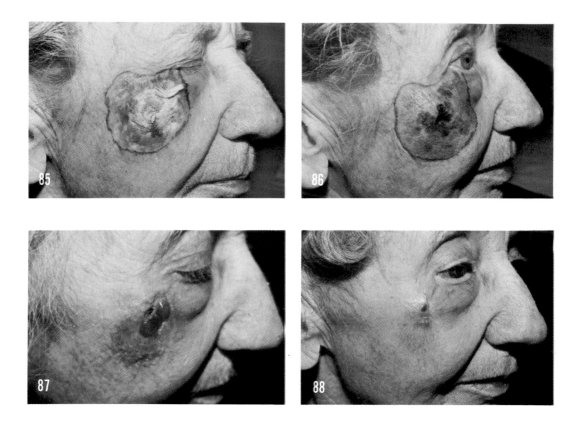

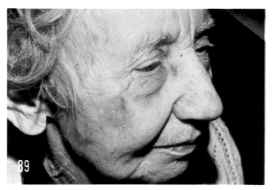

Plate 85. During the first thaw period. The initial freeze time was four minutes. A second freeze was executed after complete thawing.

Plate 86. Forty-eight hours following cryosurgery, there is some edema still present.

Plate 87. Five weeks following freezing, there is present some granulation tissue with a blue pigmented macule just above it.

Plate 88. At two months following cryosurgery, except for an area of pseudo epitheliomatous hyperplasia, the tumor is eradicated.

Plate 89. At three and one-half months, healing is complete without any clinical evidence of the lintigo maligna. Sixteen month follow-up showed no recurrence.

In the past ten years, the author has treated eight patients with lentigo maligna. At this present writing, there have been no recurrences but only five patients have been followed for over five years. The patient in Figure 5-79 was first seen four years ago with a biopsy-proven lentigo maligna situated on the malar prominence of the right cheek. This tumor was subjected to a double freeze-thaw cycle and two months later, except for some post freezing hyperpigmentation (Figure 5-80), there was no clinical evidence of the neoplasm. He has been carefully followed for four years without any evidence of a recurrence.

A recent woman patient, age 76 (Plate 83), presented a pigmented tumor of the right malar prominence of fifteen years' duration. Clinically it measured 4.5 x 5.5 cm involving the right lower eyelid and extending to the free margin of the lid. Two biopsies at separate sites histologically confirmed the diagnosis of Hutchinson's melanotic freckle (Figure 5-81). A safe margin of 6 mm was outlined outside the visible margins of the tumor (Plate 84) and the area was subjected to cryosurgery. The central and most involved site of tumor was subjected to a full minute of freezing and gradually the liquid nitrogen spray was extended to the periphery. The total freeze time was four minutes and the thaw period was seven minutes. Plate 85 demonstrates the period of thawing. After complete thawing, the tumor was completely frozen again and allowed to thaw. No local anaesthesia was used during this procedure. Forty-eight hours later (Plate 86) the patient showed considerable edema of the right cheek, but was relatively asymptomatic. Five weeks following cryosurgery, the patient presented an area of granulation healing (Plate 87) with a small 6 mm blue-pigmented macule just above and lateral to the healing wound site. At two months following cryosurgery, wound healing was about complete (Plate 88). There was a small area showing pseudoepitheliomatous hyperplasia and a persistent blue pigmented macule which was subjected to another biopsy. This area showed a collection of histiocytes with melanin pigment, deeply situated within the skin (Figures 5-81 through 5-83). This phenomenon is clearly recognized as an important sign of regression of the tumor and not to be confused as either an incomplete eradication or an early recurrence.[124, 131-133] Three and one-half months following cryosurgery, there was complete healing and complete resolution of the blue-pigmented residual macule (Plate 89).

The preliminary reports in the literature and added cases in this monograph clearly indicate the effectiveness of cryosurgery for the destruction of lentigo maligna. A larger series and a longer follow-up will be

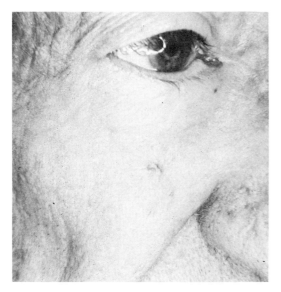

Figure 5-80. Two months following cryosurgery, the neoplasm has been eradicated. Four years' follow-up has produced no recurrences.

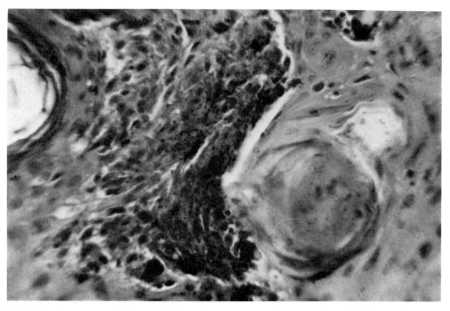

Figure 5-81. Pretreatment biopsy of lentigo maligna. Note the spindle cell malignant melanoma invading papillary corium, and the intense pigmentation of the malignant melanocytes. ×430.

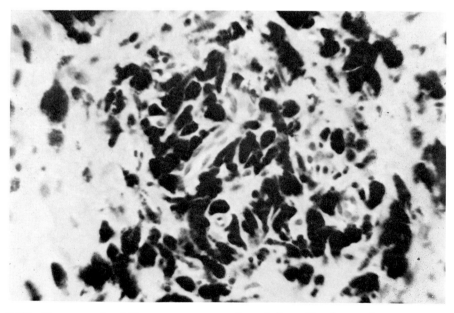

Figure 5-82. Two months following cryosurgery, a second biopsy at the residual blue-pigmented macule. The cellular detail is obscured by excess pigment. The random cluster-ing of the cells, the tendency to group around blood vessels and the absence of a consistently spindle morphology suggest melanophages. ×430.

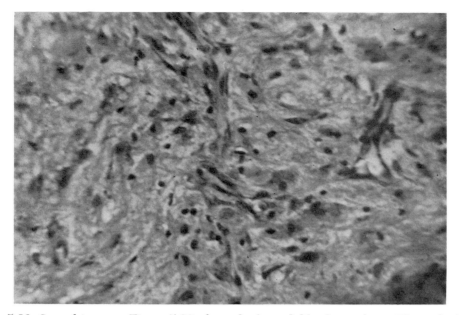

Figure 5-83. Same biopsy as Figure 5-82 after removal of the melanin discloses the histiocytic character of the cells grouped about new-ly formed blood vessels, ×430; melanin pigment removed with potassium permanganate.

needed to fully evaluate this promising new modality for Hutchinson's melanotic freckle.

III. COMPLICATIONS FROM CRYOSURGERY OF THE SKIN

As with any physical modality or therapeutic regimen, cryosurgery presents a number of complications worthy of mentioning. Table 5-III outlines them under the designation of immediate, delayed and prolonged.

1. Immediate Reactions to Freezing

Pain is a subjective reaction to freezing and differs from patient to patient. The initial pain from freezing ceases because of the analgesic effects of cold upon the superficial sensory cutaneous nerves. The pain returns during the thawing phase and is more profound. With complete thawing, pain ceases at the site of cryosurgery. The only exception to this is when freezing is directed to the forehead, temples and particularly to the scalp. Very often the patient experiences a throbbing migraine-like headache which may last from several minutes to one or two hours. The author has not been able to explain this phenomenon,

TABLE 5-III

COMPLICATIONS FROM CRYOSURGERY

Immediate
  Pain
  Edema with blister formation
  Insufflation of soft tissue
Delayed
  Inflammation
  Febrile—systemic (toxic)
  Bleeding from wound site
Prolonged
  Hypopigmentation
  Hyperpigmentation
  Atrophic scars
  Hypertrophic scars
  Neuropathy

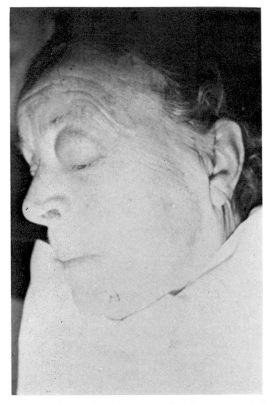

Figure 5-84. Insufflation of left upper lid which developed almost instantaneously during freezing a ulcerated tumor of the left temple. The edema persisted for several days. Courtesy of Dr. J. Stopka, Chicago.

despite diligent search and inquiry with neurologists. He has made it a rule that patients who have been subjected to cryosurgery for tumors at these sites remain in the examining room until they are symptom free, and uses local anesthesia only when inserting a thermocouple needle. Local anesthesia does not obviate the migraine-like pain.

Edema following cryosurgery is inevitable. It is usually confined to the cryosurgical site. However, whenever freezing upon the cheeks, swelling will, on occasion, manifest itself below the chin or angle of the jaw several days following the cryosurgical procedure. Tumors frozen upon the

eyelids and paranasal areas and temples will invariably produce a marked degree of periorbital edema (Figure 5-58). Tumors frozen upon the forehead and scalp will also induce periorbital edema, either singular or bilateral. This swelling may well persist for several days.

Insufflation of soft tissue from cryosurgery has been described by Torre, Lubritz and Stopka (Figure 5-84). This author has not to this writing observed this phenomenon. It is possible that an open wound site from a biopsy or an ulcerated lesion will allow free access of the sprayed cryogen to traverse through loose areolar tissue, as in the eyelids and scrotum, producing an immediate swelling and discomfort of a temporary nature.

2. Delayed Complications

Inflammation following cryosurgery is extremely rare. In the several cases encountered by this author, they have been invariably in the lower extremities where wound healing is slow with almost any modality. Two patients were diabetic which added to the complication of wound infection. Larger tumors, subjected to freezing, could be a source of secondary infection.

Febrile systemic toxic reactions following cryosurgery are indeed rare—Lubritz, Elton, and Stopka have each cited two cases. The author has frozen as many as twenty multicentric carcinomas of the chest and back at a single sitting without any sequelae. The explanation for this rare complication remains obscure; it may represent a cholinergic-like reaction or undue histamine release for reasons unknown. Lubritz further adds that the febrile reaction ceased at the end of twenty-four hours.

Postcryosurgery bleeding or hemorrhage is an extremely rare complication. It can, however, develop a few days following freezing due to rupture of an arteriole, requiring a simple suture to stop the bleeding.

3. Prolonged Complications

The loss of pigment at the frozen site is quite common following cryosurgery. Melanocytes which are highly cryosensitive are destroyed; repigmentation will take place only after several years from surrounding melanocytes which will migrate to the frozen tumor site. Hyperpigmentation is a postinflammatory response and within months, it will invariably disappear.

Atrophic scars do develop from cryosurgery but not too frequently. They appear specifically upon the forehead, lobule or tip of the nose, and the upper cutaneous aspect of the lip. The lower extremities are very prone to atrophy and occasionally the back also atrophies.

Hypertrophic scars following cryosurgery are extremely uncommon and when observed are noted on the midforehead, ala nasi, tip of the nose, vermilion aspect of the lip, chest, and back. With time, they will involute. To hasten their disappear-

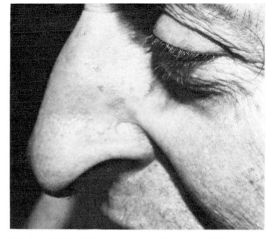

Figure 5-86. Two months after applying Cordran tape, the hypertrophic scar has all but dissolved. Intralesional triamcinolone injection will also hasten the disappearance of hypertrophic scars.

ance, intralesional injection of triamcinolone or the application of Cordran tape will effect a cure. The patient in Figure 5-85 presented an hypertrophic scar within six weeks following cryosurgery of a basal cell carcinoma at the left ala nasi. Six weeks of nightly application of Cordran tape has eliminated most of the hypertrophic scar (Figure 5-86).

Neuropathy is an extremely uncommon complication when one considers the number of patients who are subjected to freezing procedures. The first reported cases of liquid nitrogen neuropathy were observed by Nix.[134] Two patients who received liquid nitrogen applied with cotton swabs for verrucae subsequently developed anesthesia at the treated sites. The neuropathy was confined to the sensory nerves. Motor nerves were not involved. In both patients the warts were on the right hand involving fingers. In one patient the anesthesia was still present after two years.

Subsequent studies of freezing temperatures upon the sciatic and combined me-

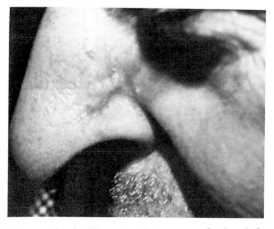

Figure 5-85. Hypertrophic scar of the left ala nasi following cryosurgery of a basal cell carcinoma.

dian-ulnar nerves of rats[135] showed no permanent damage. Their regeneration to normal function varied from several days to several weeks, dependent upon the temperatures to which the nerves were subjected (0° to −100°C). According to Carter and his associates,[136] there is no evidence to suggest that the response of sensory nerves to subzero temperatures will differ significantly from that of their motor counterparts. These studies have been recently corroborated by the work of Lenz and his colleagues.[137]

Finelli[138] reported on the first case of liquid nitrogen neuropathy in a patient subjected to cryotherapy of a common wart overlying the ulnar nerve at the elbow. He applied liquid nitrogen with a cotton swab (ten applications in a two minute period). In addition to sensory loss and motor weakness, there appeared marked atrophy of the first dorsal interosseus muscle. This report indeed concerned the author greatly and he wrote to Dr. Finelli. His reply was prompt and read in part as follows: "It has now been about two years since the patient received cryotherapy. He states the sensation has returned to normal. The wasting and atrophy of the first dorsal interosseus muscle has returned to normal and the strength and dexterity of the involved hand is almost 100 percent better."[139]

Despite the extremely rare occurrence of neuropathy following cryosurgery, it behooves us to alert the patient. From the evidence thus far, regeneration appears to follow nerve injury in time.

IV. CANCER OF THE SKIN—A CRYOSURGICAL REVIEW

In a little over twelve years, 1,801 patients with a combined total of 2,713 malignant tumors of the skin were treated by means of cryosurgery. One fourth of the patients were treated at the Western Massachusetts Hospital, Cancer Division, Westfield, Massachusetts, where this author has been a consultant. The remaining three fourths have been private patients. In the past three and one-half years, Dr. Arthur M. Sher, the author's associate, has contributed to the number of patients subjected to cryosurgery. The histological classification is 2,713 tumors presented in Table 5-IV.

Approximately 15 percent of the patients with skin cancer presented more than one tumor at the time of examination and one of every five patients treated for a skin cancer had developed a second malignant tumor of the skin within two years following the treatment of the initial tumor. This has been observed in other studies.[140] The distribution of skin cancers between sexes showed a 10 percent higher incidence in the male over the female patient.

Of the 1,801 patients with carcinoma of the skin, 240 or 14.5 percent were recurrent tumors at the time of treatment. A little over two thirds of the patients with skin cancer were between fifty and seventy years of age. Twenty percent were between seventy-one and eighty and 2.5 percent were under forty years of age. Eighty-five percent of the neoplasms were situated on the head and neck, while 38.0 percent were

TABLE 5-IV

ELEVEN YEAR STUDY OF 1,801 PATIENTS WITH 2,713 CUTANEOUS MALIGNANT TUMORS CRYOSURGICALLY TREATED

Type of Cancer	Number	Percent
Basal cell carcinomas	2,441	90.00
Epidermoid carcinomas	148	5.60
Basosquamous cell carcinomas	73	2.80
Bowen's disease (carcinoma in situ)	40	1.50
Kaposi hemorrhagic sarcomas	3	0.04
Lentigo maligna (Hutchinson's melanotic freckle)	8	0.06
	2,713	100.00

observed upon the critical areas of the face such as the nose, ears, and eyelids (Table 5-I).

Two thirds of the patients had sought medical attention within one year of the presenting symptom of the tumor growth. Approximately 15 percent had delayed treatment between three to five years. Early recognition by the patient with a growth, and continued education of the public must be sustained by both the physician and the dermatologist.

Approximately one half of the patients presented a nodular or ulcerated lesion while the remaining half were essentially superficial tumors. Only 15 percent of the patients were treated with copper discs chilled with liquid nitrogen during the first two years of the author's cryosurgical experience. This technique has been obsolete for ten years because of an unacceptable recurrence rate. There is direct relationship between the size of the tumor and its cure rate. The larger the lesion, higher

TABLE 5-V

THE FOLLOW UP OF SKIN CANCERS
SUBJECTED TO CRYOSURGERY

	Cure Rate
Of the total patients (1,801) 56 recurrences (3.4%)	96.6
Of the total combined cancers (2,713) 56 recurrences (2.2%)	97.8

In the 56 recurrences, 17 or 30% were recurrent cancers to start with.

is the incidence for recurrence. In the author's series, which may well represent the cross section of neoplasms treated by dermatologists, approximately 60 percent were between 1 to 2 cm in size while 30 percent were under 1 cm and 10 percent were over 2 cm (Figure 5-87).

The criteria of success of any modality for the treatment of cancer is the accurate follow-up and careful recording of recurrences. In the interval of eleven years, 40 percent of the patients have now been followed between three to five years; 45 percent between five to eleven years; and 15 percent under three years (Figure 5-88). Recurrences to this writing number 56. This represents a cure rate of 96.6 percent in 1,801 patients and 97.8 percent for the total of 2,713 carcinomas. The recurrences were forty-nine basal cell carcinomas, five epidermoid carcinomas, and two basosquamous cell carcinomas. Seventeen of the fifty-six recurrences or 30 percent were recurrent tumors. It has been earlier noted that the cure rate for recurrent cancer of the skin is approximately 50 percent. The 101 patients who died during this period of study and 14 lost in follow-up must be taken into account; correction is necessary in order to properly account for 115 patients from the number of carcinomas in this series. The *corrected* cure rate represents a revision of 0.3 percent less than presented in Table 5-V.

The cure rate for recurrent carcinomas

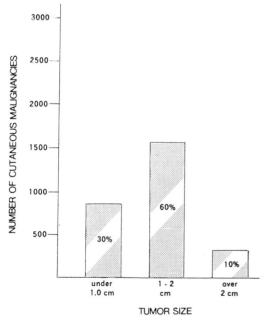

Figure 5-87. Cryosurgically treated neoplasms according to size.

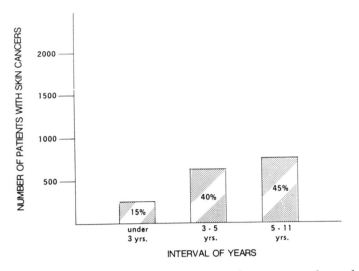

Figure 5-88. Duration of follow-up of 1801 patients with skin cancers subjected to cryosurgery.

of the skin retreated with cryosurgery stands at 75 percent. As pointed out earlier, 86.6 percent of patients demonstrated a recurrence within the first three years, the highest incidence observed during the first year numbering 43.3 percent. Double freeze-thaw cycle treatments of malignant tumors seems to offer the highest cure rates. Proper monitoring of tumors during cryosurgery in difficult areas and the execution of triple freeze-thaw cycles for neoplasms in critical areas as the eyelids, ala nasi, nasolabial fold, and the ears will salvage more malignancies of the skin. Never forget that your "initial opportunity for the treatment of skin cancer is the golden one."[41]

CRYOSURGERY IN PROPER PERSPECTIVE

In the past twelve years, the author has closely followed the management of cutaneous malignancies by means of cryosurgery. In many areas, basic laboratory experiments and animal studies have fully supported his own clinical observations.

He has also had the privilege to share the experiences of other investigators—Torre, Gage, Graham, Elton, Miller, Lubritz, and Spiller, to name a few of the early clinicians involved in cryogenics. The recent literature[142-150] in cryosurgery both in our country and abroad is ever increasing. We have gathered case histories of substantial numbers of skin cancers subjected to cryosurgery in over fifteen years, and at this time, the author is convinced that freezing skin cancers is an *established* therapeutic regimen. He is cognizant of the published report of Vistnes and his associates[151] who treated fifteen basal cell carcinomas and, three to six months following healing, found evidence of residual tumor in three. This is a high percentage of recurrence but the number of cases treated is also very small and two of the lesions were of the eyelids.

There is no single modality that is all promising and completely curative for all malignant tumors of the skin. Chemosurgery (Mohs') is the closest regimen we have for the highest cure rate. But even this modality has its drawbacks in terms of time and the necessary technical skill. Even advocates of this technique readily admit that by and large most skin cancers do not necessitate chemosurgical approach.

Each patient with skin cancer must be properly evaluated according to age, site of tumor, its histology, and most important, whether it is a primary or a recurrent tumor. The dimension of the tumor must also be considered.

Cryosurgery for skin cancers as with any modality has its limitations. The author feels that sclerosing type of tumors and those situated upon the scalp and ala nasi are difficult areas because of their depth of invasion and silent pseudopod extensions beyond measurement of the cryolesion. Adenoid tumors have been reported by Elton to be cryoresistant. Tumors just anterior to the tragus of the ear tend to be

deeply invasive and the author would be cautious to use cryosurgery. With these precautions, he would have no hesitancy to treat cancer of the skin in other locations. The expediency of time, avoidance of hospitalization, controlled monitored temperatures of the ice front, superb wound healing, avoidance of chondronecrosis of cartilage of the nose and ear, and absence of lacrimal obstruction of tumors of the medial canthus make cryosurgery a preeminent modality for the management of most skin cancers. There is also a place for cryosurgery in the treatment of the advanced skin cancer in the inoperative patient for palliation.

Cryosurgery is an added tool for the cancer therapist and when properly selected, it is extremely useful and effective.

There is a constant upgrading of instrumentations. At this writing and during the

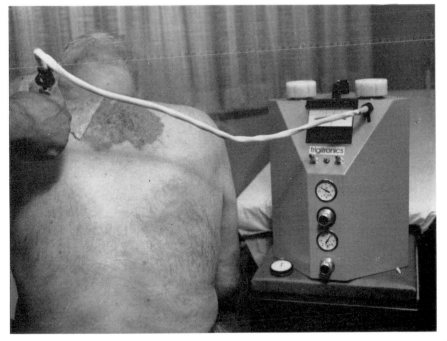

Figure 5-89. The prototype of the newest hand-held portable cryosurgical unit, the C-76. A single filling is adequate for the entire day with continuous intermittent spray of liquid nitrogen. Courtesy of Frigitronics, Inc., Shelton, CT.

period of submission of the manuscript to the publisher, this author has been working closely with the engineers at Frigitronics in the development of the C-76® cryosurgical portable unit (Figure 5-89). This nonelectric, self-pressurizing unit, with safety valves will deliver liquid nitrogen for a twelve-hour period, more than adequate for a full day's practice. It delivers an *intermittent* spray, effective for benign and malignant tumors and equally useful for acne therapy.

In addition to various gauged needles, solid probes and open cones to confine the liquid nitrogen spray are available.

BIBLIOGRAPHY

 1. Williams, A. C.: Symposium on skin cancers. *Medical Tribune,* 3, May 22, 1969.
 2. Urbach, F.: Geographic distribution of skin cancer. *J Surg Oncol,* 3:219-234, 1971.
 3. Belisario, J. C.: Effect of tropical sunlight on development of rodent and squamous cell carcinoma. *Int J Dermatol,* 11:148-155, July-Sept., 1972.
 4. Blum, H. F.: The physiological effects of sunlight in man. *Physiol Rev, 25:* 483-487, 1945.
 5. Blum, H. F.: Sunlight as a causal factor in cancer in man. *J Natl Cancer Inst,* 9:247-255, 1948.
 6. Mackie, B. S. and McGovern, V. J.: The mechanism of solar carcinogenesis. CA study of the role of collagen degeneration of the dermis in the production of skin cancer. *Arch Dermatol,* 78:218-222, 1958.
 7. Auerbach, H.: Geographic variations on the incidence of skin cancer in the U.S. *Public Health Report,* 76:345-348, April, 1961.
 8. Robertson, D. F.: Solar ultraviolet light radiation in relation to sunburn and skin cancer. *Med J Aust,* 2:1123-1126, 1968.
 9. Anderson, N. P. and Anderson, H. E.: Development of basal cell epitheliomas as a consequence of radiodermatitis. *Arch Dermatol and Syphiligr,* 63:586-596, 1951.
10. Sulzberger, M. B., Baer, R. L. and Borato, A.: Do roentgen-ray treatments as given by specialists produce skin cancers or other sequala? Follow-up study of dermatologic patients treated with low voltage Roentgen-rays. *Arch Dermatol and Syphiligr, 65:* 639-655, 1952.
11. Zackheim, H. S., Krobock, E. and Langs, L.: Cutaneous neoplasms in the rat produced by Grenz ray and 80 KV. x-ray. *J Invest Dermatol, 43:* 519-534, 1964.
12. Graham, J. H. and Helwig, E. B.: Precancerous skin lesions and systemic cancer. In U of Texas, M. D. Anderson Hospital and Tumor Institute: *Tumors of the Skin.* Chicago, Year Bk Med, 1964, pp. 209-221.
13. Graham, J. H. and Helwig, E. G.: Conference in Biology of Cutaneous Cancer (1963). Washington National Cancer Institute Monograph No. 10, 1963, pp. 323-333.
14. Graham, J. H., Mazzanti, G. R. and Helwig, E. B.: Chemistry of Bowen's disease: relationship to arsenic. *J Invest Dermatol,* 37:317-330, 1961.
15. Currie, A. N.: The role of arsenic carcinogenesis. *Br Med Bull,* 4:402-406, 1947.
16. Sommers, S. C. and McManus, R. G.: Multiple arsenical cancers of the skin and internal organs. *Cancer,* 6:347-351, 1953.
17. Gellin, G. A. and Possick, P. A.: Occupational cancer of the skin. *Cutis,* 5 (5):543-548, 1969.
18. Byrd, B. F., Munol, A. J. and Ferguson, H.: Carcinoma of the skin following acute and chronic trauma. *South Med J,* 54:1262-1264, 1960.
19. Dix, C. R.: Occupational trauma and skin cancer. *Plast Reconstr Surg, 26:* 546-549, 1960.
20. Dobson, R. L. and Griffin, M.: *The Histochemistry of Cutaneous Carcinogenesis-I. The Dermis.* Presented at the Soc Inv Meeting, June, 1962.
21. Pap, G. S. and Orlow, W. O.: Squamous cell carcinomas in a burn scar (Marjolin's ulcer). *Cutis,* 9:70-72, 1972.
22. Zelickson, A. S.: Basal cell epithelioma at site and following smallpox vacci-

nation. *Arch Dermatol, 98:*35-36, 1968.

23. Reed, W. B. and Wilson, J. E.: Malignant tumors as a late complication of vaccination. *Arch Dermatol, 98:* 132-135, 1968.

24. Marmelzat, W. W.: Malignant tumors in smallpox vaccination scars, a report of 24 cases. *Arch Dermatol, 99:* 400-406, 1968.

25. Friedman, M. M. and Miller-Cranko, J. A. W.: Malignancy in a smallpox vaccination. *Cent Afr J Med, 18* (7): 142, July, 1972.

26. MacDonald, E. J. and Bubendorf, E.: Some epidemiologic aspects of skin cancer. In U of Texas, M. D. Anderson Hospital and Tumor Institute: *Tumors of the Skin.* Chicago, Year Bk Med, 1964, pp. 23-65.

27. Spoor, H. J.: Skin cancer: Relationship to topically applied hormones. *Cutis, 9:*335-342, 1972.

28. Epstein, Ernst: Value of follow-up after treatment of basal cell carcinoma. *Arch Dermatol, 108:*798-800, 1973.

29. Schrek, R. and Gates, O.: Cutaneous carcinoma. *Arch Pathol, 31* (4):411-421, 1941.

30. Peck, G. T. and LeFevre, R. G.: Age and sex distribution and incidence of neoplastic diseases at Memorial Hospital, N.Y.C. with comments of cancer ages. *J Cancer Res, 14:*167-174, 1930.

31. Lund, H. C.: *Tumors of the Skin; Atlas of Tumor Pathology,* Section I, Fascicle, 2. Washington, Armed Forces Institute of Pathology, 1957.

32. Macomber, B. W., Wang, M. K. H. and Sullivan, J. G.: Cutaneous epithelioma. *Plast Reconstr Surg, 24:* (6): 545-562, 1959.

33. Griffith, B. H. and McKinney, P.: An appraisal of the treatment of basal cell carcinoma of the skin. *Plast Reconstr Surgery, 51:*565-571, 1973.

34. Owen, M.: Basal cell carcinoma: a study of 836 cases. *Arch Pathol, 10:*386-391, 1930.

35. Ward, G. E. and Hendrick, J. W.: *Tumors of the Head and Neck.* Baltimore, Williams & Wilkins, 1950, p. 120.

36. Lawrence, E. A., Dickey, J. W. and Vellios, F.: Malignant tumors of soft tissues of the extremities. *Arch Surg, 67:*392-399, 1953.

37. Conley, J. J.: Malignant tumors of the scalp. *Plast Reconstr Surg, 33* (1): 11-15, 1964.

38. Cotran, R. S.: Metastisizing basal cell carcinomas. *Cancer, 14:*1036-1038, 1961.

39. Wermuth, B. M. and Fajardo, L. F.: Metastatic basal cell carcinoma. *Arch Pathol, 90:*458-462, 1970.

40. Dahlgren, S. and Matensson, B.: Metastasizing basal cell carcinoma. *Acta Pathol Microbiol Scand, 59:*335-340, 1963.

41. Raitscher, R. and Stojanov, A. U.: Metastasizing basal cell carcinoma. *Hautarzt, 12:*320-323, 1961.

42. Lattles, R. and Kessler, R. W.: Metastasizing basal cell epitheliomas of the skin, report of 2 cases. *Cancer, 4:* 866-878, 1951.

43. Stell, J. S., Moyer, D. G. and Dehne, E.: Basal cell epithelioma metastatic to the bone. *Arch Dermatol, 98:*338-340, 1960.

44. Goldberg, L. C.: Metastasizing basal cell carcinoma. *Cutis, 2* (6):402-405, 1966.

45. Cranmer, L., Reginald, I. M. and Wilson, J. W.: Basal cell carcinoma of the skin metastatic to bone. *Arch Dermatol, 102:*337-339, 1970.

46. Mikhail, G. E., Kelley, A. P., Jr. and Elmquist, J. E.: Metastatic basal cell epithelioma discovered by chemosurgery. *Arch Dermatol, 105:*103-104, 1972.

47. Rueckert, F.: The malignant potential of face cancer. *Plast Reconstr Surg, 32:*21-29, 1963.

48. Warren, S. and Hoerr, S. A.: Study of pathologically verified epidermoid carcinoma of the skin. *Surg Gynecol Obstet, 69:*726-737, 1939.

49. Ackerman, L. V. and del Regato, J. E.: *Cancer Diagnosis and Treatment and Prognosis,* 3rd Ed. St. Louis, Mosby, 1947, pp. 1167 ff.

50. Katz, A. D., Urbach, F. and Lilienfeld, A. M.: The frequency and risk of metastasis in squamous cell carcino-

ma of the skin. *Cancer, 10:*1162-1166, 1957.

51. Epstein, Ervin, Epstein, N. N., Bragg, K. and Linden, G.: Metastases from squamous cell carcinomas of the skin. *Arch Dermatol, 97:*245-251, 1968.

52. Lund, A. Z.: How often does squamous cell carcinoma of the skin metastasize? *Arch Dermatol, 92:*635-637, 1965.

53. Bowers, R. F. and Young, J. M.: Carcinoma arising in scars, osteomyelitis and fistula. *Arch Surg, 80:*564-570, 1960.

54. Macomber, W.: Irradiation injuries, acute chronic and sequela. *Plast Reconstr Surg, 19:*9-10, 1957.

55. Neumann, Z.: Relationship between injury to the skin and subsequent malignant change. *Surg Gynecol Obstet, 117:*559-569, 1963.

56. Crissey, J. T.: Curettage and electrodesiccation as a method of treatment for epitheliomas of the skin. *J Surg Oncol, 3* (3):287-290, 1971.

57. Gooding, C. A., White, G. and Yatsuhashi, M.: Significance of marginal extension in excised basal cell carcinomas. *N Engl J Med, 273:*923-924, 1965.

58. Pascal, R. R., Hobby, L. V., Raffaele, L. and Crikelair, G. F.: Prognosis of "incompletely excised" basal cell carcinoma. *Plast Reconstr Surg, 41* (4): 328-332, 1968.

59. Grover, R. W.: Basal cell carcinoma. *Arch Dermatol, 107:*138, 1973.

60. Lauritzen, R. E., Johnson, R. E., and Spratt, J. S.: Pattern of recurrence in basal cell carcinoma. *Surgery,* 813-816, June, 1965.

61. Ebbehoj, E.: Experiences in the treatment of skin cancer with ultrasoft roentgen rays, 1933-1936. *Acta Radiol, 36:*1-17, 1951.

62. Newell, G. B.: Depth of basal cell epitheliomas. Personal communication, May 15, 1968.

63. Borel, D. M.: Cutaneous basosquamous carcinoma; A review of the literature and report of 35 cases. *Arch Pathol, 95:*293-297, 1973.

64. Epstein, Ernst: How accurate is the visual assessment of basal cell carcinoma margins? *Br J Dermatol, 89:*37-43, 1973.

65. Cooper, I. S.: Cryogenic cooling or freezing of basal ganglia. *Clin Neurol, 22:* 336-379, 1962.

66. Cooper, I. S.: Cryogenic Surgery; New method of destruction of extirpation of benign or malignant tumors. *N Engl J Med, 268:*747-749, 1963.

67. Cooper, I. S.: Cryogenic surgery for cancer. *Fed Proc, 24* (2):S237-S240, 1965.

68. Cahan, W. G.: Cryosurgery of malignant and benign tumors. *Fed Proc, 24* (2):S241-S248, 1965.

69. Gage, A. A. and Emmings, F.: Treatment of human tumors by freezing. *Cryobiology, 2:*14-18, 1965.

70. Gage, A. A., Koept, S., Wehrle, D. and Emmings, F.: Cryotherapy for cancer of the lip and oral cavity. *Cancer, 18:*1646-1650, 1965.

71. Torre, D.: New York; Cradle Cryosurgery. *N Y State J Med, 67:*465-667, 1967.

72. Torre, D.: Cutaneous Cryosurgery. *J Cryosurgery, 1:*202-209, 1968.

73. Torre, D.: Cryosurgery in Dermatology. In Von Leden, H. and Cahan, W. G. (Eds.): *Cryogenics in Surgery.* Flushing, NY, Med Exam, 1971, pp. 500-529.

74. Torre, D.: Freezing with freons. *Cutis, 16:*437-445, 1975.

75. Graham, G. F.: Cryosurgery of skin tumors. *N C Med J, 32* (3):81-87, 1971.

76. Graham, G. F.: Papers presented at the Cryosurgical Seminars in Dermatology I and II, New Orleans, October, 1974 and October, 1975.

77. Lubritz, R. R.: I and II Cryosurgical Seminars, October, 1974 and October, 1975, New Orleans, La. and personal communication, December, 1975.

78. Elton, R. F.: Cryosurgery of difficult basal cell epitheliomas. *Cutis, 16* (3):474-476, 1975.

79. Spiller, W. F. and Spiller, R. F.: Cryosurgery in dermatologic office practice with special reference to basal cell carcinoma. *Tex Med, 68:*84-88, 1972.

80. Miller, D. and Metzner, D.: Cryosurgery for tumors of the head and neck. *Trans Am Acad Ophthalmol Otolaryngol, 73*:300-309, 1969.

81. Miller, D.: Three years' experience with cryosurgery in head and neck tumors. *Ann Otol Rhinol Laryngol,* 786-791, 1969.

82. Miller, D., Silverstein, H. and Gacek, R.: Cryosurgical treatment of carcinoma of the ear. *Trans Am Acad of Ophthalmol Otolaryngol,* 1363-1367, Sept.-Oct., 1972.

83. Goldstein, J. C.: Cryotherapy of head and neck cancer. *Laryngoscope, 80:* 1046-1052, 1972.

84. Myers, R. S., Hammond, W. G. and Ketchum, A. S.: Cryosurgery of experimental tumors. *J of Cryosurgery,* 2:225-228, 1969.

85. Neel, H. Bryan, III, and Ketchum, A. S.: Requisites for successful cryogenic surgery of cancer. *Arch Surg, 102:* 45-48, 1971.

86. Zacarian, S. A. and Adham, M. I.: Cryotherapy of cutaneous malignancy. *Cryobiology,* 2:212-218, 1966.

87. Zacarian, S. A.: Cryotherapy of cutaneous malignancy: a two-year study of 220 patients. *J St. Barnabas Med Center, 4* (1):298-301, 1967

88. Zacarian, S. A.: Cryosurgery in dermatology. *Int Surg, 47* (6):528-534, 1967.

89. Zacarian, S. A.: Cryosurgery of cutaneous carcinoma. In *Cryosurgery of Skin Cancer and Cryogenic Techniques in Dermatology,* Springfield, Thomas, 1969.

90. Zacarian, S. A.: Cryosurgery of malignant tumors of the skin. In *Cryosurgery of Tumors of the Skin and Oral Cavity.* Springfield, Thomas, 1973.

91. Zacarian, S. A.: Cryosurgery of skin cancer: fundamentals of technique and application. *Cutis, 16*:449-460, 1975.

92. Zacarian, S. A.: Cryosurgery of skin cancer—in proper prospective. *Am J of Dermatologic Surgery, 1* (3):33-37, October, 1975.

93. Zacarian, S. A.: Recent trends in the management of skin cancer. *Comprehensive Therapy, 1* (4):60-64, 1975.

94. Harold, W. C. and Nelson, L. M.: Pseudoepitheliomatous reaction (pseudorecidive) following radiation therapy of epithelioma. In Hellerstrom, S. (Ed.): Proceedings of the 11th Congress of Dermatology. Stockholm, *Acta Derm Venereol,* 2:426, 1959.

95. Baer, R. L. and Kopf, A. W.: *The Year Book of Dermatology.* Chicago, Year Bk Med, 1964-65, p. 23.

96. Gonzalez-Ulla, M. and Flores, E. S.: Senility of the face. *Plast Reconstr Surg, 36* (2):239-246, 1965.

97. Taylor, G. A. and Barisoni, D.: Ten years' experience in the surgical treatment of basal cell carcinoma. *Br J Surg, 60* (2):522-525, 1973.

98. Conley, J.: Cancer of the skin of the nose. *Am Otology Rhinology and Laryngology,* 83:2-8, 1974.

99. McKee, D. M.: Treatment of basal cell carcinoma. *South Med J,* 57:209-215, 1964.

100. Payne, M. J.: Recurrent cancer of the skin. *Dermatol Digest,* 63-67, 1966.

101. Young, R.: The treatment of persistent recurrent basal cell epithelima of the face. *Surg Gynecol Obstet, 73*:152-164, 1965.

102. Mohs, F. F. and Lathrop, T. A.: Modes of spread of skin cancer of the skin. *Arch Dermatol and Syphiligr, 66:* 427-439, 1952.

103. Zacarian, S. A.: The cryogenic approach to the treatment of lid tumors. *Ann Ophthalmol,* 706-713, 1970.

104. Zacarian, S. A.: Cancer of the eyelid: a cryosurgical approach. *Ann Ophthalmol,* 473-480, 1972.

105. Shulman, J.: Cancer of the eyelids. *Br J Plast Surg,* 15:37-41, 1961.

106. Birge, H. L.: Cancer of the eyelids. *Arch Ophthalmol,* 19:700-704, 1938.

107. Cole, J. G.: Histologically controlled excision of eyelid tumors. *Am J Ophthalmol,* 70:240-245, 1970.

108. Domonkos, A. N.: Treatment of eyelid carcinoma. *Arch Dermatol 91*:364-371, 1965.

109. Rakofsky, S. I.: The adequacy of the surgical excision of basal cell carcinoma. *Ann Ophthalmol,* 596-600, May, 1973.

110. Payne, J. W., Duke, J. R., Butner, R.

and Eifrig, D. E.: Basal cell carcinoma of the eyelids. *Arch Ophthalmol,* 81:553-558, 1969.

111. Einaugler, R. B. and Henkind, P.: Basal cell epithelioma of the eyelid: apparent incomplete removal. *Am J Ophthalmol,* 413-417, March, 1969.

112. Abraham, J. C., Jabaley, M. E. and Hoopes, J. E.: Basal cell carcinoma of the medial canthal region. *Am J Surgery, 126:*492-495, 1973.

113. Wilder, L. W. and Smith, B.: Determination of the tumor margin in the excision of basal cell epitheliomas of the eyelids. *Ann Ophthalmol, 2:*887-888, 1970.

114. Robbin, P.: Chemosurgery. In Fox, S. A. (Ed.): *Ophthalmic Plastic Surgery.* New York, Grune, 1970, pp. 569-576.

115. Beard, C.: Observations of the treatment of basal cell carcinoma of the eyelids. *Trans. Am. Acad. Ophth & Otol., 79:* OP664-0068, Feb., 1975.

116. Bullock, J. D.: Personal communication, October 9, 1975, Dayton, Ohio.

117. Fraunfelder, F. T., Farris, H., Howard M. and Ray, M. L.: New therapy method for cancer eye in cattle. *Arkansas Farm Research, 22* (6): Nov.-Dec., 1973.

118. Farris, H. E., Fraunfelder, F. T. and Frith, C. H.: A simple cryosurgical unit for treatment of animal tumor. *Veterinary Medicine, 70:*299-302, March, 1975.

119. Farris, H. E., Fraunfelder, F. T. and White, G. L.: Cryosurgery of Ocular Squamous Cell Carcinoma of Cattle, *JAVM Assoc., 168*(3):213-216, Feb. 1, 1976.

120. Bullock, J. D.: Paper presented to the Society of Ophthalmic Surgery, October, 1975, Dallas Texas. In press.

121. Clark, W. H., From, L., Bernardino, E. and Mihm, M. C.: Histogenesis and biological behaviour of primary human malignant melanomas of the skin. *Cancer Res,* 1969.

122. Jackson, R., Williamson, G. S. and Beattie, W. G.: Lentigo maligna—a malignant melanoma. *Can Med Assoc J, 95:*846-851, 1966.

123. Hutchinson, J.: Senile freckles. *Arch Surg,* 3:319-322, 1891-1892.

124. Dubreuilh, W.: De la melanose circonscrite precancerous. *Ann Dermatol Syphiligr (Paris), 3* (Ser. 5):129-151, 205-230, 1912.

125. Wayte, D. M. and Helwig, E. B.: Melanotic freckle of Hutchinson. *Cancer, 21:*893-911, 1968.

126. Costello, M. J., Fisher, S. B. and DeFeo, C.: Melanotic freckle. *Arch Dermatol, 80:*153-171, 1959.

127. Clark, W. H. and Mihm, M. C.: Lentigo maligna and lentigo maligna melanoma. *Am J Pathol,* 55:39-69, 1969.

128. Petratos, M. A., Kopf, A. W., Bart, B. S. et al.: Treatment of melanotic freckle with X-rays. *Arch Dermatol 106:* 189-193, 1972.

129. Lindo, S. D. and Daniels, F., Jr.: Cryosurgery of junction nevi. *Cutis, 16:* 492-496, 1975.

130. Lorenc, E., Wooldridge, W. E. and Huewe, D. A.: The melanotic freckle of Hutchinson: preliminary report. *Cutis, 16:*485-486, 1975.

131. Miescher, G.: Precanceroeses Vortstadium des Melanoms, Precanceroeces Melanose. In Jadassoh, J. (Ed.): *Handbuch der Hautund Geschlechts Krankheiten,* Vol. 12, No. 3. Berlin, Springer-Verlag, 1933, pp. 1005-1135.

132. Mishima, Y.: Prophylaxis of malignant melanomas—melanosis circumscripta precancerosa. Dubreuilh distinct from junction nevus. *Cutis, 2:*588-591, 1966.

133. Justitz, H.: Melanotische Precancerose Dissertation. Druckereigenossenschaft Aarau, Zurich, 1935.

134. Nix, T. E., Jr.: Liquid nitrogen neuropathy. *Arch Dermatol, 92:*185-187, 1965.

135. Gaster, R. N., Davidson, T. M., Rand, R. W. and Fonkalsrud, E. W.: Comparison of nerve regeneration rates following controlled freezing or crushing. *Arch Surg, 103:*378-383, 1971.

136. Carter, D. C., Lee, P. W. R., Gill, W. and Johnston, R. J.: The effect of cryosurgery on peripheral nerve function. *J R Coll Surg Edinb, 17:*25-31, 1972.

137. Lenz, H., Goertz, W. and Preussler, H.:

The freezing threshold of the peripheral motor nerve: an electrophysiological and light microscopical study on the siatic nerve of the rabbit. *Cryobiology, 12:*486-496, 1975.

138. Finelli, P. F.: Ulnar neuropathy after liquid nitrogen cryotherapy. *Arch Dermatol, 111:*1340-1342 (Oct), 1975.

139. Finelli, P. F.: Personal correspondence, dated November 19, 1975, from the Veterans Administration Hospital, Providence, Rhode Island.

140. Bergstessor, P. R. and Halperin, K. M.: The sequential skin cancers: The risk of skin cancer in patients with previous skin cancer. *Arch Dermatol, 11:*995-996, 1975.

141. Young, R.: The treatment of persistent recurrent basal cell epithelioma of the face. *Surg Gynecol Obstet, 73:* 152-164, 1965.

142. Gill, W., DaCosta, J., Fraser, J. and Beazley, R.: The cryosurgical lesion. *Am Surg,* 437-445, 1970.

143. Gill, W., Da Costa, J. and Fraser, J.: The control and predictability of a cryolesion. *Cryobiology, 6* (4):347-353, 1970.

144. Neel, Bryan H., III, Ketcham, A. S. and Hammond, W. C.: Requisites for successful cryogenic surgery of cancer, *Arch. Surg., 102:*45-48, 1971.

145. Spiller, W. F. and Spiller, R. F.: Cryosurgery in dermatologic office practice with special reference to basal cell carcinoma. *Tex Med, 68:*84-88, 1972.

146. Miller, D., Silverstein, H. and Gacek, R.: Cryosurgical treatment of carcinoma of the ear. *Trans Am Acad Ophthalmol Otolaryngol,* 1363-1367, Sept. & Oct., 1972.

147. Wooldridge, W. E., Lorenc, E. and Huewe, D.: Treatment of skin cancer by cryosurgery. *Mo Med, 72* (1): 28-34, 1975.

148. Hopkins, P.: A preliminary study of the application of cryosurgery in general practice. Personal communication, October 18, 1974, and in press.

149. Berthier, DePedro Vivas: Cryosurgery of precancerous and cancerous lesions of the skin and oral cavity. Personal communication, December 8, 1975. Cuello del Institute of Oncology, Luis Razetti, de Caracas. In press.

150. Rothenburg, H. W.: Cryogenics as a tool: Aiding the Surgeon. *Cryogenics,* 3-8, January, 1975.

151. Vistnes, L. M., Harris, D. R. and Fajardo, L. F.: An evaluation of cryosurgery for basal cell carcinoma. *Plast Reconstr Surg, 55* (1):71-75, 1975.

CHAPTER SIX

Cryosurgery of Advanced and Difficult Cancers of the Skin

RICHARD F. ELTON, M.D.

THE DESTRUCTION of malignant tissue by freezing was established as a science more than a decade ago.[1-3] Cryosurgery now provides dermatologists and other physicians concerned with the treatment of skin cancer an alternative to surgical excision, electrodesiccation and curettage, chemosurgery, and irradiation. Zacarian has aptly demonstrated the destructive effects of subzero temperature on malignant cells and the vascular alterations which promote necrosis following freezing.[4,5] In many cases cryosurgery may be the treatment of choice for advanced or difficult skin cancers.

GENERAL CONSIDERATIONS

Basal cell epitheliomas (BCE) are the skin tumors with which the therapist will be most concerned, but squamous cell carcinomas may also be treated successfully with cryosurgery (Figure 6-1). The cryosurgical treatment of melanoma will not be discussed as the bulk of these tumors are probably best treated by excision.

Cryosurgery may be used alone or may be used in combination with electrodesiccation and curettage, excision, or chemosurgery. For large fungating tumors, cryosurgery may be preceded by electrodesiccation and curettage; this will thus enable the freezing to extend deeper into the tissue. This can also be advantageous when treating large penetrating BCEs of the face and trunk. Cryosurgery may also ei-

ther precede or follow surgical excision of skin cancer. When cryosurgery precedes excision, the tumor will have either been

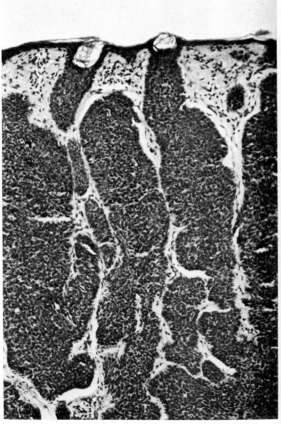

Figure 6-1. Typical histologic picture of nodular basal cell epithelioma showing masses and nests of small dark staining cells (basalioma cells) arranged in a mesodermal stroma. The peripheral cell layer of the tumor masses shows the characteristic palisading. ×150.

completely or nearly completely removed, making surgical excision of the lesion easier. Cryosurgery may follow excision in those cases in which the pathologist tells us that excision was not complete. However cryosurgery should not be considered an alternative to Mohs' chemosurgery. In many cases of tumors adjacent to or involving vital structures, there can be no alternative to Mohs' chemosurgery, although cryosurgery may be useful in some cases preceding chemosurgery for especially large tumors.

A skin cancer may be classified as advanced or difficult depending upon the area of the body involved, its histologic type, the size of the particular lesion, and whether or not it has been previously treated.[6]

AREA INVOLVED. The eyelids, nose, and ears each have their own particular problems and these areas can be particularly difficult to treat depending on the extent of involvement. For example, the tarsal plate can be easily damaged and ectropion can be the result of treating eyelid tumors with radical surgery. Zacarian feels that cryosurgery is the treatment of choice for basal cell epitheliomas of the eyelids.[7] Lesions on the ears and nose are difficult to treat, because damage to the cartilage often occurs with surgical excision, and radionecrosis of the cartilage may occur after X-ray therapy. With cryosurgery, damage to the cartilaginous structures is usually spared unless the cartilage itself has been invaded by tumor. The cosmetic result of treating tumors of these areas cryosurgically is often superior to other forms of treatment.

HISTOLOGIC TYPE. Sclerosing basal cell epitheliomas or those of the morphea type are well known to dermatologists to be extremely difficult to treat (Figure 6-2). This type of lesion is characterized by tumorous strands of basal cells embedded in a dense fibrous stroma (Figure 6-3). The borders of such a lesion are difficult to define and excision of such a lesion may leave nests of tumor at the edges of the lesion. These

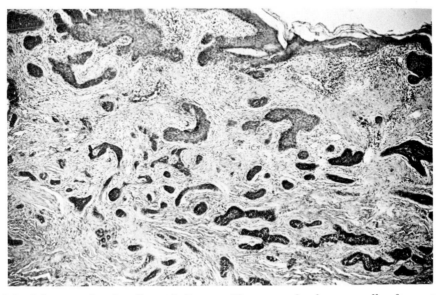

Figure 6-2. Sclerosing basal cell epithelioma showing small groups and thin cords of tumor cells embedded in a dense fibrous stroma. These strands of tumor cells often extend deep into the dermis. ×60

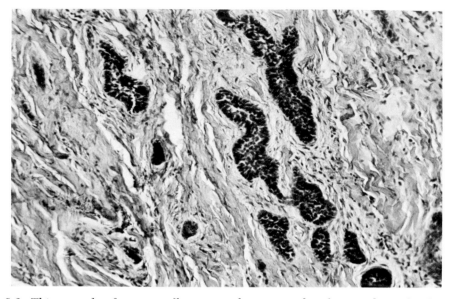

Figure 6-3. Thin strands of tumor cells as in this sclerotic BCE often extend deep into the dermis and far beyond the obvious margins of the tumor, therefore, making this lesion difficult to treat. These tumors must be frozen widely and deeply. ×150.

tumors also tend to be more radioresistant than other types and heretofore Mohs' chemosurgery has been one of the best forms of treatment. The author has found this type must be *vigorously* treated with a triple freeze of −35° to −40°C with a border of at least 1 cm.

SIZE. Cryosurgery offers an alternative treatment for large tumors of the face and trunk that one would not ordinarily want to excise or remove by electrodesiccation and curettage. We have arbitrarily chosen to classify tumors greater than 2 cm in diameter as advanced lesions. Zacarian noted in his classic monograph that, over an eight year period, 175 or 10.2 percent of the 1,720 skin cancers he had treated cryosurgically were greater than 2 cm in diameter.[8] Very large lesions may be treated cryosurgically either in one sitting or in some cases may be better treated in several stages. Mohs' chemosurgery may still be the treatment of choice for many of these le-

sions. Chemosurgery has proven to be very reliable with a 99 percent cure rate.[9]

RECURRENT LESIONS. It is well accepted by those who commonly treat skin cancer that the cure rate following therapy of a recurrent skin cancer is substantially lower than for lesions not previously treated. In the author's experience, skin cancer is much more likely to recur in the first two years following treatment. Dr. Zacarian also shares this experience.[10] Skin cancers, especially BCEs, which have been treated previously by electrodesiccation and curettage, excision, or irradiation but have recurred, often after several such treatments, respond well to cryosurgical therapy given an adequate margin and frozen vigorously.

TECHNIQUE. Whereas most simple basal cell epitheliomas respond well to a double freeze-thaw cycle frozen to −25°C, advanced and difficult BCEs will usually require a triple freeze-thaw cycle frozen to

−25° to −40°C. A double freeze-thaw cycle has been demonstrated to be more injurious to tissue than a single freeze-thaw cycle, while a triple freeze-thaw has been shown to be more destructive on tumor transplants than a double freeze-thaw.[11, 12] When the author initially began to treat large and difficult skin tumors cryosurgically, he was using a double freeze-thaw cycle at −20° to −25°C. He now feels that with a lower temperature and using a *triple* freeze-thaw cycle he is less likely to have recurrences and is less likely to have to repeat the cryosurgical procedure. Before any procedure is started, preoperative photographs should be taken. These will serve the dual purpose of legal documentation and a clinical record much better than any narrative. Photographs should also follow the healing in various stages and the final postoperative result should be similarly documented. Unless a biopsy was previously taken, a specimen should be taken from the lesion by means of a punch, curette, or incision and read by a competent dermatopathologist. The entire procedure from the initial freezing to the final healing should be explained to the patient as thoroughly as possible. This should preferably be done in advance of the actual procedure so that the patient will have time to formulate his own specific questions. The patient is usually told that the only pain he will feel is from the Xylocaine® at the point of insertion of the thermocouple needles and a burning pain at the beginning of the cryosurgical procedure and for up to two hours following the procedure. Some patients will develop a headache following treatment of lesions on the temple and forehead. Thus far, it has not been necessary to give a single patient an analgesic because of pain. Following cryosurgery, swelling can be expected in the operative area from a minimal

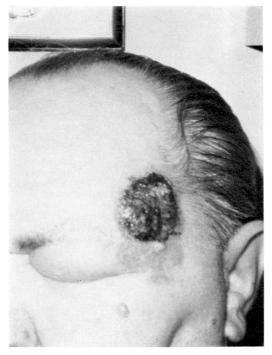

Figure 6-4. Postoperative cryosurgical patient demonstrating swelling around the eye which routinely occurs following freezing in this area. Note that the left eye is completely swollen shut following cryosurgery of a BCE of the left temple.

amount to very substantial swelling which may close one or both eyes (Figure 6-4). This swelling may persist from a few days to a few weeks. A large bulla frequently forms over the cryosurgical site. At times this bulla may be hemorrhagic and quite disturbing in appearance (Figure 6-5). Drainage of a serous to serosanguinous discharge will begin from the cryosurgical site in one to two days. Although hemorrhage is a frequent complication following cryosurgery of the oral cavity, it rarely happens following cryosurgery of the skin.[13] Large arteries appear to be resistant to freezing injury.[14] Necrotic material which at times exudes from the wound must not be confused with infection. Al-

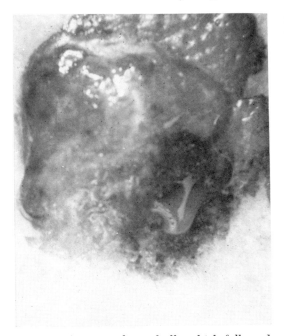

Figure 6-5. Hemorrhagic bulla which followed by one day the freezing of a BCE. Appearance, unless expected by the patient, could be quite disturbing.

though a possibility, infection following cryosurgery for skin cancer is probably a very rare finding. Drainage will persist until a firm crust has formed over the area— usually in two to four weeks. The area should be covered only by a loose gauze dressing and antibiotic ointments should not be used over the wound. After crust formation, final healing time will vary widely from a few weeks to a few months depending on the area frozen.

Although local anesthesia is not routinely used, local Xylocaine has been injected into the area of the tumor in a few very sensitive individuals. When this is done the freezing time appears to be shorter and the thaw period is prolonged, due probably to ice crystal formation and vasoconstriction of the microvessels in the area. This does not seem to have affected the postoperative

result and local anesthesia is not routinely used.

Cryosurgery of malignant tumors may be accomplished either using a cryoprobe or by the direct application of liquid nitrogen spray. Torre pioneered the first liquid nitrogen spray unit in 1965, and was one of the pioneers in its use for a variety of lesions.[15, 16] The author has been routinely using the C-21® spray unit made by Frigitronics for most work. This self-pressurizing unit has a capacity of about 250 cc and allows for continual spraying for roughly five minutes. The author employs two of these units and, although the five minute spray is adequate for most work, both units have been used several times. The area to be treated should first be marked with a skin marking pen, for in many lesions the outlines are blurred once freezing has started. Thermocouple needles should next be inserted into the predetermined areas (Figure 6-6).

Although the patient may be treated in a prone position, in general it is much easier to have the patient seated, especially for facial lesions. This enables the head to be moved to any desired position. The needle must be inserted from outside the marked area in a subcutaneous position below the tumor. Caution should be used so that the needle itself is not sprayed, resulting in a false temperature. Spraying of the area is then started. Spraying of the tumor should be done on an intermittent basis. When continual spraying is done in one area, the ice front tends to spread laterally without being deep enough. Spraying on an intermittent basis allows one to get adequate depth both in the center and laterally as measured by the thermocouple needle. The necessary thermal gradient is extremely important in achieving an adequate temperature in malignant tumors.[17] One should *always* measure the temperature of each skin cancer treated except in those areas where the tumor is quite shallow and overlying bone or cartilage. In those cases the tissue must be frozen through the cartilage to the other side or must be frozen until adherent to the underlying bone. Even though with experience one can often sense the adequacy of the freeze, one should not depend on this sense when treating a larger skin cancer. After complete thaw of the frozen area, this procedure should be repeated two more times. As previously mentioned a triple freeze-thaw cycle of $-35°$ to $-40°C$ is advised for advanced and difficult skin cancer. Postoperatively, the author tries to see all patients one day, three days, and one week following the procedure. In some cases the patient may be seen either more or less often the first week. After this the patient is seen at weekly intervals and then at biweekly intervals until the crust has fallen off. The patient is checked at three months and then at six month intervals. Very large skin cancers may need to be treated in stages. Much will depend on the size and location of the tumor in addition to the tolerance of the patient. After complete healing has taken place, it is often wise to rebiopsy the postoperative site at about six months. This is especially true in large lesions and for sclerotic BCEs. In some cases more than one area will need to be biopsied, especially at the periphery of the postoperative site where most tumors recur. One should not confuse pseudoepitheliomatous hyperplasia, which occurs very often following cryosurgery, with a recurrence. This phenomenon disappears within a very few months while a recurrence obviously will continue to enlarge. Formation of a pyogenic granuloma at the site of cryosurgery for a BCE has been re-

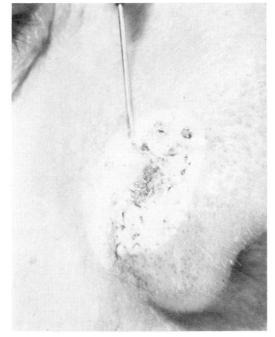

Figure 6-6. Thermocouple needle in place during cryosurgery for a BCE of the right ala nasi.

ported.[18] Milia formation which may persist for several weeks is also seen often at the postoperative site. In the event of a recurrence, cryosurgery may have to be repeated. This should not discourage you anymore than a recurrence following electrodesiccation and curettage. If there is doubt in your mind concerning the ability of cryosurgery to control the tumor, the patient should be referred for additional treatment such as Mohs' chemosurgery.

One of the advantages of cryosurgery is the excellent scar formation and good cosmetic postoperative result which usually occurs. Occasionally one will get some hypertrophic or contracted scar formation; this is most likely to occur following a very deep freeze (Figure 6-7). This needs to be corrected by a plastic surgeon only in an extremely small percentage of cases. There

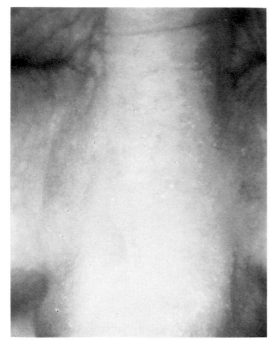

Figure 6-7. Superficially contracted scar of the nose following a deep freeze for a BCE. Although probably not necessary in this case, contracted scars following cryosurgery can be surgically revised if disfiguring.

are certain areas of the body which do not respond well to cryosurgical treatment. The scalp is very vascular and does not freeze well; recurrences can be expected in this area and cryosurgery should probably not be used. Lesions of the extremities may be very slow to heal, especially those on the legs when there is some compromise in circulation. Lesions of the lower legs may take as long as one year to heal, so it is best, if possible, to avoid cryosurgery for skin cancer in these areas.

Cryosurgery may not always be a curative procedure. As stated before it may be combined with other forms of treatment in especially large skin cancers. Andrew Gage reported a patient in whom cryosurgery was used following excision for squamous cell carcinoma of the ear canal with

apparently good results.[19] Cryotherapy, which has been used as a palliative measure in the treatment of other cancers, is also a useful tool for the palliative treatment of skin cancer, especially in the very old or the debilitated person in whom it is not wise to use a routine surgical procedure and in whom it is wise to treat the tumor because of discomfort in the area involved.[20, 21] Thus cryosurgery appears to be a useful modality for skin cancer treatment in several aspects, both as a curative procedure for advanced or difficult cancers and as an adjuvant treatment either combined with another form of therapy or as a palliative procedure.

CANCER OF THE NOSE

The cryosurgical removal of large skin cancers of the nose presents its own set of problems. Cryosurgery lends itself especially well to larger lesions in this area because it usually produces less distortion than other techniques. Because much of the nose is predominantly cartilaginous, the final outcome of the surgery will essentially depend upon how much of the cartilage has been eroded by the skin cancer. Cartilage that is not involved with tumor can be expected to survive cryosurgical destruction. The remainder of the cosmetic result will depend upon the distortion produced by the contraction of scar tissue in the area. Shallow subcutaneous tissue on the nose does not allow as much flexibility of the final scar as on other areas of the face with the exception of the ears.

As in most other areas of the face, it is suggested that a triple freeze-thaw cycle be used. The tissue should be frozen to $-30°$ to $-40°C$. The placement of the thermocouple needles is very important and the finger should be placed inside the nostril to enable one to more accurately place the needle. Tumors which involve the skin over the bony surface of the nose should have their needles placed in a subcutaneous position. Tumors over or involving the cartilaginous areas should have the needles placed in the cartilaginous tissue, guided by the finger inside the nose. In large lesions a second needle should be placed at the periphery of the tumor. During the initial freeze a finger placed inside the nose will help determine if the depth of the freeze is adequate. Freezing should extend throughout. The thaw time will vary, depending upon the vascularity of the nose. In general it can be said that those persons having a rosacea picture on the nose will have a faster thaw time and may have to be frozen for a longer period of time. In addition, patients having this rosacea picture can be expected to heal more quickly after cryosurgery.

As previously indicated, the cosmetic result will depend upon the size of the tumor as well as on scar formation and cartilage involvement. Several cartilaginous defects may occur. When the tumor has invaded the cartilage along the margin of the nostril, notching or irregularity of the nostril margin can be expected for a final result. Although the author has not yet experienced this, perforation of the nose would seem a distinct possibility in selected cases. If this possibility is entertained before surgery, the patient should be so informed and it should be explained that plastic surgery might be necessary after the cryosurgical procedure. Although more likely to occur on the ear, bare cartilage may be exposed on the nose. If this occurs, an additional surgical procedure will be necessary to correct this.

In addition to physical defects which may persist after cryosurgery to the nose, a persistent crust and a feeling of tender-

ness inside the nose on the involved side may persist for several months. Physical inspection of the nasal mucous membrane will reveal a moderate erythema surrounding scar formation.

A special reference must be made about tumors involving the ala nasi and the nasolabial folds. Tumors in this area have a very high recurrence rate and lesions in this area can be expected to recur after cryosurgery. To minimize this, the thermocouple needle should be placed quite deep and a wide margin of tissue should be frozen around the original tumor.

Case 1

A forty-three-year-old white female gave a history of having had a skin cancer of the left nasolabial fold removed three times previously by electrodesiccation and curettage. This tumor measured about 2

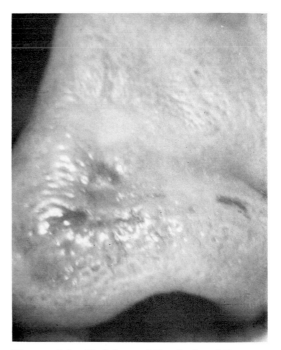

Figure 6-8. Nodular BCE of the left nose measuring 2 cm in diameter. Extent of penetration is sometimes difficult to determine.

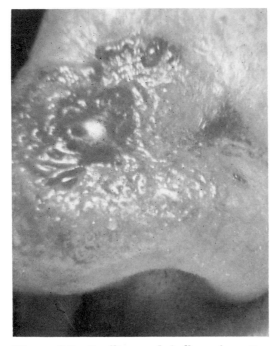

Figure 6-9. Swelling and bullous formation occurring one day following a double freeze of a BCE of the left nose.

cm in diameter (Plate 90). Biopsy revealed a sclerotic basal cell epithelioma. This tumor was treated with a double freeze-thaw cycle frozen to −20°C. Plate 91 shows the lesion three days postoperative with blister formation while Plate 92 shows crust formation present at the end of two weeks. Plate 93 shows the smooth scar six weeks following cryosurgery. This is one of the author's earlier cases using only a double freeze-thaw. There has been no recurrence four years following the treatment.

Case 2

Over a period of three to four years a seventy-eight-year-old white male developed a large 1.5 cm penetrating basal cell epithelioma of the left side of the nose. This lesion was ulcerated and showed evidence of deep penetration and cartilage involvement (Plate 94). This lesion was

treated with a triple freeze-thaw cycle and frozen to −30°C. One week following the freeze, the edge of the nose was already notched and the tumor mass was very necrotic (Plate 95). Plate 96 shows a good postoperative scar but with obvious notching of the cartilage indicating previous tumor involvement.

Case 3

A sixty-six-year-old white male presented a large nodular biopsy-proven basal cell epithelioma of the left side of the nose. This lesion measured just under 2 cm in diameter (Figure 6-8). The tumor was treated with a double freeze-thaw cycle frozen to −20°C. Figure 6-9 illustrates the area one day after freezing while Figure 6-10 demonstrates *pseudoepitheliomatous* hyperplasia of the lesion five weeks fol-

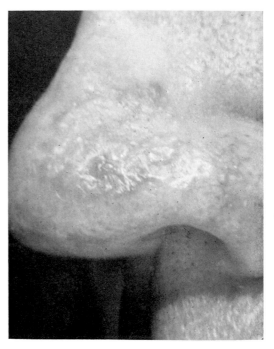

Figure 6-10. Pseudoepitheliomatous hyperplasia five weeks following cryosurgery of a BCE of the left nose. This should not be confused with a recurrence.

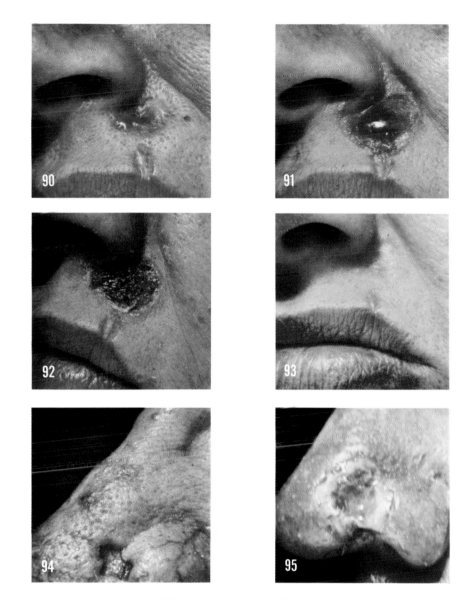

Plate 90.* Recurrent sclerotic BCE of the left nasolabial area had been removed three times previously by electrodesiccation and curettage.

Plate 91. Sclerotic BCE 3 days after cryosurgery to the area.

Plate 92. Drainage has stopped and a crust has appeared over the area frozen two weeks previously for a sclerotic BCE.

Plate 93.* Good postoperative scar formation six weeks following cryosurgery of a sclerotic BCE of the left ala nasi.

Plate 94.* Deep penetrating BCE of the left nose measuring 1.5C. Although not evident from the photograph, evidence of cartilage involvement was present on physical examination.

Plate 95. Necrotic tumor mass one week following cryosurgery. Notching of the edge of the nose was evident very early in the postoperative course.

*From R. F. Elton, Cryosurgery of difficult basal cell epitheliomas, *Cutis, 16*:475-476, Sept. 1975. Courtesy of Yorke Medical Journals, Dun Donnelley Publishing Corp.

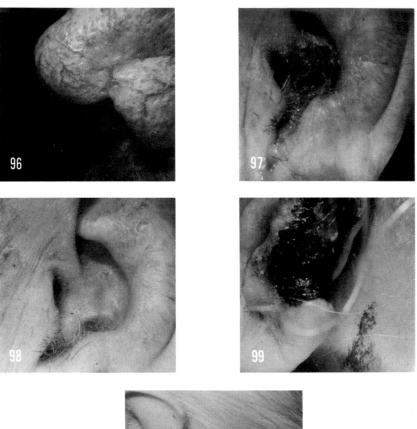

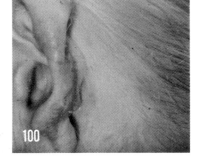

Plate 96. Good postoperative scar formation but with dramatic notching of the left side of the nose seven weeks following cryosurgery of a deep destructive BCE. From R. F. Elton, Cryosurgery of difficult basal cell epitheliomas, *Cutis, 16*:475, September 1975. Courtesy of Yorke Medical Journals, Dun Donnelley Publishing Corp.

Plate 97. BCE's of the ear canal such as in this eighty-one-year-old white male may present difficult therapeutic problems.

Plate 98. Following a triple freeze of the ear canal tumor, a good postoperative scar resulted. Freezing in the area is often very painful.

Plate 99. Dramatic erosion of the cartilage is evident in this large BCE involving over one half of the entire left ear.

Plate 100. Cryosurgery prevented further destruction of the left ear in this eighty-one-year-old white female. A triple freeze was used in treating this lesion.

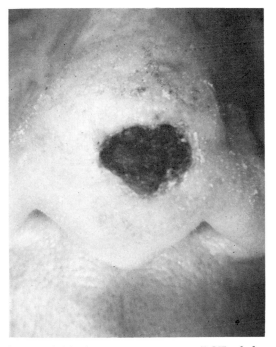

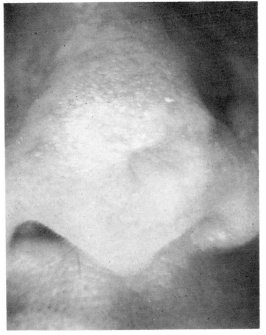

Figure 6-11. An erosive recurrent BCE of the tip of the nose in a seventy-three-year-old white female. A triple freeze was used to treat this lesion.

Figure 6-12. Eight weeks following cryosurgery, a very acceptable hypopigmented scar of the tip of the nose was evident.

lowing the initial freeze. This is a temporary condition and should not be confused with a recurrence.

Case 4

A seventy-three-year-old white female presented a 1.8 cm erosive BCE of the tip of the nose which had been treated previously by electrodesiccation and curettage (Figure 6-11). The tumor was frozen to $-40°C$ using a triple freeze-thaw cycle. Figure 6-12 reveals a good postoperative scar with minimal scar contracture.

CANCER OF THE EAR

Whereas cartilaginous defects following cryosurgery to the nose are unusual, defects appear to occur more often following cryosurgery to large skin cancers of the ear. These defects usually appear as irregular shapes on the ear margin. Just as exposed areas of cartilage may occur on the nose, these also occur more frequently on the ear. Thus it is very important to advise a patient about to have cryosurgery on the ear that a possible defect may occur, and in the case of more advanced skin cancers of the ear, that a defect will probably occur. It is the author's experience that patients are more sensitive about a defect on the ear than on the nose; this is especially true of male patients. Patients who have been advised ahead of time of the probability of having a defect of the ear are usually well satisfied with the cosmetic result. When one is speaking of very large tumors of the ear, the alternative of having part of an ear is better than having none.

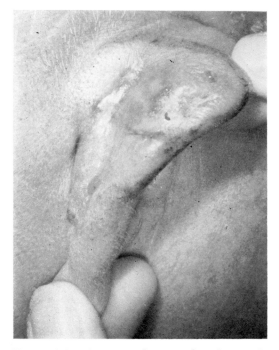

Figure 6-13. A sixty-eight-year-old white male with tumorous involvement of the entire upper half of the right ear.

As with lesions of the ala nasi, large tumors of the ear appear to recur more frequently than tumors on other areas of the face. Thus it is important that both proper technique and adequate freezing be done in such lesions. Thermocouple needles should be placed in several areas if the entire tumor is to be frozen at one sitting. The needles should be placed deep in the cartilaginous tissue and at the margin of the tumor. A triple freeze-thaw cycle frozen to −30° to −40°C should be used. When adequate freezing of the pinna has been accomplished, the ear will be frozen throughout. In other words, freezing throughout should be a normal procedure when dealing with large tumors of the pinna. Freezing in or near the external auditory canal can be extremely painful and in this case local anesthesia may be de-

sirable. Lesions which appear to have eroded deeply into the auditory canal might better be treated by a combination of cryosurgery and Mohs' chemosurgery or in many cases by Mohs' chemosurgery alone. When spraying the ear canal, one should protect the ear drum from sudden exposure to liquid nitrogen. Although not reported from liquid nitrogen, sudden exposure of the ear drum to extreme cold could produce sudden death.

Tumors about the ear which are frozen very deeply may result in facial nerve paralysis. Regeneration of nerve tissue thus frozen can be expected to occur.[22, 23]

One last point to remember is that healing of the external ear may be very slow and it is not unusual for such a lesion to take three to four months to completely

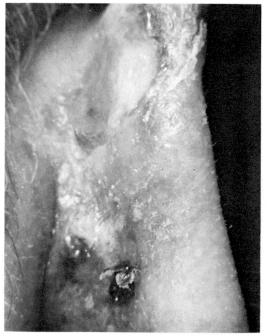

Figure 6-14. One day following cryosurgery, the upper half of the right ear appeared raw and exudative. Bare cartilage can be seen in the upper portion of the ear.

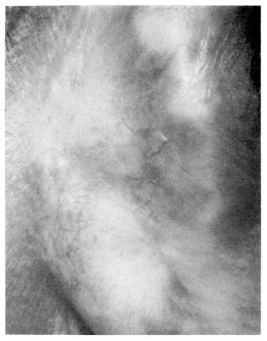

Figure 6-15. Six months following cryosurgery, a good postoperative scar is present. The area over the bare cartilage has epithelialized.

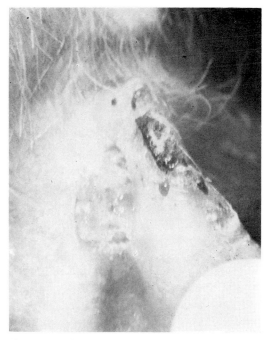

Figure 6-17. Posterior view showing extensive tumor involvement.

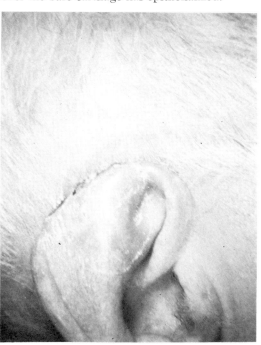

Figure 6-16. This very large erosive BCE which had been treated previously by X-ray has destroyed the upper third of the right ear.

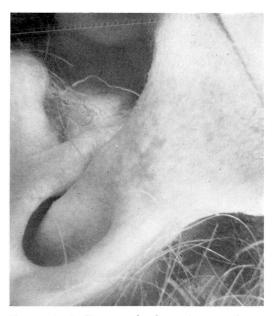

Figure 6-18. Despite the loss of a significant portion of the upper half of the right ear, the patient was satisfied with the final postoperative result.

heal. Patients should be advised of this before the cryosurgical procedure so that undue concern about healing does not lead
to needless anxiety.

Case 1

A sixty-eight-year-old white male with
tumorous involvement of the entire upper
half of the right ear was seen with a biopsy-proven sclerotic basal cell epithelioma
(Figure 6-13). This tumor was treated
with a double freeze-thaw cycle frozen to
−30°C. Figure 6-14 shows the area one day
after cryosurgery. Figure 6-15 shows the
area six months after the initial freeze.
This lesion recurred and it was necessary
to freeze the margins of the tumor two
more times.

Case 2

An eighty-four-year-old white male presented a large erosive basal cell epithelioma involving the upper third of the right
ear with additional involvement behind
the ear. This lesion had been previously
treated with X-ray. A double freeze to
−20°C was performed. Figure 6-16 and 6-17
show the extensive involvement, while Fig-

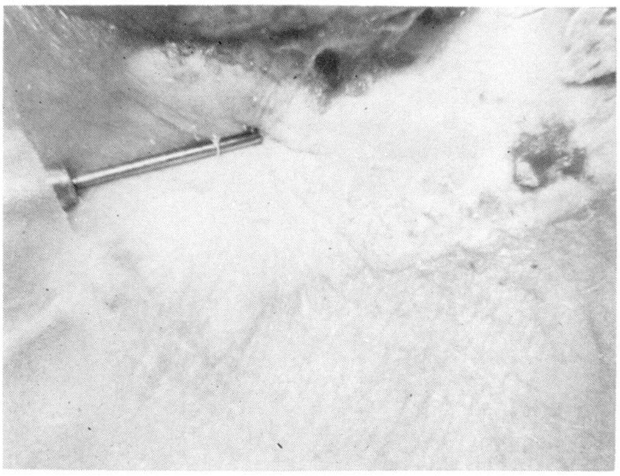

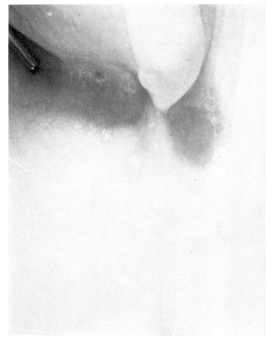

Figure 6-20. Thermocouple needle in place
during a triple freeze of the 2.3 cm tumor.

ure 6-18 demonstrates the area six months
following cryosurgery.

Case 3

An eighty-seven-year-old white female
gave a history of having a large 2.3 cm

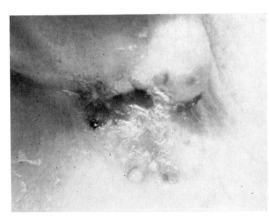

Figure 6-19. BCE involving the right ear lobe
and adjoining area which had previously been
treated several times by electrodesiccation and
curettage.

Figure 6-21. Good postoperative scar eight
weeks following cryosurgery of the right ear
lobe. This tumor recurred two years after
cryosurgery.

basal cell epithelioma of the right earlobe and adjoining area treated several times previously by electrodesiccation and curettage. This lesion was painful and frequently bled. Figure 6-19 shows the extensive involvement. Figure 6-20 shows the thermocouple needle in place after a triple freeze-thaw cycle to −40°C. Figure 6-21 indicates a good postoperative result, but the tumor did recur two years later. No further treatment was done due to the patient's age and deteriorating physical condition.

Case 4

An eighty-one-year-old white male presented a 1.8 cm basal cell epithelioma involving the left ear canal. This lesion had not previously been treated. He had several other large skin cancers of the face which had previously been treated cryosurgically. Plate 97 shows the tumor on the edge of the ear canal, while Plate 98 shows the result six weeks following the surgery.

Case 5

An eighty-one-year-old white female presented a huge basal cell epithelioma involving over one half of the entire left pinna. Much of the ear tissue had already been eroded away by the tumor. A triple freeze-thaw cycle to −30°C was done to the entire tumor at a single sitting. Plates 99 and 100 show the pre- and postoperative results. The tumor recurred on one margin a year later and cryosurgery was repeated.

Case 6

A sixty-nine-year-old white male with a basal cell epithelioma involving the entire left posterior ear had been aware of the

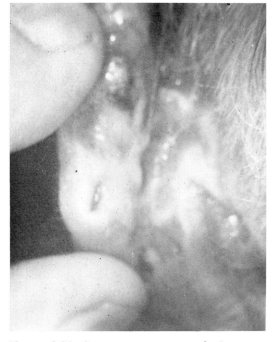

Figure 6-22. Over a ten year period, this BCE had involved the entire left posterior ear. Fear of loosing his ear prevented this man from seeking treatment.

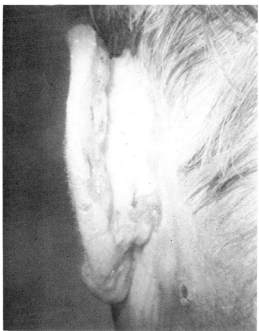

Figure 6-23. Much necrotic tissue was evident three days following cryosurgical treatment of this advanced BCE.

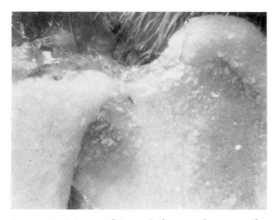

Figure 6-24. Notching of the cartilage on the superior portion of the pinna followed cryosurgical destruction of the BCE.

tumor for more than ten years before seeking treatment. Figure 6-22 shows the tumor before freezing, while Figure 6-23 shows the area three days following a triple freeze to −40°C. Figures 6-24 and 6-25 demonstrate the notching of the carti-

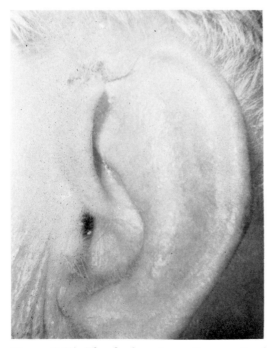

Figure 6-25. The final postoperative result of this huge BCE was cosmetically acceptable.

lage which occurred after the freezing. This tumor recurred at the margin and required two more treatments.

CANCER OF THE EYELID

Although skin cancer involving the eyelid does not constitute a very large percentage of cancers of the face, these cancers are among the most difficult to treat. Zacarian has studied these tumors thoroughly and has become an expert in their cryosurgical therapy.[4] Although most of these tumors will involve the inner canthus and lower eyelid, the upper eyelid is much more difficult to treat. Basal cell epitheliomas will be the tumors most often seen and treated in these areas.[24] It is wise in very large lesions of the inner canthus to obtain sinus X rays in order to rule out invasion of the underlying bone. Cryosurgery appears to have a distinct advantage in treating skin cancer of the eyelids, for not only does it avoid destructive surgery, especially in the aged, but unless the cancer has invaded the tarsal plate of the upper lid or the nasolacrimal duct, it appears to spare these structures.

The author also uses a triple freeze-thaw cycle for skin cancer in this area but the freeze time is usually quite short for lesions of the upper eyelid due to the thinness of the skin in this area. For lesions of the upper eyelid and lower lid margin it is necessary to retract the lid away from the globe. After insertion of the thermocouple needle subcutaneously, Pontocaine is dropped into the eye to topically anesthetize the conjunctiva. The eyelid is pulled away from the globe using a chalazion forcep and the globe can be protected from liquid nitrogen spray using a portion of a styrofoam cup cut to the necessary size and shape. Postoperatively the patient can expect a great deal of swelling with the eye usually swollen shut for sev-

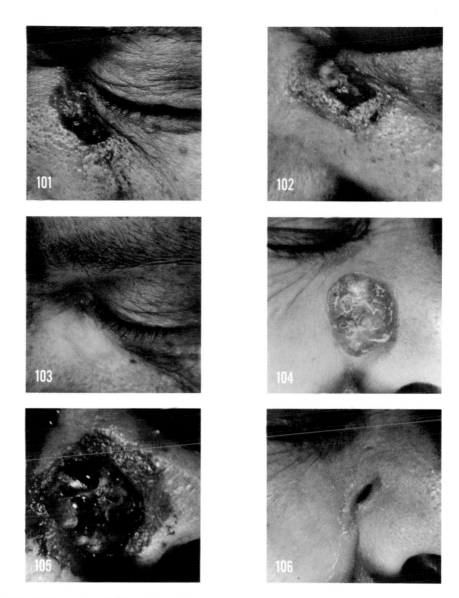

Plate 101. This erosive BCE of the left inner canthus was slightly greater than 2C in diameter. From R. F. Elton, Cryosurgery of difficult basal cell epitheliomas, *Cutis, 16*:475, September 1975. Courtesy of Yorke Medical Journals, Dun Donnelley Publishing Corp.

Plate 102. Much swelling can be expected following cryosurgery about the eye as in this illustration. Tearing may occur for several days secondary to the swelling which compresses the nasolacrimal duct.

Plate 103. Postoperative scar four years following cryosurgery of the tumor of the left inner canthus.

Plate 104. Very large nodular deeply penetrating BCE of the right cheek and adjacent nose.

Plate 105. One day after freezing a large hemorrhagic bulla is present with an even wider area of tissue reaction. The patient was experiencing no pain in spite of the appearance.

Plate 106. A deep hole was the final cryosurgical result. This area was excised but the tumor had eroded so deeply that the patient was referred for Mohs' chemosurgery.

eral days. It is extremely important that the patient be made aware that the severe swelling will persist for several days to allay the almost certain apprehension that occurs from any procedure done about the eyes. Postoperative healing in this area is no different and follows the outlined pattern. In large tumors of the lower lid, contraction of the scar produces the possibility of ectropion. This has been a rare occurrence in the author's practice.

Case 1

A fifty-one-year-old white male presented a 2.2 cm basal cell epithelioma of the left inner canthus and lower eyelid (Plate 101). Plate 102 shows the area one day following a double freeze and Plate 103 indicates the postoperative result two months later.

CANCER OF OTHER AREAS OF THE FACE AND THE TRUNK

There are few special problems in treating lesions on other areas of the face. Skin cancer of the lips will respond to cryosurgical treatment but does need to be vigorously frozen because of the vascularity of this tissue. Much swelling of the lips can be expected postoperatively. Lesions of the mid forehead often result in tremendous postoperative swelling with both eyes being swollen shut at times.

Hypopigmentation in the postoperative area of cryosurgery is a very common finding in the author's experience. This hypopigmentation may be temporary, but at times has been a permanent finding. Alopecia occurs often in the area of deep cryosurgery. This is an expected postoperative finding after the freezing of large or deep skin cancers of the face. This author has one case where there is a permanent alopecia of one half of the eyebrow following treatment for a large basal cell epithelioma in that area.

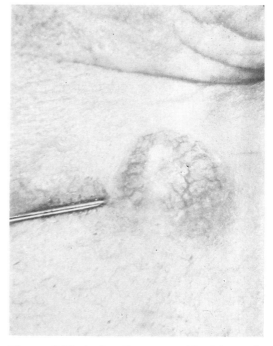

Figure 6-26. A sixty-three-year-old white male with an adenoid BCE of the right upper cheek. The thermocouple needle is situated subcutaneously.

Cryosurgery offers a useful approach for treating multiple skin cancers of the face and trunk at a single sitting. Although not considered different or advanced in their nature, multiple basal cell epitheliomas may be treated successfully in this manner with a minimal amount of scarring and time lost from work.

Case 1

A sixty-three-year-old white male presented a 2.0 cm adenoid basal cell epithelioma of the right upper cheek. Figure 6-26 shows the tumor with thermocouple needle in place before freezing. Figure 6-27 demonstrates the tremendous tissue reaction still present one week after freezing, while Figure 6-28 shows the very acceptable postoperative scar two months after freezing.

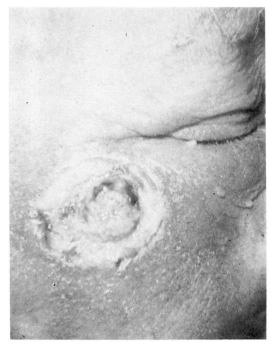

Figure 6-27. Tremendous swelling and tissue reaction still present one week after freezing.

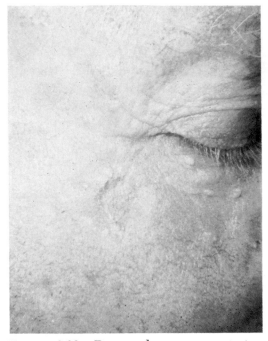

Figure 6-28. Depressed scar present two months following cryosurgery of an adenoid BCE.

Case 2

A fifty-nine-year-old white female presented a 3.0 cm basal cell epithelioma of the right cheek and adjacent nose (Plate 104). This tumor was treated with a triple freeze to −40°C. Plate 105 shows the area one day postoperative. The patient was left with a deep hole lateral to the nose (Plate 106). This area was excised deeply but there was still tumor penetrating to the margin of the excision and the patient was then referred for Mohs' chemosurgery.

Case 3

A forty-four-year-old white male with a sclerotic basal cell epithelioma, 2.8 cm in diameter, anterior to the left ear, was treated with a triple freeze to −30°C. Figure 6-29 shows the preoperative area, while Figure 6-30 demonstrates the area two days after cryosurgery. Figure 6-31 shows the area two and one-half months following the

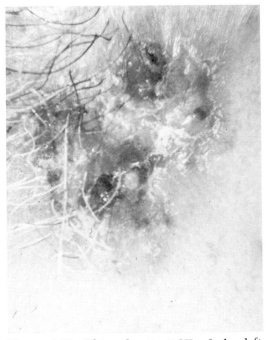

Figure 6-29. This sclerotic BCE of the left temple was treated by means of a triple freeze to −30°C.

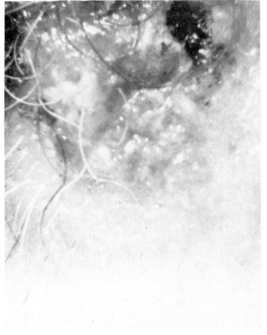

Figure 6-30. Two days following cryosurgery, much necrotic material was present over the surface of the tumor.

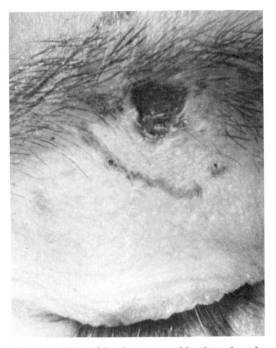

Figure 6-32. A fifty-four-year-old white female with an erosive BCE of the right eyebrow. The area to be frozen has been outlined by a skin marker.

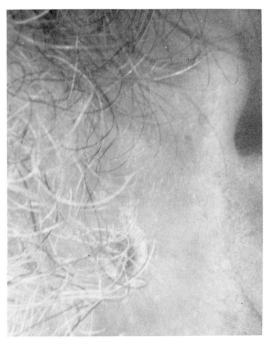

Figure 6-31. Two and one-half months following cryosurgery the area appeared well healed but the tumor had to be re-treated because of a recurrence at both upper and lower poles.

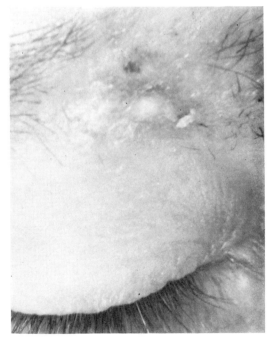

Figure 6-33. Permanent alopecia of the eyebrow resulted following cryosurgery.

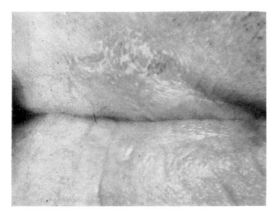

Figure 6-34. This recurrent BCE of the left upper lip had been treated twice previously by electrodesiccation and curettage.

initial freeze. This tumor recurred at both the upper and lower poles and had to be re-treated.

Case 4

A fifty-four-year-old white female presented a 1.5 cm erosive basal cell epithelioma of the right eyebrow which was treated with a triple freeze to −40°C. Figure 6-32 demonstrates the area outlined for freezing by a skin marker, while Figure 6-33 shows the alopecia occurring as part of the postoperative result.

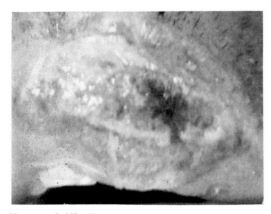

Figure 6-35. Dramatic tissue reaction often follows freezing of the lip as seen four days after cryosurgery.

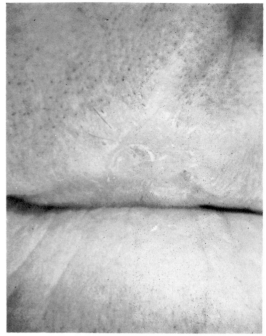

Figure 6-36. Only a small crust remained six weeks following cryosurgery of a BCE of the upper lip.

Case 5

A fifty-two-year-old white male presented a recurrent basal cell epithelioma of the left upper lip approximately 2.0 cm in length (Figure 6-34). This lesion had been removed twice previously by electrodesiccation and curettage. The area was treated with a double freeze to −30°C and Figure 6-35 shows the area four days postoperative. Six weeks after the initial freeze, the area was nearly completely healed (Figure 6-36).

ANALYSIS OF TREATED CASES

Zacarian recently reported that he had cryosurgically treated 2,193 carcinomas in the past ten years with a recurrence rate of 2 percent.[25] The author has treated ninety-five advanced and/or difficult skin cancers as previously defined and followed them

TABLE 6-I

CLASSIFICATION BY SITE OF 95 DIFFICULT
CUTANEOUS MALIGNANCIES TREATED
CRYOSURGICALLY BETWEEN 1971-1974

Site	1971-72	1973	1974
Nose	6	11	10
Ear	4	3	6
Eyelid	2	4	3
Face	11	16	12
Neck and trunk	3	1	3
TOTAL	26	35	34

over a three and one-half year period
from 1971 to 1974. These lesions were at
least 2 cm in size or were located in a difficult area to treat. Table 6-I classifies these
lesions by site. Thirty-seven, or 38.9 percent, of these ninety-five lesions were recurrent, i.e. treated previously by means
other than cryosurgery. Table 6-II classifies
these ninety-five lesions by histologic type.

After initial cryosurgical treatment of
these ninety-five lesions, eighteen or 19
percent recurred. Of these eighteen recurrences, seven were from the original
group of thirty-seven recurrent skin cancers. Four lesions were subsequently treated by Mohs' chemosurgery; the remaining
fourteen were successfully treated by repeat cryosurgery or surgical removal of the
remaining malignancy. Table 6-III classifies these recurring lesions as to site and
histologic type.

Most of the early tumors were treated

TABLE 6-II

CLASSIFICATION BY HISTOLOGIC TYPE
OF 95 DIFFICULT CUTANEOUS
MALIGNANCIES TREATED
CRYOSURGICALLY

Type	1971-72	1973	1974
Nodular BCE	21	33	31
Sclerotic BCE	4	2	2
Squamous cell	1	0	1
TOTAL	26	35	34

TABLE 6-III

CRYOSURGICALLY TREATED RECURRENT
SKIN CANCERS CLASSIFIED BY SITE
AND HISTOLOGIC TYPE

	1971-72	1973	1974	Total
Site				
Nose	1	3	1	5
Ear	2	1	3	6
Eyelid	0	0	1	1
Face	3	2	1	6
Neck and trunk	0	0	0	0
Type				
Nodular BCE	3	5	6	14
Sclerotic BCE	3	1	0	4

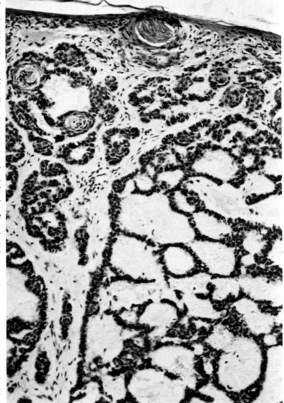

Figure 6-37. Basal cell epithelioma of the
adenoid type showing the characteristic mucin
filled spaces surrounded by dark staining epithelial cells. ×150.

with a double freeze-thaw cycle but later tumors were treated with a triple freeze-thaw cycle. The author felt more secure in doing this as he tended to treat larger and more difficult tumors.

One of his recent observations is that the adenoid type of basal cell epithelioma may be more resistant to cryosurgical destruction than the nodular type. This tumor characteristically shows cells arranged somewhat regularly around numerous small mucin-filled spaces. The adenoid appearance is due to accumulation of mucin between epithelial cells[26] (Figure 6-37). This tumor tends to behave more like the sclerosing type of BCE.

Cryosurgery is still a relatively new tool and definite parameters of treatment are still not completely established. It is hoped that as more physicians use this technique, we will be able to establish more definite guidelines for the treatment of skin cancer.

BIBLIOGRAPHY

1. Cooper, I.: Cryogenic surgery. A new method of destruction or extirpation of benign or malignant tissues. *N Engl J Med, 268*:743, 1963.
2. Cooper, I.: Cryogenic surgery for cancer. *Fed Proc, 24*:S237, 1965.
3. Gage, A. A. and Emmings, F.: Treatment of human tumors by freezing. *Cryobiology, 2*:14, 1965.
4. Zacarian, S. A.: *Cryosurgery of Tumors of the Skin and Oral Cavity.* Springfield, Thomas, 1973.
5. Zacarian, S. A., Stone, D. and Clater, M.: Effects of cryogenic temperatures on microcirculation in the golden hamster cheek pouch. *Cryobiology, 7*:27, 1970.
6. Elton, R. F.: Cryosurgery of difficult basal cell epitheliomas. *Cutis, 16*:474, 1975.
7. Zacarian, S. A.: Cancer of the eyelid. A cryosurgical approach. *Ann Ophthalmol, 4*:473, 1972.
8. Zacarian, S. A.: *Cryosurgery of Tumors of the Skin and Oral Cavity.* Springfield, Thomas, 1973, p. 231.
9. Mohs, E. E.: Chemosurgery for the microscopically controlled excision of skin cancer. *Medical Tribune, 15:* March 31, 1969.
10. Zacarian, S. A.: Personal communication.
11. Gage, A. A. et al.: Cryotherapy for cancer of the lip and oral cavity. *Cancer, 18:* 1646, 1965.
12. Myers, R. S. et al.: Cryosurgery of experimental tumors. *J Cryosurgery, 2*:225, 1969.
13. Gage, A. A.: Cryosurgery for tumors of the oral cavity. In Zacarian, S. A.: *Cryosurgery of Tumors of the Skin and Oral Cavity.* Springfield, Thomas, 1973, p. 268.
14. Cooper, I., Samra, K. and Wisniewska, K.: Effects of freezing on major arteries. *Stroke, 2*:471, 1971.
15. Torre, D.: New York: Cradle of cryosurgery. *N Y State J Med, 67*:465, 1967.
16. Torre, D.: Cutaneous cryosurgery. *J Cryosurgery, 1*:202, 1968.
17. Smith, J. J. and Fraser, J.: An estimation of tissue damage and thermal history in the cryolesion. *Cryobiology, 11*:137, 1974.
18. Greer, K. E. and Bishop, G. F.: Pyogenic granuloma as a complication of cryosurgery. *Arch Dermatol, 111*:1536, 1975.
19. Gage, A. A.: Cryosurgery for difficult problems in cutaneous cancer. *Cutis, 16*:465, 1975.
20. Gage, A. A.: Cryotherapy for inoperable cancer. *Dis Colon and Rectum, 2*:36, 1968.
21. Beggs, J. H.: Cryotherapy as a palliative maneuver. *JAMA, 206*:1570, 1968.
22. Gaster, R., Davidson, T., Rand, R. and Fonkalsrund, E.: Comparison of nerve regeneration rates following controlled freezing or crushing. *Arch Surg, 103:* 378, 1971.
23. Carter, D., Lee, P., Gill, W. and Johnston, R.: The effect of cryosurgery on peripheral nerve function. *J R Coll Surg, 17*:25, 1972.
24. Shulman, J.: Treatment of malignant tumors of the eyelids by plastic surgery. *Br J Plast Surg, 15*:37, 1961.
25. Zacarian, S. A.: Cryosurgery of skin cancer: Fundamentals of technique and application. *Cutis, 16*:449, 1975.
26. Pinkus, H. and Mehregan, A. H.: *A Guide to Dermatohistopathology.* New York, Appleton, 1976, p. 563.

CHAPTER SEVEN

Cryosurgery for Tumors of the Oral Cavity

ANDREW A. GAGE, M.D.

BENIGN AND MALIGNANT tumors as well as precancerous conditions of the oral cavity constitute a group of diseases singularly suitable for treatment by cryosurgery. Except perhaps for the skin, cryosurgical techniques are more easily used in the oral cavity than in any other part of the body. Although the full potential of cryosurgery for oral disease has not yet been realized, its considerable advantages are already in evidence. First, the oral cavity is easily accessible to treatment. Second, cryosurgery is given with little risk, little discomfort, commonly under local anesthesia, and the effect of treatment is readily observed in the postoperative period. Third, treatment can be repeated whenever necessary with a minimum of preparation and risk. Fourth, cryosurgical techniques offer excellent suitability for high-surgical-risk patients. Fifth, cryosurgery offers the outstanding advantage of permitting conservation of bone of the oral cavity so that bone-sacrificing operations and their attendant ill effects on form and function may be avoided. As is true with all methods of treatment, cryosurgery for benign and malignant lesions of the oral cavity yields satisfactory results only if careful attention is given to *selection* of cases and to use of proper technique. The information in this chapter is based largely on thirteen years' personal experience with cryosurgery for tumors in diverse areas of the body.[1-3]

EQUIPMENT

Cryosurgery for the treatment of tumors requires the use of equipment utilizing liquid nitrogen ($-196°C$). The apparatus originally developed by Cooper[4] for neurosurgical purposes and later adapted to the treatment of tumors[5-9] has been supplemented by other types of cryosurgical equipment using liquid nitrogen or other cryogenic agents. Some cryogenic agents, such as liquid nitrous oxide ($-80°C$), providing warmer temperatures, do not have sufficient freezing capability to cope with large volumes of tissue. Extensive freezing requires the use of liquid nitrogen-cooled apparatus which is now available in several types that are much less sophisticated and expensive than Cooper's original equipment. Details regarding the construction and operation of various types of cryoinstrumentation have been described by Garamy.[10]

Experience with different cryosurgical apparatus using liquid nitrogen has shown similarities in use, function, and freezing capabilities, but at times certain reasons dictate choice of one in preference to another. The Linde CE-4® cryosurgical apparatus (Frigitronics) functions only as a closed system with freezing via cryoprobes so that liquid nitrogen is not released on the tissues but rather, after change of phase, the gas is returned to the equipment cabinet for venting. The flexible feed shaft is vacuum insulated. Controls on the console make possible reasonably accurate control of the temperature of the probe tip. At termination of freezing, a heater in the probe near its tip speeds release from the tissue. The Linde CE-8® cryosurgical unit (Frigitronics) and

171

the Brymill Model SP-5® unit can be used either as closed systems with cryoprobes or as open systems spraying liquid nitrogen directly on the tissues. Neither feedline is vacuum-insulated. The probes lack controls for temperature and cannot be heated. These units do not function as efficiently as the CE-4 unit and the lack of a heater is inconvenient, but on the other hand, the capability of use as a spray device is of considerable advantage in certain situations. With all units, a variety of cryoprobes are available.

In choosing cryosurgical equipment, the surgeon must consider the nature of the lesions to be treated. Large tumors require considerable freezing capability which can be provided only by the liquid nitrogen units mentioned. Small tumors can be treated with small hand-held units using liquid nitrogen. When only superficial inflammatory or other benign conditions of the skin and mucous membranes are to be treated, the surgeon can choose from other types of apparatus that use cryogenic agents other than liquid nitrogen.

TECHNIQUE

The objective in cryosurgery is to produce local necrosis of tissue by freezing in situ. Preferably nothing is excised, thus avoiding hemorrhage. The devitalized tissue becomes liquefied and is absorbed or sloughs. Healing of the wound follows. Careful application of the technique is necessary to be certain that the desired result is achieved.

Treatment is given by the application of liquid nitrogen either as a spray or via a cryoprobe. Tumors in the oral cavity are preferably treated by closed systems. The choice of cryoprobe depends in part on the size and location of the lesion, but large tumors require large probes for effective freezing. The end of the probe is pressed firmly on the tumor. The greater the area of contact with the tissue, the greater will be the extent of freezing. If the contact is poor, as might be the case if the tumor overlies bone, then a small amount of water-soluble hospital lubricating jelly should be placed about the probe tip. If the tumor is soft and bulky, the cryoprobe may be inserted into it to obtain greater contact with the tissue and to produce more extensive freezing. More commonly in the oral cavity, only surface contact freezing is used without tissue penetration. Surface contact freezing, as compared to penetration freezing, has several advantages: no tissue wound is caused, chance of bleeding is lessened, tissue planes are not disrupted, and dissemination of tumor cells is minimized.

With the probe carefully placed to prevent movement once freezing starts, liquid nitrogen is allowed to flow and produce freezing. The instrument is always used as cold as possible in order to produce a maximal temperature gradient, a prime factor controlling rate of freezing. The larger the gradient, the more rapid the enlargement of the frozen area. As the frozen tissues turn white and hard, the extent of freezing is judged by inspection and palpation. With surface contact freezing, the shape of the frozen volume of tissue is roughly hemispheric, so the depth of freezing can be judged to be about the same as the lateral spread of freezing from the site of the probe. Freezing is continued until the frosted appearance encompasses the entire lesion plus a generous margin of apparently normal tissue. The same amount of tissue must be frozen that would be removed in a local excision. Tumors too large to be frozen with a single application of the probe are treated by immediate successive applications overlapping frozen areas. After a thawing period

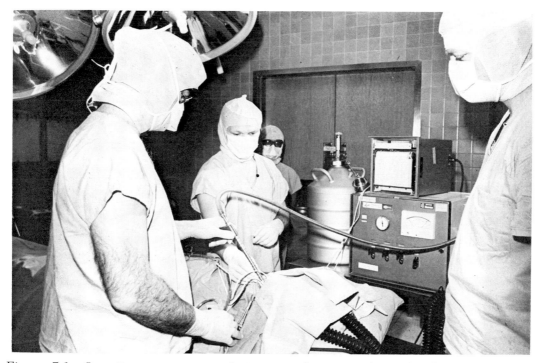

Figure 7-1. Operating room scene during freezing of an oral cancer. Though nothing is excised and there is little chance of causing infection, sterile technique is followed. The Linde CE-4 cryosurgical apparatus and a PR-5 cryoprobe are being used. Two thermo-couples are in place. Also shown is a Honeywell recorder on which the thermocouple temperatures are traced. The treatment is being given under general anesthesia, which commonly is advisable for large tumors.

of about ten minutes, the entire tumor is again frozen. Repetition of freezing is recognized by cryosurgeons as being essential to insure destruction of tissue. Most tumors of moderate size require about thirty minutes for completion of treatment (Plate 107).

Duration of freezing time of each application varies, since the progress and extent of freezing are dependent upon variable factors mentioned later. Freezing is allowed to continue until the desired amount of tissue is frozen or, in the case of large lesions, as long as the frosted edge advances. As time passes, the rate of expansion of the frozen area slows as equilibrium is established between heat lost from the tissues via the cryoprobe and heat brought to the area by circulation of the blood. Seldom is a freezing time of longer than seven minutes practical because the rate of enlargement of the frozen area slows considerably after that time. If after about five to seven minutes, the entire tumor is not yet included in the freezing, the probe is thawed and moved to another site for successive overlapping applications.

Each cryoprobe has its own characteristics of freezing. Some knowledge of the function of a cryoprobe can be obtained by experimental use to determine how large a frozen lesion will form in any chosen time-temperature freezing cycle.

For example, with a 9.5 mm cryoprobe*
used at −180°C, it is possible to create a
roughly hemispheric frozen lesion 3 cm in
diameter in three minutes. If probe contact is maintained for five minutes, the
area frozen is about 4 cm in diameter. On
continued contact, the ice ball grows very
slowly, and for practical purposes, it soon
is pointless to continue freezing. If additional freezing is required, the cryoprobe
should be moved to a new unfrozen site.
Successive adjacent applications improves
the width of the frozen area but only
slightly increases the depth of freezing. In
the tissues adjacent to the probe, the closed
systems almost always produce tissue temperatures colder than −80°C in less than
a minute and commonly produce tissue
temperatures as cold as −170°C in this
time. The apparatus with vacuum-insulated feedline functions better than the less
expensive apparatus with less efficient
feedline insulation. However, with any
equipment, the necessity of freezing large
volumes of tissue may pose problems.

Formulas may be used to predict the
thermodynamic growth of ice balls around
cryoprobes,[11, 12] but they are not practical
for use in cryosurgery.[13] In clinical practice, there are too many complicating variable factors to permit anything better than
rather crude estimation of the size of the
frozen area. Fortunately since osmolality
and thermal characteristics of various tissues show only minimal differences, tissue
resistance to freezing is rather uniform
and only little variation of the cryolesion
will result if freezing conditions are kept
constant. However, standard freezing conditions are not always easy to achieve. Variations in blood supply, especially the proximity of a major blood vessel, may profoundly alter the size and shape of the

frozen area. Apart from this, the single
most important variable factor in freezing
tissue is technique. Removal of heat from
the tissues largely depends upon the temperature of the cryoprobe, the area and
quality of contact between the cryoprobe
and the tissue, and the duration of freezing. Heat sources and shape of probe contact also modify the volume and shape of
the frozen area. Unless careful attention
is given to these factors, apparently identical therapy conditions will yield variation in tissue freezing. It is of extreme importance to maintain good contact between
cryoprobe and the tissue. This is not always easy because slight movement of the
probe can cause fracture in the bond between tissue and probe and interfere with
heat exchange; then reduced heat loss to
the probe will result in deficient freezing.
When this happens, it is usually best to
thaw the probe and start freezing over
again. The important point is that careful
attention to technique and correct use of
the instrument is vital to success in cryosurgery.

Thermocouples *must* be used in freezing
tumors to control the correctness of technique. Thermocouples mounted in needles
are inserted into the tissues to record temperatures beneath the tumor and in apparently normal tissue at the periphery of the
tumor. Only in this way is it possible to be
reasonably certain that lethal temperatures
are achieved deep in the tissues. The goal
in treatment should be to reach at least
−40°C at the periphery of the tumor during each freezing cycle. Temperatures commonly are expressed as maximal freezing
temperature achieved. It is however more
meaningful and instructive to examine the
temperature profile shown by a thermocouple during freezing. This requires recording the temperatures during treatment. Thermocouples have other uses.

---

* PR-5® cryoprobe, Frigitronics, Inc., Shelton,
Connecticut.

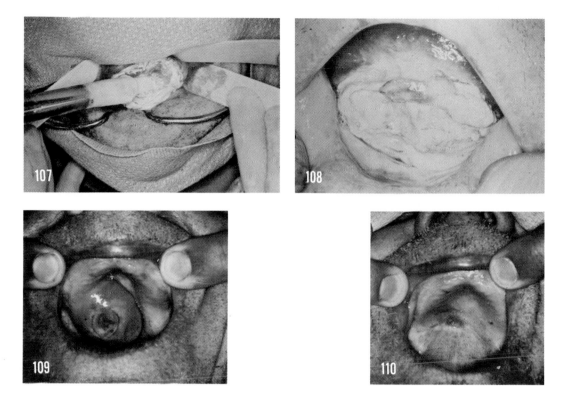

Plate 107. This photograph shows a stage in the freezing of the carcinoma of the anterior part of the floor of the mouth. Using a 9.5 mm cryoprobe at -180°C in a surface contact application, after about three minutes the entire tumor has been frozen. Two thermocouples are obscured by the cryoprobe. A margin of apparently normal tissue will be included. After a period of thawing which requires about ten minutes, the tumor area will be frozen again.

Plate 108. Ten days after freezing, the tumor shown in Figure 7-2 is a mass of malodorous necrotic tissue. It slowly separates in small pieces or is gradually absorbed over a three-week period. When the wound clears of necrotic tissue, adequacy of treatment is checked by biopsy, looking for persistent cancer.

Plate 109. The rounded tumor of the palate is a mixed tumor, present for eighteen months and enlarging slowly. The patient is a cachectic old man unable to withstand general anesthesia or major surgery. The lesion was easily frozen under local anesthesia. From J Oral Surg, 25:323, July 1967.

Plate 110. Three months after freezing the mixed tumor, the palate is almost healed and functionally intact. Healing was complete in another month. From *J Oral Surg*, 25:323, July 1967.

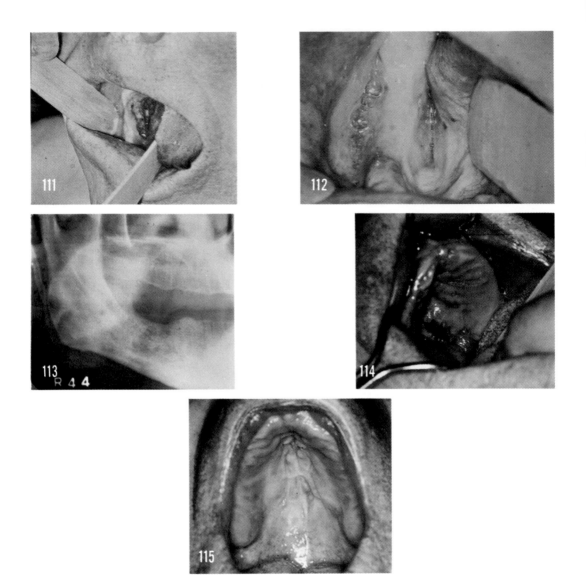

Plate 111. Elderly white male with an ulcerating squamous cell carcinoma over the inner alveolar ridge extending onto the gingiva and into the floor of the mouth for a small extent. There is no enlargement of the cervical lymph nodes. This is an ideal case for cryosurgery. Because of heart failure and angina, the patient is a high surgical risk. The cancer is of moderate size and the underlying bone limits depth penetration. The lesion was frozen using local anesthesia. The soft tissue sloughed and exposed the underlying bone. From *Cancer*, *18*:1649, December 1965.

Plate 112. Two years after freezing, soft tissue coverage of the mandible has been completed. There has been no bony loss. The treated area is healed with some gingival loss. The tongue is mobile. The patient has a useful mandible and no disturbance of speech or swallowing.

Plate 113. Radiograph of mandible at the same time as photograph in Plate 112. There is only slight bony resorption at the site of the treated area.

Plate 114. Adenocystic carcinoma of the palate. This is a tumor of low grade malignancy but prone to recurrence after conservative surgical excision, perhaps because the palate is penetrated by many bony foramina into which tumor can grow. The lethal effect of freezing extends into the bone and increases the chance of cure. From *Cancer*, *18*:1648, December 1965.

Plate 115. Three months after cryosurgery to the palate, the area is well healed and there has been no recurrence of the disease. From *Cancer*, *18*:1648, December 1965.

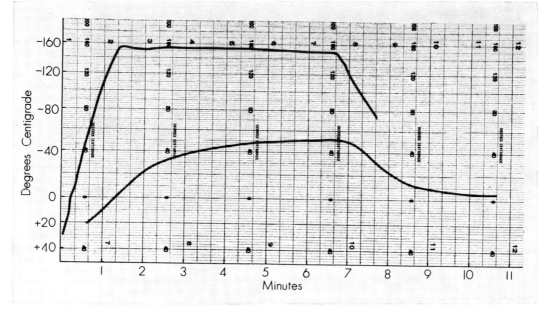

Figure 7-2. Temperatures recorded during freezing of a moderate-sized oral cancer with a large cryoprobe. Two thermocouples were used. One, situated on the surface of the tumor, between the probe and the tissue, shows a fall in temperature to nearly −160°C in eighty seconds and remained close to this temperature during the seven minute freezing period. The other thermocouple, placed at the periphery of the tumor, about 1.5 cm away from the probe contact area, formed the lower tracing on the recording paper. Here freezing was slower and −40°C was reached only after three minutes of freezing. In an additional four minutes, temperature fell to −52°C and freezing was discontinued. Note that the slow warming process continues the tissue in the frozen state for additional minutes.

They can be placed to insure that important tissues are not frozen, and hence prevent unwanted destruction of normal tissue at the periphery of lesions. Furthermore, a thermocouple placed in the tissues close to the probe or between the tissue and the probe will quickly reveal fault in the maintenance of an adherent bond. If the bond is fractured, this thermocouple will fail to show satisfactory freezing.

Extreme gradients in temperature develop in the frozen area during cryosurgical treatment. Rate of freezing decreases with increasing distance from the probe and expansion of the frozen area gradually slows. The coldest temperatures, therefore the most extensive freezing damage, occur close to the site of probe-tissue contact. Remote from the probe, freezing is slower, tissue temperatures are higher, and the probability of cell survival increases. The temperature at the border of the frozen zone is about zero and here cell survival is possible. Since a thermocouple shows temperature only in its own location, it is practically impossible to know what temperature is achieved everywhere in a lesion. The cryosurgeon, knowing the distance of the thermocouple from the probe, must use this evidence along with the knowledge of the expected temperature gradients under a particular set of conditions, to be as certain as possible that a lethal temperature was achieved.

The exact lethal temperature is difficult to define. Though ice crystals begin to form in tissue at −2.2°C, under certain conditions temperatures as low as −20°C may be reached before ice crystals appear. Since this temperature is close to the eutectic point of sodium chloride solution, a common electrolyte in the body, it is commonly cited as that which must be achieved in order to be certain of cell death. However, the evidence suggests that success in cryosurgery requires considerably colder temperatures. In freezing animal tissues under cryosurgical conditions, temperatures much colder than −20°C must be achieved in order to produce cell death in single freeze-thaw cycles. Even at temperatures of −50°C, single freezing episodes are uncertainly destructive. Temperatures of −60°C and colder are certainly lethal, even with single freezing episodes, and predictable areas of necrosis are produced. Under clinical conditions, especially in the treatment of cancer, such considerations become important. Emphasis should be placed on producing temperatures at least as cold as −60°C in all of the tumor area.[14] This requires at least −40°C in the normal tissue at the tumor periphery. This deep freezing is not easy to achieve in a large volume of tissue. Fortunately repetition of freezing increases the lethality of the freezing process so that there is no survival even at −20°C.[15] The importance of this to the cryosurgeon is that everything visibly frozen will die, excepting only a narrow margin at the periphery.

Since the goal of cryosurgery is the production of a desired area of tissue necrosis, in the treatment of tumors it is important to use techniques that achieve maximal lethal effect. The important points in technique may be summarized as follows: (1) use a large cryoprobe cooled by liquid nitrogen; (2) maintain good tumor-probe contact; (3) use the probe as cold as possible; (4) control freezing procedure with thermocouples; (5) freeze as quickly as possible; (6) thaw slowly and unassisted; (7) overlap frozen area; (8) repeat freezing after thawing; and (9) include a margin of normal tissue.

USE OF LIQUID NITROGEN AS SPRAY. Direct application of liquid nitrogen is also an effective way of destroying tissue. Spray technique has slightly greater freezing capability then the cryoprobe technique because the cryogen is being used at the coldest possible temperature and is being applied to the tissues directly. The nozzle of the spraying device can be moved readily over the tissues to produce tissue freezing over a wide surface area, yet not freeze deeply, which is not easily possible with a cryoprobe. The more superficial the lesion, the more suitable is the use of a liquid nitrogen spray. Therefore in the oral cavity, spray technique has proven useful for oral mucosal lesions such as leukoplakia and dyskeratotic lesions. The hand-held cryosurgical apparatus, especially with curved spray nozzles to reach certain areas, is highly satisfactory for non-neoplastic oral mucosal lesions. Treatment should be conservative because it can always be repeated if disease persists and because extensive tissue destruction is usually unnecessary. Measurement of tissue temperatures by thermocouples is not necessary in these applications, but still may be desirable for training purposes.

In contrast to skin disease, where liquid nitrogen spray is an excellent choice, the technique is not as well suited to the oral cavity where the use of the spray is accompanied by the production of a cloud of frozen vapor which obscures vision. Sucker systems are required to remove the cloud to permit good vision. There are additional problems. Use of the spray has a disadvantage that conversion of liquid nitrogen to gas becomes less efficient as the tissue becomes frozen. Therefore the spray works well for moderate freezing, but in extensive freezing, phase transition may be incomplete. Then a common problem is liquid nitrogen run-off, which occurs when the apparatus cools and the tissue freezes. Liquid nitrogen droplets form, strike the cold tissue without vaporizing, and run off the tissue to freeze in undesirable areas. Control of tissue freezing and liquid nitrogen run-off problems are more difficult in spray apparatus which has considerable pulsatile increase in liquid nitrogen flow, as phase transition occurs in the feedline. Variation in flow may occur also from partial occlusion of the aperture in the spray nozzle. When the aperture is blown open by pressure, then greatly increased flow suddenly follows. In most apparatus, as the spray nozzle cools, drops of liquid nitrogen may form at the nozzle tip and precautions against their falling in unwanted areas must be taken. Because of these problems, there is the same limitation on extensive deep freezing of tissues with the use of liquid nitrogen spray as with a cryoprobe technique.

Choice of spray or cryoprobe depends on the type of oral lesion under treatment and on personal preference. For tumors, a cryoprobe is preferable because it produces a deeper and more predictable area of necrosis. On the other hand, for the extensive superficial freezing required for non-neoplastic oral mucosal lesions, the spray technique is better.

POSTOPERATIVE CARE

Principal requirements of postoperative care are related to edema which begins to form after thawing and increases to a maximum within a day. It is associated with excessive salivation and interferes with deglutition to some extent, depending upon the amount of swelling and the area frozen. Although some liquids can usually be swallowed, often intravenous fluids are given for the first day or two. Thereafter patients are gradually able to ingest a soft diet. An occasional patient, such as one who has extensive carcinoma in the posterior part of the oral cavity, requires a nasogastric tube for feeding for several days. Serious feeding problems generally do not occur in patients with lesions of moderate size, especially those in the anterior part of the oral cavity. Respiratory difficulty is not a problem after freezing lesions in the anterior part of the oral cavity, but it may be a serious threat to life after extensive freezing to the base of the tongue or tonsillar region. In such patients, a tracheostomy is done at the time of freezing in order to avoid any difficulty in the postoperative period.

Postoperative pain is usually minimal and only analgesics are required for the discomfort caused by swelling of tissues in the oral cavity. Some fever and leukocytosis always develop. A reasonable precaution is to give a prophylactic broad spectrum antibiotic, such as ampicillin, for several days after treatment. As edema subsides over several days, the previously frozen tissue becomes necrotic and a mass of malodorous tissue develops in the oral cavity. The use of pleasant tasting mouth washes is helpful during this period. The partially necrotic liquefying tissue sloughs in small pieces over a three-week period until the wound has a clean granulating base (Plate 108). Separation of the necrotic tissue may be aided by careful debridement and irrigation during this period. After about three weeks, the wound is usually sufficiently clear of necrotic tissue to permit close examination and biopsy of areas of suspected persistent tumor. In cases where tumor is still present, treatment with cryosurgery is repeated. Most soft tissue wounds in the oral cavity heal remarkably well with little scarring in about four weeks. When bone is exposed by loss of the overlying soft tissue, soft tissue repair and final healing require many months. Devitalized bone in the frozen area requires as long as two years to repair.

COMPLICATIONS

The complications which follow cryosurgery are related to the mass of necrotic tissue in the oral cavity. Potential danger to the airway is preventable by preliminary tracheostomy in those patients in whom extensive freezing is required in the posterior part of the oral cavity. Lesser degrees of freezing, or freezing in the anterior part of the oral cavity, do not necessitate tracheostomy. However, all patients should be observed very carefully in the first postoperative hours to be certain that no respiratory difficulty develops.

Later complications are parasthesias, trismus, hemorrhage, and sequestration. Although most patients have only minimal discomfort after operation, parasthesias caused by freezing the inferior alveolar nerve usually subsides in a few days. Sensory loss in the lower lip and chin and part of the tongue may occur and persist for months before slow improvement and perhaps complete recovery occurs. Fortunately nerves commonly regenerate after freezing injury.[16, 17] For example, facial nerve paralysis following cryosurgery to tumors about the ear has been observed to be followed by *restoration* of nerve function about three months after freezing. This surprisingly rapid return of function is an indication that cryosurgery may be the best choice of treatment in situations where there is risk of undesired major neurologic

damage from conventional surgical excision.

A frequent complication after cryosurgery is hemorrhage from the treated area about seven to ten days after freezing when the necrotic tissue begins to slough. It occurs in about 10 percent of patients with carcinoma of the floor of the mouth and the tongue and much less often elsewhere in the oral cavity. The lingual artery is the usual origin of hemorrhage and bleeding is controlled by suture-ligatures or electrocoagulation. Though it is well known that large blood vessels resist freezing injury,[18, 19] whenever necrotic tissue of any cause begins to slough, there is risk of hemorrhage.

Trismus is a more serious postoperative problem. It occurs only after freezing tumors in the retromolar area and probably is caused by edema, partial destruction, and later fibrosis of the pterygoid muscles. Prevention of the disability by exercise of the jaw in the postoperative period must be encouraged.

Sequestration has not been a problem, although freezing of bone commonly occurs during treatment of tumors. When treatment is for cancer overlying bone, then extensive areas of bone are deliberately frozen and devitalized. The sequence of events following devitalization is well known as a result of animal experimentation and clinical observation.[20–23] The devitalized bone remains fixed perfectly in place and repair requires many months, perhaps as long as two or three years, depending upon the volume of bone frozen. The bone exposed in the oral cavity becomes yellowish in color due to collection of surface debris. It is not painful. Slowly, as blood supply is restored, soft tissue covers the exposed bone again. Bone heals far more kindly after freezing injury than after injury by radiotherapy.

BENIGN TUMORS

Benign tumors of the oral cavity are often ideal for treatment by cryosurgery.[24, 25] Local or topical anesthesia is adequate for most benign lesions and treatment can often be given on an outpatient or ambulatory basis. Especially noteworthy is the fact that treatment can be conservative so that normal tissue is not necessarily destroyed. If the lesion is not destroyed on the first application, then freezing can be repeated within a few weeks to complete destruction. Almost any benign tumor of the oral cavity can be treated by freezing in situ. Especially suitable are tumors that occur on the palate because of their location over bone (Plate 109-110).

In dealing with such tumors, cryosurgery offers considerable advantage over excision in terms of operative blood loss, postoperative pain, risk of infection, and probability of cure. It affords the significant advantage of penetration of the bony palate with lethal thermal effects. Mixed tumors may penetrate their capsules and involve periosteum and bone, which is responsible for the high recurrence rate after conservative excision. Bone sacrifice, necessary with radical surgery, can be avoided by cryosurgery because the lethal effect of freezing extends into the bone and obviates the need for excision.

HEMANGIOMA: Hemangiomas of the oral cavity are particularly suitable for treatment by freezing. Usually they are small in size, elevated, superficial, and well circumscribed, so that conditions for freezing in situ are ideal. Since they usually present a typical appearance, preliminary identification by biopsy is often unnecessary. Usually a cryoprobe is employed because the pressure of probe application empties blood from the hemangioma and facilitates freezing. In order to cure the lesion, freezing must extend into the normal tissue around the tumor. Hemangiomas of the buccal mucosa, gingiva, and tongue have been easily cured with minimal scarring, minimal loss of normal tissue, and excellent healing. Large hemangiomas may present a considerable problem in surgical removal, but in selected cases freezing in situ affords the possibility of safe removal without loss of blood.[26, 27] Extensive vascular lesions of the oral cavity, which present a problem for any method of treatment, have occasionally been successfully managed by cryosurgery. The experience of Goldwyn, reported in chapter ten of this volume, describes the treatment of hemangiomas elsewhere in the body, as on the skin or in the pharynx and larynx, and should be reviewed.

Lymphangiomas of the oral cavity have seldom been treated by cryosurgery but present problems in management similar to hemangiomas. For this reason, mention of the tumor is made at this point.

PRECANCEROUS LESIONS: The various types of white patches occurring on the mucous membrane of the oral cavity are easily treated by cryosurgery under local anesthesia in an oral surgical clinic or similar facility. Papillary epithelial hyperplasia, hyperkeratosis, and leukoplakia are examples of lesions which have been satisfactorily treated by freezing.[24, 28, 29] Preliminary biopsy is necessary to differentiate between those lesions which are innocuous and those which show premalignant changes. Most such lesions are superficial, so freezing must be wide rather than deep, sometimes covering large areas. Either the cryoprobe or the spray system can be used; choice depends on the extent and location of the disease. Small lesions, especially in areas difficult to apply a liquid nitrogen spray, are better treated with a cryoprobe. Multiple applications of short duration are necessary because usually treatment need be given to a depth of only 2 to 3 mm. For most superficial lesions, use of the liquid nitrogen as a spray to freeze the area is preferred. Caution must be observed that undesirable run-off of droplets of liquid nitrogen into other areas does not occur. Ordinarily there need be little concern for dental structures, although minor changes are known to occur.[30] The amount of freezing used for benign disease is not sufficient to cause permanent tooth damage. Since freezing is superficial, the edema which occurs after operation is not troublesome. The patient is able to eat a soft diet and healing is ordinarily rapid and completed in two weeks or less. About 20 percent of patients, usually those with rather extensive lesions, have healing delayed beyond two weeks. Occasionally repetition of treatment is needed to completely eliminate the disease.

ORAL CANCER

Oral cancer is commonly treated by surgical excision or radiotherapy. Chemotherapy is commonly used as an adjunct to the more effective methods of treatment, especially as the disease persists or develops metastatic spread and passes beyond the possibility of control by local means. With any method of treatment, the overall survival rate is low. Only about one third of patients survive five years. In addition, the patient faces a number of problems related either to neglect of the cancer, to failure of treatment to cure, or to the effects of treatment even when the cancer is cured. For example, problems may be caused by radical surgery, such as loss of form and function of a part, or by the deleterious effect of radiotherapy on bone. As a result, there are a variety of patients with oral cancer in whom cryosurgery may be used for widely different reasons. The goal of treatment may be palliation of in-

curable cancer, attempt at salvage of advanced cancer still localized and hence potentially curable, or it may be used as primary treatment for cancer. The goal of treatment should be decided before freezing in order to facilitate later evaluation of results.

PALLIATION OF ADVANCED ORAL CANCER: Advanced oral cancer causes pain and bleeding and interferes with mastication and deglutition. The bulk of the tumor as it occupies space and ulcerates is primarily responsible for these symptoms. When palliation of symptoms is intended, there are no special criteria for case selection except that the tumor is obviously incurable by any method of treatment. The goal of treatment is not necessarily to freeze the entire tumor but certainly most of it should be frozen in order to attain considerable reduction in size. Some lesions, even though small, are painful and these should be frozen thoroughly in order to desensitize the nerve supply which may be infiltrated by cancer at some distance from the ulcerated area. During the first days after freezing large bulky tumors, nutrition by nasogastric tube or parenteral route is needed. However, rapid reduction in tumor size usually permits ingestion of food within a few days. Relief of pain is occasionally immediate and complete, but more often only partial. When tumor slough has been completed, oral hygiene is improved.

In most cases radiotherapy is used in followup care because its diffuse effect usually provides additional benefit. In patients in whom radiotherapy is not used, tumor growth will recur in three to four months. It may then be frozen again to maintain control. Radiotherapy extends control of recurrence for several months, so it appears advisable to combine radiotherapy with freezing. In certain patients, chemotherapy may be combined with cryosurgery as well.[31] At this time it is not possible to say whether freezing potentiates response to either drug treatment or radiotherapy.

Although palliation of symptoms of advanced oral cancer can be provided, this is difficult to achieve in large bulky tumors. The massive necrosis which follows freezing is difficult for the patient to manage. With palliation as a goal, the best reason to use cryosurgery is for relief of pain. However, in general, when the amount of cancer is large, and if pain is not a prominent symptom, radiotherapy is usually a better choice for palliation.

ORAL CANCER PERSISTENT AFTER EXCISION OR RADIOTHERAPY: Some patients are seen with oral cancer persistent after radiotherapy or surgical excision. The diseased area may appear to be small, still localized and potentially curable. Often the lesion is painful. Usually such patients have had both surgical excision and radiotherapy; further surgery is not possible, and further radiotherapy is considered inadvisable because of tissue tolerance. Such patients are potentially good candidates for cryosurgical treatment since the risk is small and chance of benefit reasonably good. The patients must be carefully selected so that the possibility of cure is recognized and treatment is sufficiently aggressive. Ordinarily the cryoprobe technique is best suited to the lesions, although commonly the mandible is involved or exposed and maintenance of good contact between cryoprobe and tumor is not easy. In such instances, if exposure permits, a spray technique may be used. In well chosen cases, cryosurgery can destroy the residual cancer and relieve pain. Occasional long-term survival of patients is an indication of the usefulness of cryosurgery as a method of salvage when disease is persistent after other methods of treatment.[32]

Even those who are not cured may be provided with striking relief of pain. More often only partial relief of pain and palliation of other symptoms can be provided.

ORAL CANCER—PRIMARY TREATMENT BY CRYOSURGERY

The use of cryosurgery for the primary treatment of oral cancer with the object of cure requires careful selection of patients. It is a departure from standard methods of treatment and chance of cure must not be compromised by faulty judgment as to extent of disease or faulty application of a new technique. The technique must be learned through animal trials and use in benign tumor or palliative treatments before use as the sole method for primary cure of cancer. After this experience has been gained, certain patients can be chosen for cryosurgery as the primary method of treatment of their cancer.[33-35] Selection of patients is based on the following criteria:

1. the cancer is on or adjacent to bone so that excision would require removal of a portion of mandible or palate,
2. the patient has extensive cardiopulmonary disease so that the risk of extensive operation is prohibitive.

In some patients, both reasons may be present but one is sufficient. In addition, some patients may be chosen for cryosurgery even when conservation of bone is not a factor in operative treatment and even when the risk of major operation is acceptable. These generally are those who refuse the suggested radical excision or radiotherapy for various reasons (Plates 111-113).

When first seen the extent of the lesion is carefully determined and staged by the TMN classification of the American Joint Committee of Cancer Staging and End Results Reporting. The presence or absence of enlarged cervical lymph nodes is of considerable importance in planning treatment. Patients without enlarged cervical lymph nodes are treated only by cryosurgery to the primary lesion and radical neck dissection is deferred indefinitely. Prophylactic lymph node dissection is not practiced, but rather radical neck dissection is performed later if cervical lymph nodes enlarge. Oral cancer patients in whom the cervical lymph nodes are enlarged at the time of first examination are treated by cryosurgery to the primary lesion, followed by radical neck dissection about a month later. This interval is necessary to be certain that the primary lesion is controlled, which cannot be done until the necrotic tissue in the primary site is sloughed to permit examination and biopsy of the clean wound. Evidence of persistent disease requires further treatment of the involved area. As experience with the technique improves, the need for repetition of treatment decreases due to more aggressive initial freezing. It is difficult to freeze too much in the treatment of cancer.

Results in terms of survival are best shown by the fate of forty-four patients who underwent cryosurgery as primary treatment for oral cancer in the year 1964-1968, providing a follow-up period of more than five years.[36] The series was comprised of forty-three men and one woman, consistent with our hospital population of military service veterans. Women generally have a better prognosis in oral cancer, so this male preponderance has a bearing on survival. Most patients were over sixty years of age (Table 7-I), many with severe disease of heart, lungs, or other important organs. All had squamous cell carcinoma in various stages of the disease. The sites of origin of the cancer were buccal mucosa—2, floor of mouth—21, an-

terior two thirds of tongue—6, posterior one third of tongue—2, soft palate—1, hard palate—2, lower alveolar ridge—9, and upper alveolar ridge—1.

Thirty-six patients had no cervical adenopathy when first seen and only cryosurgery to the primary lesion was done. During this period, a decision was made not to perform prophylactic neck dissections in order to preserve the option of surgical excision if cryosurgery failed. Early satisfactory results and reluctance to perform extensive operations on aged patients led to a continuation of this practice during this period of study. Eight patients had enlargement of cervical lymph nodes, apparently from metastatic cancer, when first seen. These patients were treated by cryosurgery to the primary lesion, followed in about a month by radical neck dissection.

Five-year survival is shown in Table 7-II. The data are presented by the staging system of the American Joint Committee on Cancer Staging and End Results Reporting, which provides for the clinical categorization of the primary lesion, its extensions and metastases. In stage 1 disease, the table shows thirteen survivors among fourteen patients treated. In stage 2 disease, there are seven surviving out of nineteen treated five years earlier. In stage 3 and stage 4 disease, which represents ad-

TABLE 7-I

AGE RANGE OF 44 PATIENTS WITH CANCER
OF THE ORAL CAVITY TREATED
PRIMARILY BY CRYOSURGERY IN THE
YEARS 1964-1968

Age Range	Number of Patients
40-49 years	7
50-59 years	12
60-69 years	10
70-79 years	14
80-89 years	1

TABLE 7-II

FIVE-YEAR SURVIVAL OF PATIENTS WITH ORAL
CANCER PRIMARILY TREATED BY CRYOSURGERY
IN YEARS 1964-1968

	NO	N1	N2	N3
T1 Stage 1	13/14			
T2 Stage 2	7/19	2/3	0/1	
T3 Stage 3	0/3	1/3	0/1	
			Stage 4	

Classification by TNM staging system of the American Joint Commission on Cancer Staging and End Results Reporting.

The fractions indicate patients shown as:

$$\frac{\text{number of patients living five years}}{\text{total number of patients in group}}$$

Primary Tumor:

T1 indicates a tumor 2 cm or less in greatest diameter.

T2 indicates a tumor greater than 2 cm but not yet 4 cm in greatest diameter.

T3 indicates a tumor larger than 4 cm.

Cervical Lymph Node Metastases:

N0 means that cervical lymph nodes are not palpable.

N1, N2, and N3 indicate progressive extent of enlargement and involvement of cervical lymph nodes and suspected metastatic disease.

vanced disease with lymph node extension, there is the expected low survival rate.

Five years after treatment by cryosurgery, twenty-three of forty-four patients are alive. These are apparently free of tumor, although two have been treated for a second primary oral carcinoma. Eight have died of unrelated disease, usually heart failure or coronary thrombosis, but there was no evidence of cancer at the time of death. The mean survival of nineteen months in this group of eight reflects the serious nature of their associated disease. Nine patients with metastatic tumor have died from unrelated disease, usually heart disease, or from metastatic cancer,

but the primary area was healed and apparently free of disease (mean survival twenty-nine months). Four patients died with persistent cancer in the primary site and thus were clearly failures of cryosurgical technique (mean survival twenty-six months). The cancers which persisted after freezing were large tumors of the floor of the mouth and tongue, over 4 cm in greatest diameter, and already metastatic to the cervical lymph nodes when first seen. After failure of cryosurgery, which in one patient did not become obvious for nearly three years, radiotherapy was used.

Regarding the thirty-six patients who had no cervical adenopathy when first seen, from three months to two years after treatment of the primary lesion, cervical lymph nodes enlarged in twelve patients. A radical neck dissection was then done. Eight remained well and four later died with persistent cancer in the cervical region. Metastatic cancer is a common cause of death in oral cancer and might be avoided by early cervical node dissection, so this experience compels a reevaluation of prophylactic lymph node dissection in relation to cryosurgery. The incidence of later appearance of metastatic nodes in the neck, as long as two years after treatment of the primary lesion, may be sufficient reason to perform prophylactic neck dissection after cryosurgery, even though the nodes are not enlarged when first seen. However, it is necessary to defer the dissection until the primary lesion has been adequately treated.

It appears from this small series that freezing in situ is more likely to cure small cancers than large ones, but this is true of any other kind of treatment as well. In selected cases, cryosurgery can achieve a survival rate comparable to that afforded by surgical excision. Equally important, this result can be achieved at lessened cost to the patient in terms of operative mortality and postoperative functional disability. Reduced disability is due chiefly to conservation of the bony structure of the oral cavity. For this outstanding reason, cryosurgery deserves a place in surgical management of oral cancer.

Cryosurgery is particularly well applicable to tumors overlying the palate or mandible because invasion of tumor is limited by the bone (Plates 114, 115). Cancers in the anterior portion of the floor of the mouth are also suitable because of easy accessibility to treatment; this location, because of the disability caused by resection of the anterior portion of the mandible, encourages acceptance of the risk of cryo-

surgery. Tumors of the anterior portions of the tongue are easily destroyed by freezing. Cancers of the posterior third of the tongue are usually rather large, not very accessible, and few are suitable for freezing. Cancers of the tongue or floor of the mouth are not as suitable as cancers overlying bone because depth penetration may be surprisingly great and invasion via lymphatics may be early. Although the risk of failure is higher than with a lesion overlying bone, cryosurgery should be considered for small to moderate-sized cancers of tongue or floor of the mouth rather than acceptance of the disability caused by excision of generous segments of the mandible.

On the other hand, advanced cancers of the oral cavity, especially of the floor of the mouth, base of tongue and pharynx, are probably not curable by cryosurgery and the technique should not be used for extensive cancer unless necessitated by the general condition of the patient. It is preferable to use surgical excision or radiotherapy and reserve cryosurgery for adjunctive treatment if disease persists or recurs.

Cryosurgery is best reserved for patients who do not have enlarged cervical lymph nodes. However if other factors, such as high surgical risk and desire to conserve bone, dictate use of cryosurgery, then node dissection should be deferred until it is certain that the primary lesion is under control. There is always some concern about the possibility of tumor in the tissues between the primary lesion and the tissues removed in neck dissection. At the time of node dissection, if the primary lesion is in the floor of the mouth, the operative removal may include the contracted scar tissue in the floor of the mouth. If the primary lesion is in a remote site so that tissues cannot be removed in continuity, radiotherapy should be used in the postoperative period.

COMPARISON WITH OTHER METHODS OF TREATMENT

Cryosurgery for the cure of tumors is not yet generally practiced and cannot yet be considered a standard method of treatment. However, its use is gradually expanding in this country and abroad as physicians acquire the apparatus, gain experience with the technique, and acquaint other physicians with its merits. The advantages lie in simplicity of use, rather little need for anesthesia, lack of hemorrhage during freezing, and few complications in the postoperative period. Most of these advantages are due to the fact that in treatment nothing is excised but rather the tumor is allowed to become necrotic and slough.

Limitations of the technique are several, apart from the obvious fact that only local treatment is given and lymphadenopathy must be managed by an alternate treatment method. One limitation is the difficulty in evaluating the extent of freezing, especially when treatment is given via endoscopy. Determining depth of freezing is a problem even when vision is good. Another limitation is the difficulty in freezing large volumes of tissue, even though liquid nitrogen is used as the cryogenic agent. Improvements in cryosurgical apparatus are needed in order for the technique to achieve greater therapeutic usefulness.

As a form of producing local necrosis of tissue, cryosurgery must be compared with other physical-chemical methods of producing similar effects and with conservative local excision of tissue, which might be expected to achieve similar cure rates and benefits. The closest comparison must be with electrocoagulation.[37-39] Electrocoagulation is commonly used as a means of excision, a technique which may be associated with considerable bleeding, which does not occur with freezing. On the other hand, electrocoagulation can be used to cook tissue without attempting excision at the same time, which is more competitive with cryosurgery. Cold is more easily controlled than electrocautery and depth of treatment is more predictable. The use of heat for destruction is more painful than is cold, so increased anesthesia is needed. Explosion hazards must be considered in electrocoagulation but not in cryosurgery. Heat is more destructive to bone than is cold. Even though healing is delayed, the end result is better after freezing than after cauterization. With cryosurgery, scar formation is often surprisingly little. Though electrocoagulation has proven its usefulness under many clinical conditions, freezing is the preferred treatment in the types of lesions described in this chapter.

Local surgical excision cannot compete successfully with cryosurgery in selected patients. It requires more anesthesia, causes bleeding, and cannot deal satisfactorily with lesions that rest on underlying bone. Excision of the bone increases the scope of the operation and produces undesirable and unnecessary postoperative disability. On the other hand, the lethal effect of freezing extends into the bone and destroys any tumor cells which might be there while permitting the bone to remain behind for revitalization while maintaining function. The outstanding reason for the preference of cryosurgery in oral tumors is the possibility of conserving bone.

SUMMARY OF CURRENT PRACTICE AND EXPERIENCE OF OTHER SURGEONS

Acceptance of cryosurgery for palliation of incurable oral cancer has been good. Although some surgeons are firm advocates,[40-43] others,[39] including this author, have valued its merit for palliation as limited and have found that it may cause problems unless used very carefully. It is generally agreed that relief of pain may be excellent. With regard to its use for cure of cancer, cryosurgery is not yet generally practiced by surgeons and it cannot be considered a standard method of treatment. Few physicians object to its use for inoperable radioresistant tumors or for cancers in which other methods of treatment have failed. As a primary method of treating oral cancer, there is reason to be cautious, even though cryosurgery is recognized to have considerable potential.[31, 32, 34, 40] Caution of quick acceptance is justified by the realization that tissues resist freezing injury, the extent of the cancer is always uncertain, and cryosurgical technique and equipment need improvement. The author's view on the prospects of cryosurgery for cancer is one of cautious optimism.[44] In some aspects, its advantages exceed those of electrocoagulation. It is likely that its suitability for high surgical risk patients will lead to wide use in oral cancer and to selective use to manage problems not easily solved by other methods.

REFERENCES

1. Gage, A.: Cryosurgery for diverse human tumors. *Panminerva Medica, 13:*475, 1971.
2. Gage, A.: Cryosurgery for oral and pharyngeal carcinoma. *Panminerva Medica, 13:*488, 1971.
3. Gage, A.: Cryosurgery for difficult problems in cutaneous cancer. *Cutis, 16:* 465, 1975.
4. Cooper, I.: Cryostatic congelation: a system for producing a limited controlled region of cooling or freezing of biologic tissues. *J Nerv Ment Dis, 133:* 259, 1961.
5. Cooper, I.: Cryogenic surgery. A new method of destruction or extirpation of benign or malignant tissues. *N Engl J Med, 268:*743, 1963.
6. Cooper, I.: Cryogenic surgery for cancer. *Fed Proc, 24:*S237, 1965.
7. Cahan, W.: Cryosurgery of malignant and benign tumors. *Fed Proc, 24:*S241, 1965.
8. Gage, A., Koepf, S., Wehrle, D. and Emmings, F.: Cryotherapy for cancer of the lip and oral cavity. *Cancer, 18:* 1646, 1965.
9. Gage, A., Gonder, M., Soanes, W. and Emmings, F.: Cancer cryotherapy. *Milit Med, 132:*550, 1967.
10. Garamy, G.: Engineering aspects of cryosurgery. In Rand, R., Rinfret, A. and Von Leden, H. (Eds.): *Cryosurgery.* Springfield, Thomas, 1968.
11. Cooper, T. and Trezek, F.: Analytical prediction of the temperature field emanating from a cryogenic surgical cannula. *Cryobiology, 7:*79, 1970.
12. Cooper, T. and Trezek, G.: Rate of lesion growth around spherical and cylindrical cryoprobes. *Cryobiology, 7:*183, 1971.
13. Gill, W., DaCosta, J. and Fraser, J.: The control and predictability of a cryolesion. *Cryobiology, 6:*347, 1970.
14. Neel, H., Ketcham, A. and Hammond, W.: Requisites for successful cryogenic surgery of cancer. *Arch Surg, 102:*45, 1971.
15. Smith, J. and Fraser, F.: An estimation of tissue damage and thermal history in the cryolesion. *Cryobiology, 11:*139, 1974.
16. Gaster, R., Davidson, T., Rand, R. and Fonkalsrud, E.: Comparison of nerve regeneration rates following controlled freezing or crushing. *Arch Surg, 103:* 378, 1971.
17. Carter, D., Lee, P., Gill, W. and Johnston, R.: The effect of cryosurgery on peripheral nerve function. *J R Coll Surg Edinb, 17:*25, 1972.
18. Gage, A., Fazekas, G. and Riley, E.: Freezing injury to large blood vessels in dogs, with comments on the experimental freezing of bile ducts. *Surgery, 61:*748, 1967.
19. Cooper, I., Samra, K. and Wisniewska, K.: Effects of freezing on major arteries. *Stroke, 2:*471, 1971.
20. Gage, A., Greene, G., Neiders, M. and Emmings, F.: Freezing bone without

excision. An experimental study of bone-cell destruction and manner of regrowth in dogs. *JAMA, 196*:770, 1966.

21. Emmings, F., Neiders, M., Greene, G., Koepf, S. and Gage, A.: Freezing the mandible without excision. *J Oral Surg, 24*:145, 1966.

22. Gage, A. and Erickson, R.: Cryotherapy and curettage for bone tumors. *J Cryosurgery, 1*:60, 1968.

23. Emmings, F., Gage, A. and Koepf, S.: Combined curettage and cryotherapy for recurrent ameloblastoma of the mandible; report of case. *J Oral Surg, 29*:41, 1971.

24. Emmings, F., Koepf, S. and Gage, A.: Cryotherapy for benign lesions of the oral cavity. *J Oral Surg, 25*:320, 1967.

25. Van Leden, H.: Cryosurgery of the head and neck. *Tex Med, 68*:108, 1972.

26. Henderson, R.: Cryosurgical treatment of hemangiomas. *Arch Otolaryngol, 93:* 511, 1971.

27. Hansen, J.: Cryosurgical therapy for benign lesions of the skin and mucous membranes. *Int Surg, 56*:401, 1971.

28. Goode, R. and Spooner, T.: Office cryotherapy for oral leukoplakia. *Trans Am Acad Ophthalmol Otolaryngol, 75:* 968, 1971.

29. Sako, K., Marchella, F. and Hayes, R.: Evaluation of cryosurgery in the treatment of intra-oral leukoplakia. *J Cryosurgery, 2*:239, 1969.

30. Natiella, J. Gage, A., Armitage, J. and Greene, G.: Tissue response to cryosurgery of oral cavity in rhesus monkeys. *Arch Pathol, 98*:183, 1974.

31. Benson, J. W.: Regional chemotherapy and local cryotherapy for cancer. *Oncology, 26*:134, 1972.

32. Chandler, J. and Hiott, C.: Cryosurgery

in the management of tumors of the head and neck. *South Med J, 64*:1440, 1971.

33. Gage, A.: Cryotherapy for oral cancer. *JAMA, 204*:565, 1968.

34. Gage, A.: Cryosurgery for oral and pharyngeal carcinoma. *Am J Surg, 118*:669, 1969.

35. Weaver, W. and Smith, D.: Cryosurgery for head and neck cancer. *Am J Surg, 128*:466, 1974.

36. Gage, A.: Cryosurgery for oral cancer—technique and five-year survival. *Panminerva Medica, 17*:376, 1975.

37. Poswillo, D.: A comparative study of the effects of electrosurgery and cryosurgery in the management of benign oral lesions. *Br J Oral Surg, 9*:1, 1971.

38. Poswillo, D.: Cryosurgery and electrosurgery compared in the treatment of experimentally induced oral carcinoma. *Br Dent J, 131*:347, 1971.

39. Ostergard, D., Townsend, D. and Hirose, F.: Comparison of electrocauterization and cryosurgery for the treatment of benign disease of the uterine cervix. *Obstet Gynecol, 33*:58, 1969.

40. Miller, D.: Three years experience with cryosurgery in head and neck tumors. *Ann Otol Rhinol Laryngol, 78*:786, 1969.

41. Beggs, J.: Cryotherapy as a palliative maneuver. *JAMA, 206*:1570, 1968.

42. Goode, R., Breitenbach, E. and Cox, D.: Cryosurgical treatment of head and neck tumors—a comparative study. *Laryngoscope, 84*:1950, 1974.

43. Holden, H. and McKelvie, P.: Cryosurgery in the treatment of head and neck neoplasia. *Br J Surg, 59*:709, 1972.

44. Gage, A.: Cryosurgery for cancer. An evaluation. *Cryobiology, 5*:241, 1969.

CHAPTER EIGHT

Cryosurgery of Eyelid Disorders Including Malignant Tumors

CROWELL BEARD, M.D. AND JOHN H. SULLIVAN, M.D.

CRYOGENICS HAS BECOME vital to many procedures in ophthalmic surgery. Application of the *adhesive* effect of freezing to cataract surgery was introduced by Krwawicz[1] in 1961 and has since virtually replaced all other techniques. Deutschmann[2] in 1935 reported the use of *inflammation* from freezing in the treatment of retinal detachment. This also has become a firmly established technique. In 1950, Bietti[3] reported the use of the *necrotizing* effect of freezing to partially destroy the secretory epithelium of the ciliary body in the treatment of glaucoma.

Recently, interest has been aroused in the necrotizing potential of cryosurgery on disorders of the eyelids and ocular adenexa. Zacarian[4] reported cryosurgical destruction of 730 malignant skin tumors, of which 40 involved the eyelids. Following this work, the authors began using cryosurgery for various disorders of eyelids and conjunctiva.

BASAL CELL CARCINOMA OF THE EYELIDS

The eyelid is a relatively uncommon site for skin cancer. According to Brodkin,[5] only 5 percent of all basal cell carcinomas occur in this region. Still, as with other cutaneous malignancies, more than 90 percent of tumors of the lids are basal cell epithelioma. The lower lid is involved in 53 percent of cases, and the medial canthal region in 27 percent. Tumors are much less frequent in the upper lid and lateral canthal region.[6]

Despite its infrequency, basal cell carcinoma of the eyelid is responsible for a disproportionate morbidity and mortality. Relatively inconspicuous lesions may have significant extension into periocular and lacrimal tissues. Neglect or inadequate treatment may result in osseous and cerebral involvement. The mortality of periocular basal cell carcinoma is between 2 and 11 percent.[7, 8] Enucleation or exenteration of the orbit is sometimes necessary for survival.[8, 9]

It is, therefore, of some importance to accurately diagnose and treat eyelid tumors. Few areas demand more exacting skill for successful repair than the eyelid. The integrity of the cornea, and vision itself, is dependent upon preservation of the function of the eyelids. Malposition or destruction of the lid can result in exposure keratopathy or disturbance of the lacrimal system. This may cause disfigurement and epiphora or even xerophthalmia and blindness. There are many successful methods for treatment of basal cell carcinoma. Each, when properly performed, results in a high cure rate, and consequently, proponents of each method tend to have a dogmatic therapeutic approach.

Surgery

Excision of a tumor, the extent of which has been clinically estimated at the time of surgery, is associated with a high recurrence rate. Rakofsky[10] reported on ninety-five basal cell lesions of the eyelids and found 50 percent of the specimens submitted showed inadequate excision. The rate of recurrence during the period studied was 12 percent. Payne[7] found a similar rate in a study of 273 cases. Incomplete excision was discovered in 23.3 percent of 129 cases described by Aurora and Blodi.[11] Einaugler and Henkind[12] reported 50 percent incomplete excision in forty specimens; Wilder and Smith[13] had a similar experience in reviewing seventy cases.

A more certain method for complete eradication of the tumor is excision combined with meticulous histological examination of the surgical margins. The Mohs technique uses the application of a fixative paste to the skin for a layered removal of specimens which are microscopically examined. This requires an extended period of treatment which is tedious to the surgeon and patient. Modification by "Fresh Tissue Chemosurgery,"[14] utilizes surgical excision with immediate frozen section examination of specimens. This principle has been practiced for many years,[15] using the services of skilled and cooperative pathologists. Older et al.[6] reported a 0 percent recurrence rate in a study of 157 patients with basal cell carcinoma in the eyelids treated in this manner.

Although unquestionably efficacious in eradicating tumor, the classic Mohs technique has limited usefulness in the mobile region of the eyelids. Chronic cicatricial changes following open granulation of large lesions usually lead to disfigurement and disability. However, when this principle of eradication is combined with skilled surgical reconstruction, the results are most gratifying.

Radiation

Domonkos[16] found a 2 percent recurrence rate in 142 patients with basal cell carcinoma treated by irradiation. Lederman[17] reported 194 patients with basal cell carcinoma of the eyelids treated by radiation with recurrence in 9.3 percent. Complications occurred in 10.5 percent of the patients. Keratitis, keratinization of the conjunctiva, keratoconjunctivitis sicca, corneal opacification, cataract, obliteration of the secretory and excretory lacrimal apparatus, and skin necrosis are among the most serious complications of radiation. Skillful radiation with shielding and fractionation reduce the rate of complications, but loss of lashes, obliteration of canaliculi, radiodermatitis, conjunctival epidermalization, and alteration of lid contour are frequent side effects. A unique problem with this method is that of recurrences. Further treatment by radiation is not possible, and reconstructive surgery is very difficult. Complications are inevitable from any form of therapy. Those resulting from radiation are more serious than from other types of treatment.

Cryosurgery

Cryosurgery has been used in the treatment of benign and malignant cutaneous lesions for many years. Only in recent years has it been used upon the eyelids in a sophisticated manner with predictable results. The pathophysiology of the cryogenic reaction and instrumentation were considered in chapters one and two of this volume and will not be reviewed. Liquid nitrogen, because of its low boiling temperature, is the preferred freezing agent for malignant lesions. It is best applied by direct cutaneous spray or by a probe cooled with continuous circulation of liquid nitrogen. Application by cotton-tipped swabs and frozen metal discs is somewhat effective but unpredictable, and cannot be recommended for treatment of malignant lesions of the eyelids. Nitrous oxide has a higher boiling point than liquid nitrogen, yet possesses sufficient freezing capacity to treat most superficial lesions. Availability and storage is an advantage of nitrous oxide, but it has limited ability in the treatment of large tumors. Direct spray of liquid nitrogen is the most effective means of achieving an adequate cryogenic lesion to the base of such tumors.

The recurrence rate following cryosurgery for basal cell carcinoma is similar to that of radiation. Zacarian[4] reported on the treatment of forty malignant skin tumors involving the eyelids. The recurrence rate in this series was 7.5 percent. Recurrence is the result of persistent viable tumor cells following incomplete treatment. This is the inevitable consequence of the inability to histologically examine the margins of the tumor. It is possible, however, to insure the generation of an adequate cryosurgical lesion by tissue temperature monitoring. Unfortunately, one cannot be certain the thermocouple sensor is beyond the border of the tumor.

In many respects, cryosurgery is ideally suited for eyelid tumors. *Advantages of cryosurgery for selected basal cell eyelid tumors include:*

Effective

Lid function and appearance preserved

Canaliculi and punctae spared

Few complications

Inexpensive and convenient

Single outpatient treatment

Re-treatment by any means uncompromised

Patients generally present at an early stage, because eyelid tumors are so obvious. Such small tumors are well suited for cryosurgical destruction. The relative absence of cicatrization minimizes deformity of the lid contour. The sparing effect on the conjunctiva and lacrimal canaliculi result in maximum functional result.

Effect of Freezing on Lacrimal Canaliculi

In collaboration with John Bullock, M.D.,[18] experiments were performed to determine the effect of freezing on the lacrimal excretory apparatus of rabbits. Canaliculi and punctae were treated separately using a double freeze-thaw cycle with liquid nitrogen at various temperatures. The patency of the lacrimal system was determined pre- and postoperatively by inspection and irrigation with aqueous fluorescein solution. Tissue temperature was determined by implantation of a microthermocouple within the lumen of the canaliculus and beneath the conjunctiva of the punctum. Using a metallic probe cooled by circulating liquid nitrogen, lesions were made at $-10°C$, $-30°C$, $-50°C$, and $-70°C$. After eight weeks, sections were made through the canaliculi and punctae, and each specimen was studied microscopically. The effects of freezing on the punctum are shown in Table 8-I. Figure 8-1a shows the lacrimal punctum of a control animal with nonkeratinized, stratified, squamous epithelium overlying the substantia propria. Treatment to $-30°C$ resulted in no clinical or histological changes. Figure 8-1b is a photomicrograph of the punctum after freezing to $-50°C$ and demonstrates irregularity of the epithelium. After treatment to $-70°C$ (Figure 8-1c), marked thin-

TABLE 8-I

PATENCY OF RABBIT LACRIMAL PUNTAE EIGHT WEEKS FOLLOWING CRYOSURGERY

Temperature (°C)	Number Observations	Cases Patent (%)
+37 (control)	2	100
−10	3	100
−30	2	100
−50	3	100
−70	3	67

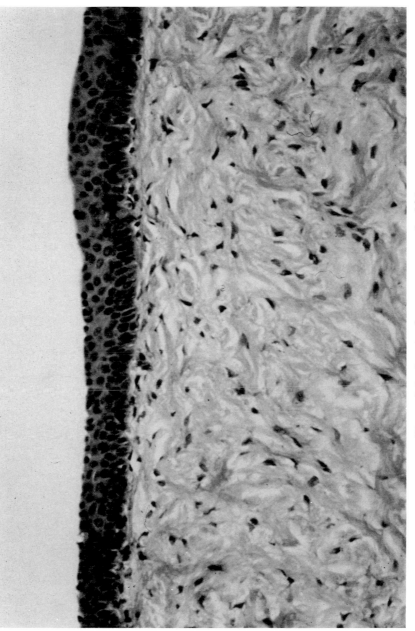

Figure 8-1a. Lacrimal punctum, control rabbit.

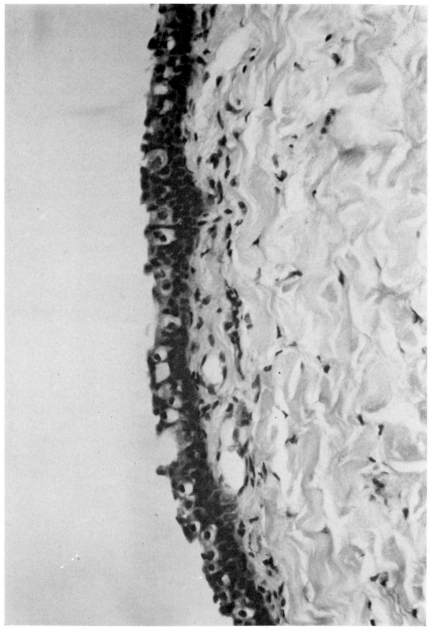

Figure 8-1b. Rabbit punctum, −50°C.

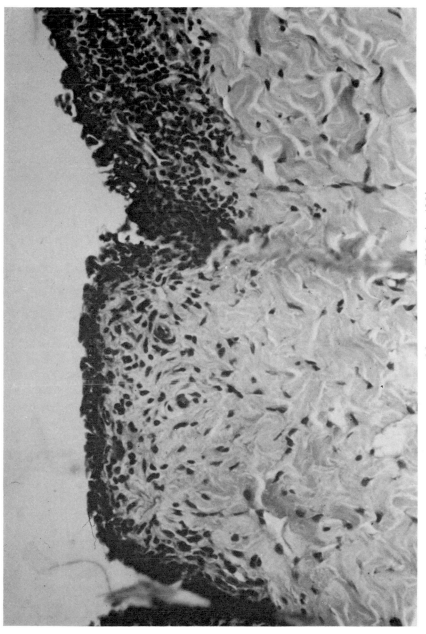

Figure 8-1c. Rabbit punctum, −70°C (×400).

TABLE 8-II

PATENCY OF RABBIT CANALICULI
EIGHT WEEKS FOLLOWING
CRYOSURGERY

Temperature (°C)	Number Observations	Cases Patent (%)
+37 (control)	2	100
–10	3	100
–30	3	67
–50	2	50
–70	3	33

ning and irregularity of the epithelium is observed with infiltration of chronic inflammatory cells in the substantia propria.

The effects of freezing on the canaliculus are shown in Table 8-II. Figure 8-2a shows the canaliculus of a control animal lined with columnar epithelium. No changes were evident following treatment to −10°C. One of three canaliculi treated at −30°C was obstructed (Figure 8-2b). The specimen demonstrated stenosis and loss of epithelium. After −70°C, occlusion of the canaliculus occurred as a result of marked fibrosis (Figure 8-2c).

This data indicates the rabbit punctum is generally resistant to freezing up to −70°C. The canaliculus is somewhat more susceptible to freezing, and obstruction can result with temperatures as low as −30°C. Animals treated at −70°C were more likely to show permanent stenosis of the canaliculi than of the punctae.

This apparent difference in susceptibility may be a result of the differences between the stratified, squamous epithelium of the punctum and the columnar epithelium of the canaliculi. The design of the experiment may also have been a factor. Punctae were frozen by direct application of the probe to the epithelium. The result was a high velocity freeze and thaw. To treat canaliculi, the probe was applied through the skin of the lower eyelid, and the thawing time was markedly prolonged. The effect of increased inflammatory reaction from cryonecrosis of adjacent lid tissue is speculative.

This study demonstrates the sparing effect of cryosurgery on the rabbit lacrimal excretory apparatus. It implies that lesions of the medial canthal region can be treated in the temperature range sufficient for tumor cryonecrosis without damage to the lacrimal drainage system. This is confirmed in the clinical series presented below.

Clinical Experience

Forty-five patients with forty-nine basal cell carcinomas of the eyelid were included in this prospective study. The patients ranged in age from 34 to 82, with an average age of 64. Periodic reexamination was conducted for two to forty-one months after treatment. The mean follow-up period was thirteen months. The protocol included a preoperative biopsy, treatment with liquid nitrogen, either circulating within a metal probe or as a direct spray, tissue temperature monitoring to −30°C in a double freeze-thaw cycle, and a postoperative biopsy at least six weeks after treatment. After some experience with various cryosurgical units, the most reliable method of freezing was found to be by direct spray of liquid nitrogen. Tissue temperature was monitored by a thermocouple placed below the deepest extent of the tumor (Figure 8-3). With small, superficial tumors, no difficulty was encountered in delivering an adequate dose either by spray or probe. It was often impossible to freeze large lesions to −30°C using a probe. Equipment failure was sometimes responsible for inability to deliver the desired temperature. In six instances, the temperature could not be lowered to −30°C. On one occasion this resulted in obviously inadequate treatment of a large tumor.

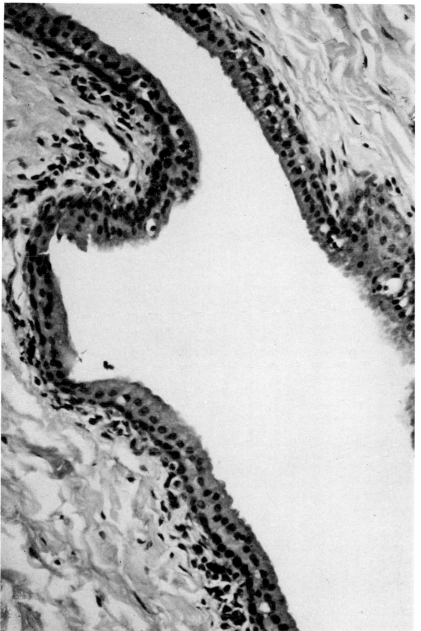

Figure 8-2a. Canaliculus, control rabbit (×400).

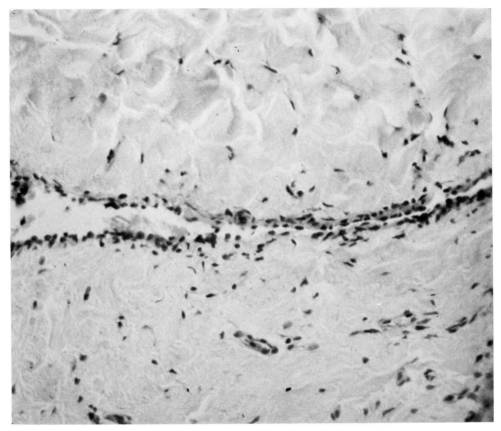

Figure 8-2b. Rabbit canaliculus, −70°C (×400).

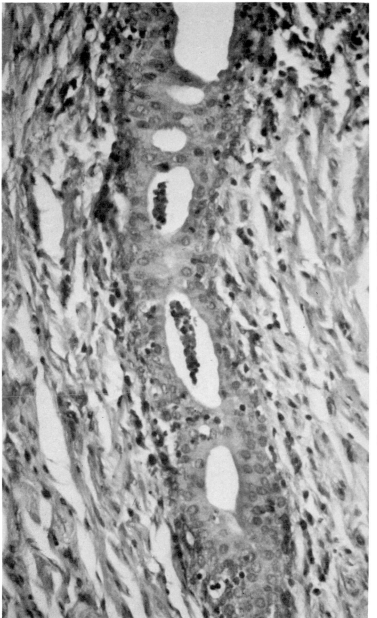

Figure 8-2c. Rabbit canaliculus, −70°C (×400).

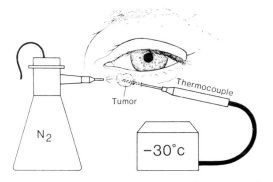

Figure 8-3. Cryosurgery spray technique with tissue temperature monitor.

Cases were not selected for cryosurgery on a random basis. Those patients with large, invasive or recurrent tumors were generally advised to have surgical excision. Those with small, clinically superficial lesions were encouraged to have cryosurgery. In several instances, surgery was advised but either the patient's general health was a contraindication or he refused to undergo a surgical procedure, and cryosurgery was performed. Of forty-nine lesions treated, there was one recurrence and one treatment failure. The recurrence occurred in a sixty-three-year-old man with a large (3×10 mm) lesion of the lower lid, below the lid margin. Initial treatment with liquid nitrogen was monitored to $-30°$C by subcutaneous thermocouple beneath the center of the tumor. Recurrence was observed seven months later at the medial border. Re-treatment by cryosurgery was successful. The treatment failure occurred in a seventy-nine-year-old man with an 8×8 mm tumor involving the lower punctum. Equipment malfunction resulted in what was believed at the time of surgery to be an inadequate freeze. Tissue temperature was lowered to $-26°$C only with difficulty, and the resultant necrotizing reaction did not destroy the tumor. Re-treatment three months later was successful, and the punctum remained patent.

Elderly patients, poor surgical risks and those who refuse surgery may be treated by cryosurgery. Three patients in this series were septuagenarians in poor health following major surgery. There was reluctance on the part of physician and patient to undertake further surgery or a prolonged course of treatment. Two additional patients had uncomplicated cryosurgery while receiving anticoagulation therapy. Multiple basal cell tumors of the eyelids were treated with cryosurgery in two patients with basal cell nevus syndrome. Both were grotesquely disfigured as a result of multiple operations.

Recurrence of basal cell carcinoma following irradiation creates a difficult therapeutic problem. Further radiation is usually not possible and, because of compromised vascularity, surgery is often inadvisable. Two patients in this series are successful examples of cryosurgery in post-radiation recurrence.

Nine of the forty-nine lesions treated were located in the region of the inferior punctum and canaliculus. The customary double freeze-thaw cycle to $-30°$C was employed. Epiphora was not noted, and in all instances, the patency of the lacrimal system was maintained as determined by irrigation.

Few complications were observed in this series of patients. Intense inflammatory reaction with hypertrophic scar formation occurred in one instance (Figure 8-4). Tissue temperature was monitored to $-30°$C, yet the patient had a severe reaction with pain, swelling, and ulceration persisting six weeks. Keloid formation ensued which gradually subsided, leaving a flat depigmented region one year after treatment. In several patients, swelling of the lid and cheek occurred, which subsided within two weeks. Keratoconjunctivitis and chemosis were observed infrequently. Transient entropion of the lower lid was noted in one patient. Loss of pigmentation and eyelashes was a consistent finding.

The primary consideration in the treatment of basal cell carcinoma is complete eradication of the tumor. This principle is especially important in tumors of the eyelids because of their potential for orbital and intracranial involvement. Complete eradication by cryosurgery relies, in part, on clinical estimation of the extent of the tumor. Large and morpheaform tumors are more likely to be incompletely removed by any technique which does not permit the borders to be histologically defined. Incomplete excision of basal cell tumors is often not associated with recurrence[19] and the same is true of cryosurgery. The disappearance of tumor following incomplete excision or cryosurgery has not been fully explained. An immunizing effect has been demonstrated after cryosurgery and may contribute to destruction of residual tumor cells.[20]

The cure rate in this series of forty-nine basal cell lesions of the eyelid treated by cryosurgery was 96 percent. Excluding one failure which was suspected at the time of surgery, the cure rate was 98 percent. These statistics are biased by selection of the most favorable patients for treatment and by the relatively brief mean follow-up period of thirteen months.

The proper use of cryosurgery is an effective technique for treatment of basal cell carcinoma in selected patients. It has special application to many of the multiple tumors that occur in patients with basal cell nevus syndrome. Surgery, radiation, chemosurgery, and cryosurgery each have specific advantages. The selection of any one modality should be determined by multiple factors, including the size and location of the tumor, previous treatment, the patient's age and general health, and the facilities available to the physician.

TREATMENT OF TRICHIASIS BY CRYOSURGERY

Trichiasis refers to the apposition of cilia against the globe. It may occur with or without entropion of the lid margin. The cilia involved may be eyelashes misdirected from their normal position or may be aberrant lashes originating from the posterior lid margin. In congenital hereditary distichiasis, an accessory row of cilia arise from the stomas of meibomian glands and are directed toward the cornea. Following injury or chronic irritation, trichiasis may result from inflammatory metaplasia. Lanugo hairs from skin may

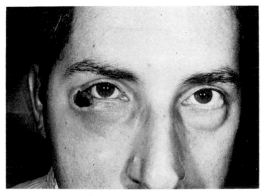

Figure 8-4. Ulceration following cryosurgery.

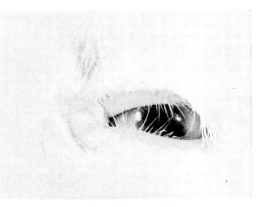

Figure 8-5a. Rabbit eyelid, −5°C.

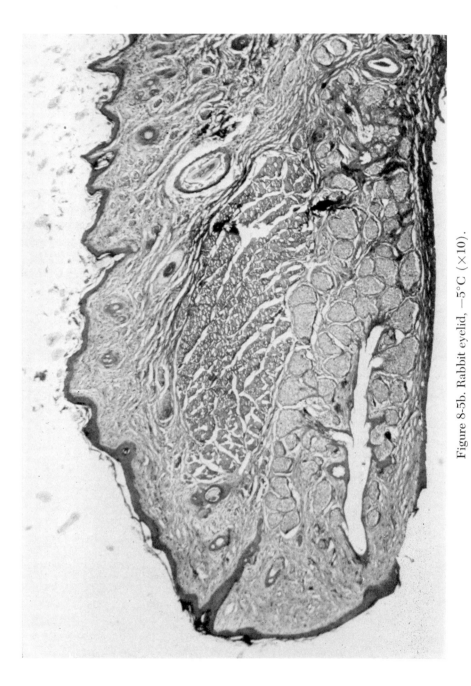

Figure 8-5b. Rabbit eyelid, −5°C (×10).

cause trichiasis following major reconstructive surgery of the lid margin. Chronic irritation from trichiasis, whatever its origin, is usually associated with considerable discomfort and may result in keratitis of varying severity.

Mechanical epilation provides only temporary relief from trichiasis. A permanent effect can be expected with proper use of electrolysis when only a few lashes are involved. For electrolysis to be effective, the base of the lash follicle must be destroyed by current from the electrode tip. It is an impossible task to direct an electrolysis needle to the base of an eyelash follicle when the aberrant cilia are of small caliber and exit in varying directions. In the case of multiple lashes, galvanic or diathermy current may result in cicatrization of the lid margin and induce additional aberrant cilia growth.

Many operations have been described for trichiasis. Tarsal fracture[21] is one of the simplest. Wedge resection of the eyelid can be used in certain situations. Transplantation of the ciliary bed[22] or transposition techniques[23, 24] are often complicated by trichiasis from lanugo hairs. Interposition of mucous membrane,[25] nasal septal cartilage,[26] or tarsoconjunctiva[27] is more effective. Mucous membrane grafting with tarsal advancement[28] is useful to prevent complications of graft contraction. These procedures are time consuming and involve surgical skills of varying complexity. The functional and cosmetic results are often less than optimum, and recurrence of trichiasis is a common problem.

Cilia Destruction

The basic construction of a hair follicle consists of a tubular invagination of epidermis surrounded by connective tissue. The cilia itself is produced from mitotic activity within the small mass of epidermal cells at the base of the follicle. During periods of growth, there is a high metabolic requirement to support mitotic activity and protein synthesis. During the growth cycle, connective tissue elements beneath the bulb of the follicle enlarge to form the highly vascularized dermal papilla. This structure is essential to the regrowth of hair, and its destruction results in permanent loss of the cilia.

Permanent destruction of hair can result from a variety of physical stresses, including freezing. Taylor[29] was first to describe loss of hair and pigmentary changes in rat skin following freezing. The relative sensitivity of eyelash follicles to the effects of freezing became apparent in the author's observations of patients after cryosurgery of the eyelid margin for tumors. As a side effect, it was noted that the eyelashes included in the frozen area failed to regenerate. It became obvious that cryosurgery could be used in the treatment of the vexing problem of trichiasis. To investigate this possibility, experiments were performed on rabbits, and this information was used in a clinical study of selected patients with trichiasis.

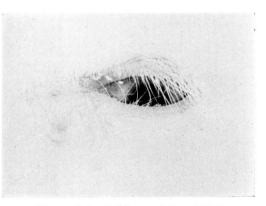

Figure 8-6a. Rabbit eyelid, −15°C.

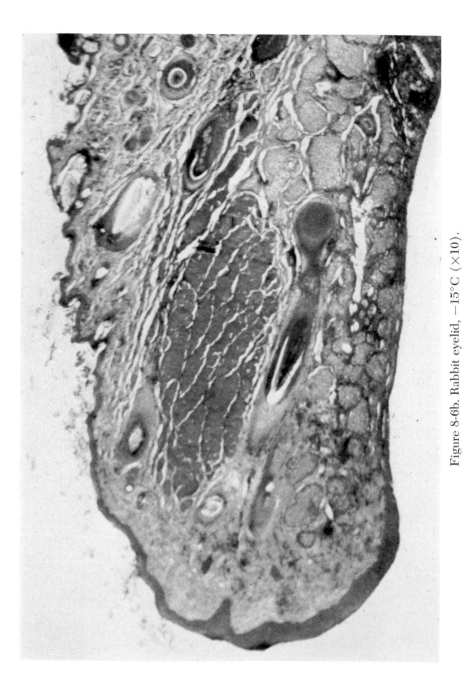

Figure 8-6b. Rabbit eyelid, −15°C (×10).

Experimental Eyelash Destruction

Eleven adult male and female albino rabbits were the subjects of one experiment.[30] A segment of the lid margin of both upper eyelids in each rabbit was treated by cryosurgery at one of four temperatures: $-5°C$, $-15°C$, $-30°C$, and $-70°C$. Tissue temperature was monitored by a thermocouple needle implanted 2 mm from the lid margin. Lesions were applied with a cryosurgical instrument utilizing liquid nitrogen circulating through a 5 mm diameter metal probe (Frigitronics CE-8). The probe was applied directly to the lid margin with minimum pressure. When the temperature fell to its designated level, the probe was removed. The tissue was allowed to return to body temperature, and the procedure was repeated.

After eight weeks, the animals were sacrificed, and specimens were taken through the eyelids in the region of treatment. Paraffin sections were stained with hematoxylin, eosin, and Masson's trichrome. Representative sections were matched with controls and compared for microscopic alteration in lid structure.

Lids treated at $-5°C$ retained a full complement of eyelashes and could not be distinguished from controls (Figure 8-5a, b). At $-15°C$, few clinical changes were apparent (Figure 8-6a). Some specimens demonstrated loss of cilia along the lid margin. Histopathology consisted of cutaneous and conjunctival epithelial hypertrophy. Minimal tissue disorganization was present. Occasional hair follicles showed vacuolization and disorganization in the bulb (Figure 8-6b).

Eyelids treated at $-30°C$ retained their general appearance, except that alopecia was present in the region treated (Figure 8-7a). Microscopic examination showed scar tissue formation in the deeper lid structures. Epithelial surfaces were hyperplastic and sebaceous glands were reduced in size (Figure 8-7b). The amount of reaction varied from one specimen to another. Regenerating cilia were observed in one specimen.

Severe reaction resulted from treatment at $-70°C$ (Figure 8-8a). Secondary infection was often present. Total loss of lashes occurred in all lids. In many specimens, lid structure appeared totally replaced by scar tissue. Sebaceous gland was frequently the only recognizable structure (Figure 8-8b).

Figure 8-9 depicts the relationship between the loss of cilia and magnitude of cryosurgery. A precise dose response curve cannot be made because of the technical difficulty in monitoring and controlling a reproducible cryogenic reaction. The results do indicate that temperatures colder than $-15°C$ are required for cilia cryoablation and that temperatures beyond $-70°C$ are unnecessary and undesirable. A temperature of $-30°C$ appears to be within the range at which irreversible follicular damage occurs, using the double rapid-freeze-slow-thaw technique. Most specimens treated at $-30°C$ appeared to have achieved the desired result of alopecia without observable alteration of lid structure or function.

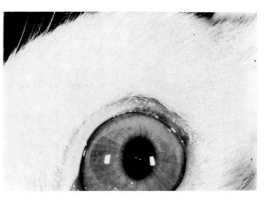

Figure 8-7a. Rabbit eyelid, $-30°C$.

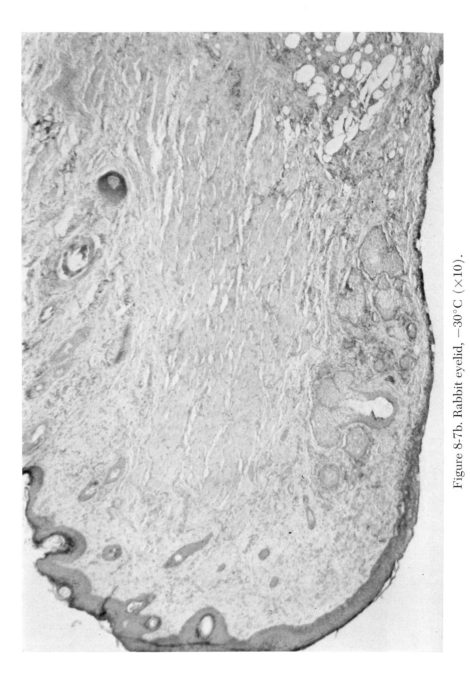

Figure 8-7b. Rabbit eyelid, −30°C (×10).

Clinical Experience

Forty-two patients were selected for cryosurgical destruction of aberrant eyelashes from a variety of causes and were followed for from two to twenty-eight months (Table 8-III). Cryosurgical lesions were generated by techniques using either liquid nitrogen or nitrous oxide. In all instances, a cutaneous application of coolant was made at the lid margin. Lidocaine (Xylocaine), 1 percent, with epinephrine, 1 : 100,000, was used routinely as an infiltration anesthetic. Liquid nitrogen was used either as a direct spray or within a contained system circulating through a metal probe. Adjacent skin surfaces were partially insulated by circumscribing the region with paper tape (3M® #1222). Tape was also used to secure a nonmetallic lid plate in the conjunctival fornix to protect the cornea (Figure 8-10). Nitrous oxide gas was used with a large diameter probe in a high-flow system (Cryomedics MT-650®) (Figure 8-11) or with an Amoils® retinal pencil.

Tissue temperature was monitored by a microthermocouple implanted in the epitarsal region 2 to 3 mm from the lid margin. Within seconds after the application of the coolant, the treated area appeared white and hard. A temperature of −20°C was usually attained in thirty to forty-five seconds, regardless of which coolant was used. Temperatures cooler than −20°C were sometimes difficult to obtain using nitrous oxide gas. Colder temperatures were readily obtained with liquid nitrogen spray. Spontaneous thawing to body temperature was allowed to proceed and sometimes required several minutes. During refreezing, the desired temperature was reached within ten to fifteen seconds.

Results

In successfully treated cases, a substantial effect was noted in the first twelve hours. This consisted of moderate edema, occasionally with bulla formation. When extensively treated, the eyelids were swollen closed in the first forty-eight hours. There was little pain associated, even with such severe responses. Maximum tissue reaction generally occurred between forty-eight and seventy-two hours. If treated cilia were grasped at this time, there was little resistance to epilation. After seven to ten days, the reaction subsided and more cilia shed spontaneously. Lashes which had been broken at the skin surface sometimes persisted in the root sheath for several months, although there was no resistance to their epilation. The reaction in most instances consisted of moderate tissue swelling and exudation on the cutaneous surfaces. A thin eschar often formed, but prompt surface epithelialization was the rule. The conjunctival surface was quick to recover and generally resistant to damage. There was minimal loss of tissue and cicatricial distortion of the lids were not observed (Figure 8-12a, b). In successfully treated areas, meibomian glands were no longer visible on slit lamp biomicroscopy.

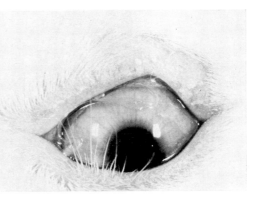

Figure 8-8a. Rabbit eyelid, −70°C.

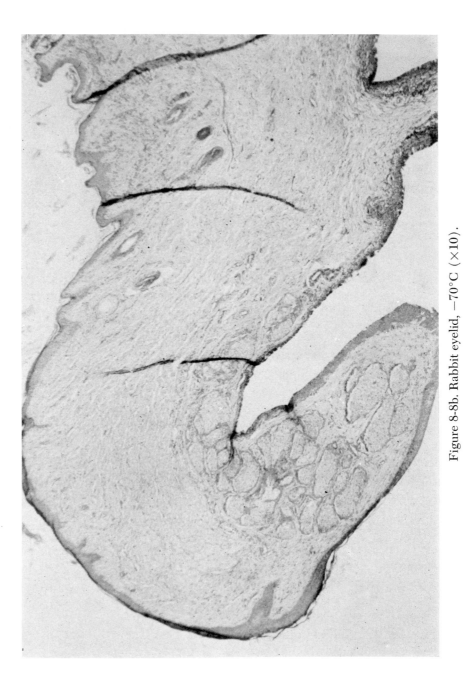

Figure 8-8b. Rabbit eyelid, −70°C (×10).

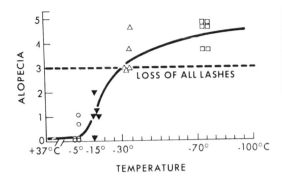

Figure 8-9. Alopecia as a function of attained temperature.

Loss of cutaneous pigmentation was a very frequent finding. Histopathologic correlation of these clinical observations was not available.

Complications

Recurrence was observed in five instances after the use of liquid nitrogen. In these cases, tissue temperature monitoring was not performed, and the end-point for the duration of application of the coolant was the appearance of the iceball. In two of these instances, a single freeze-thaw cycle, monitoring the tissue temperature to −20°C, was successful.

Notching of the lid margin occurred in

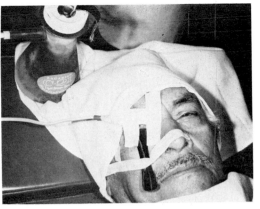

Figure 8-10. Patient prepared for liquid nitrogen spray.

one patient (Figure 8-13) following cryosurgery to −20°C, using nitrous oxide in a double freeze-thaw cycle.

Comments

Cryosurgical destruction of lash follicles is an effective technique for treatment of trichiasis. It is a significant improvement over existing methods which are difficult, laborious, and often ineffective. Cryosurgery is simple, effective, and well tolerated by the aged and infirm.

TABLE 8-III

ETIOLOGY OF TRICHIASIS TREATED
BY CRYOSURGERY

Idiopathic aberrant lashes	19
Misdirected normal lashes	4
Inflammatory metaplasia	4
Pemphigoid	4
Postoperative and traumatic	3
Chemical injury	2
Lanugo hair following lid reconstruction	2
Congenital misdirected	1
Hereditary distichiasis	1
Trachoma	1
Erythema multiforme	1

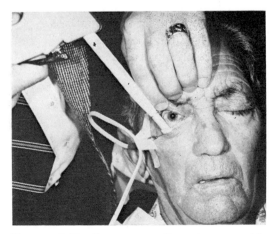

Figure 8-11. Preparation for nitrous oxide probe.

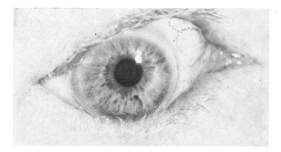

Figure 8-12a. Trichiasis, twenty years duration.

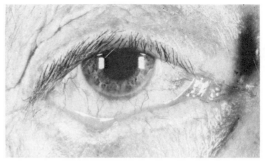

Figure 8-13. Notching of lid margin following cryosurgery.

Cryonecrosis is a complex biophysical reaction caused by changes in tissue solute concentration, ice formation and vascular stasis (see chapter one of this volume). The lesion is somewhat unique both in its pathogenesis and repair. Its benign healing process is due in part to specific tissue susceptibility to irreversible damage from freezing.[31-33] A spectrum of survival thresholds to freezing exists among the various cell types. Melanocytes are among the most sensitive cells to cryonecrosis. Yet, not all melanocytes react identically. Lynn[32] reported a difference in the susceptibility of perifollicular melanocytes between species and even between different types of hair on the same animal. Epidermal melanocytes were more resistant to the effects of freezing than those in hair follicles. Arrectores pilorum muscle and sweat

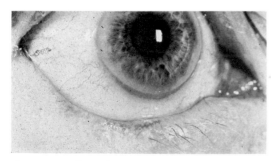

Figure 8-12b. Three months following cryosurgery.

glands were more cryosensitive than surrounding epidermis. Large blood vessels,[33, 34] peripheral nerves,[35] sebaceous glands,[33] fibroblasts, collagen, cartilage, and bone[36] are more resistant to cryonecrosis. The cause of this variability is not completely understood.

The hair follicle is relatively sensitive to the effects of freezing. Mild cryosurgical lesions are reported by Argyris[37] to stimulate hair growth in animals. This enhancement is similar to that following mild X radiation in mice, chemically induced damage, surgical wounds or damage of any sort, as long as it is of a critical intensity.[38] More intense cryosurgical lesions result in destruction of follicular melanocytes,[29] inhibition of DNA synthesis with temporary suppression of hair growth,[32, 39] and finally, complete destruction of the hair follicle. This range of effects has practical usefulness in the identification of laboratory animals by "freeze marking"[40] and as a biological marker of viability of cryopreservation of skin grants.[41]

Treatment with liquid nitrogen and nitrous oxide are equally effective in the destruction of aberrant eyelashes when adequate tissue temperature is achieved. Using the double rapid-freeze-slow-thaw cycle technique, the optimum temperature for

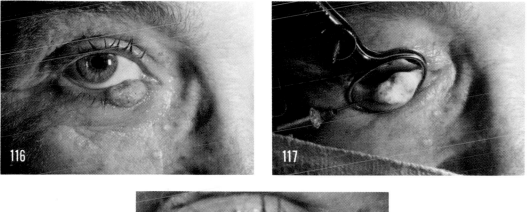

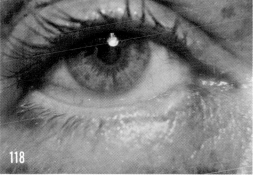

Plate 116. Keratoacanthoma.
Plate 117. Treated with liquid nitrogen.
Plate 118. Four weeks following cryosurgery.

destruction of lashes is −20°C. This temperature can easily be achieved with a high-flow nitrous oxide probe applied to the lid margin. The standard retinal pencil, when cooled by nitrous oxide gas, is also effective in small regions when the tissue temperature is properly monitored.

The critical temperature for cryonecrosis is determined by a variety of factors, including the cell type to be destroyed, velocity of freezing and thawing, and duration of freezing. Zacarian[42] has indicated −25° to −30°C as a clinically applicable range for cryosurgery.

The technique of double freeze-thaw cycles is customary in cryosurgery. It has been demonstrated that, in contrast to a single cycle, repeated freeze-thaw cycles release the enzyme content from lysosomes.[43] The effect of this and possibly other cellular alterations is marked enhancement of the necrotic reaction. In this series, lidocaine with epinephrine (1 : 100,000) was infiltrated into the eyelid prior to freezing. In addition to its anesthetic effect, it was believed that epinephrine would facilitate rapid freezing and slow thawing through vasoconstriction.[44, 45]

It is common practice to judge the adequacy of cryosurgery by physical appearance or duration of application of the coolant. Physical appearance is most deceiving as, once tissue has become frozen, its appearance does not change with further decline in temperature. A timed application is more likely to be successful, but variations in conductivity increase the likelihood of treatment failures. The recurrences reported in this series are all believed to be a result of inadequate treatment which was delivered in the manner just described.

This indicates the importance of achieving adequate tissue temperature for de-

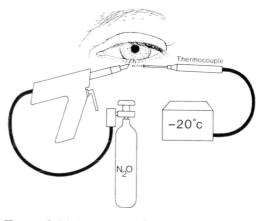

Figure 8-14. Nitrous oxide cryosurgery probe for trichiasis.

struction of the lash follicle. However, prolonged exposure to the coolant results in a larger area of damage, and tissue temperature colder than −30°C may be associated with necrosis and scar formation. To assure delivery of the minimum effective dosage, tissue-temperature monitoring is obligatory.

At the present time, the author's treatment of choice for trichiasis is cryosurgery, using a nitrous oxide gas unit (Cryomedics MT-650) with double cycle freezing to −20°C as measured in the region of the lash follicles (Figure 8-14). The convenience of nitrous oxide makes it more suitable for office procedures. Nitrous oxide systems, like liquid nitrogen probes, are *limited* in their capacity to freeze large tumors. Direct spray of liquid nitrogen is a *more effective* means to adequately freeze such lesions.

MISCELLANEOUS DISORDERS OF THE EYELIDS

Keratoacanthoma

Keratoacanthoma is a tumor of unknown etiology which rarely involves the eyelid. It is most often confused clinically and histologically with squamous cell carcinoma. The diagnosis may be suspected by its very rapid growth. It is typically dome-shaped with a central keratin core. Histologically, there is hyperplasia of prickle cells with orderly maturation to keratinization, but the features may be confused with low-grade, malignant, squamous cell carcinoma. Although self-limiting, keratoacanthoma may cause scarring and disfigurement of the eyelid.

Plate 116 shows a 7 × 5 mm tumor of the right lower eyelid margin which appeared six weeks earlier. Biopsy was consistent with keratoacanthoma. Liquid nitrogen was used to freeze the tumor to −30°C on two occasions (Plate 117). Four weeks after treatment, the tumor had completely regressed (Plate 118).

The effectiveness of cryosurgery for keratoacanthoma has previously been reported.[46] Because of its freedom from scarring, we consider cryosurgery the treatment of choice for keratoacanthoma of the eyelid.

Vernal Catarrah

Cryosurgery is useful in treating giant conjunctival papillae associated with vernal catarrah. Such papillae may be so large as to interfere with eyelid function. Application of a nitrous oxide cooled probe results in prompt involution of the papillae and relief of symptoms.[47]

REFERENCES

1. Krwawicz, T.: Intracapsular extraction of intumescent cataract by application of low temperature. *Br J Ophthalmol, 45:* 279, 1961.
2. Deutschmann, R.: Behandlung der netzhautablosung mit jodtinktur und kohensaureschnee. *Klin Monatsbl Augenheilkd, 94:*349, 1935.
3. Bietti, G. B.: Surgical intervention of the ciliary body; new trends for the relief of glaucoma. *JAMA, 142:*889, 1950.
4. Zacarian, S. A.: Cancer of the eyelid—a cryosurgical approach. *Ann Ophthalmol, 4:*473, 1972.
5. Brodkin, R. H., Kopf, A. W. and Andrade, R.: Basal cell epithelioma and elastosis: a comparison of distribution. In Urback, F. (Ed.): *The Biological Effects of Ultraviolet Radiation.* Oxford, Pergamon, 1969, pp. 581.
6. Older, J. J., Quickert, M. H. and Beard, C.: Surgical removal of basal cell carcinoma of the eyelids utilizing frozen section control. *Trans Am Acad Ophthalmol Otolaryngol, 79:*664, 1975.
7. Payne, J. W., Duke, J. R., Butner, R. and Eifrig, D. E.: Basal cell carcinoma of the eyelids. A long-term follow-up study. *Arch Ophthalmol 81:*553, 1969.
8. Birge, H. L.: Cancer of the eyelids. *Arch Ophthalmol, 19:*700, 1939.
9. Shulman, J.: Treatment of malignant tumors of the eyelids by plastic surgery. *Br J Plast Surg, 15:*34, 1962.
10. Rakofsky, S. I.: The adequacy of the surgical excision of basal cell carcinoma. *Ann Ophthalmol, 5:*596, 1973.
11. Aurora, A. L., and Blodi, F. C.: Reappraisal of basal cell carcinoma of the eyelids. *Am J Ophthalmol, 70:*329, 1970.
12. Einaugler, R. B. and Henkind, P.: Basal cell epithelioma of the eyelid: Apparent incomplete removal. *Am J Ophthalmol, 67:*413, 1969.
13. Wilder, L. W. and Smith, B.: Determination of the tumor margin in the excision of basal cell epitheliomas of the eyelids. *Ann Ophthalmol, 2:*887, 1970.
14. Tromovitch, T. A. and Stegman, S. J.: Microscopically controlled excision of skin tumors: Chemosurgery (Mohs); fresh tissue technique. *Arch Dermatol, 110:*231, 1974.
15. Beard, C.: Annual Review: Lids, lacrimal apparatus and conjunctiva. *Arch Ophthalmol, 57:*112, 1957.
16. Domonkos, A. N.: Treatment of eyelid carcinoma. *Arch Dermatol, 91:*364, 1965.
17. Lederman, M.: Discussion of carcinomas of conjunctiva and eyelid. In Boniuk, M. (Ed.): *Ocular and Adnexal Tumors.* St. Louis, Mosby, 1964, p. 104.
18. Bullock, J. D., Beard, C. and Sullivan,

J. H.: Cryotherapy of basal cell carcinoma in oculoplastic surgery: clinical and experimental considerations. To be published.

19. Gooding, C. A., White, G. and Yatsuhashi, M.: Significance of marginal extension in excised basal-cell carcinoma. *N Engl J Med*, 273:923, 1965.

20. Shulman, S.: Cryoimmunology. The production of antibody by the freezing of tissue. In Rand, R. W., Rinfret, A. P. and Von Leden, H. (Eds.): *Cryosurgery*. Springfield, Thomas, 1968, p. 78.

21. Ballen, P. H.: A simple procedure for the relief of trichiasis and entropion on the upper lid. *Arch Ophthalmol*, 72:239, 1964.

22. Jasche, E.: Jäche's operation fur entropium und distichiasis. *Klin Monatsbl Augenheilkd*, 11:97, 1873.

23. Watson, T. S.: On the treatment of trichiasis and distichiasis by a plastic operation. *Med Times*, 2:546, 1874.

24. Dianoux, E.: De l'autoplastic palpebrale par le procédé de Bayet. *Ann Ocul*, 2: 132, 1882.

25. Van Millingen, E.: De la guérison radical du trichiasis par le tarso-chiloplastie. *Arch Ophthalmol (Paris)*, 8:60, 1888.

26. Mustarde, J. C.: *Repair and Reconstruction in the Orbital Region*. Baltimore, Williams and Wilkins, 1966, p. 314.

27. Hughes, W. L.: *Reconstructive Surgery of the Eyelids*. St. Louis, Mosby, 1954, p. 103.

28. Beard, C.: Symposium—New York Society for Clinical Ophthalmology. *Am J Ophthalmol*, 53:149, 1962.

29. Taylor, A. C.: Survial of rat skin and changes in hair pigmentation following freezing. *J Exp Zool*, 110:77, 1949.

30. Sullivan, J. H., Beard, C. and Bullock, J. D.: Cryosurgery for treatment of trichiasis. *Am J Ophthalmol*: in press.

31. Athreya, B. H., Grimes, E. L., Lehr, H. B., Greene, A. E., and Coriell, L. L.: Differential susceptibility of epithelial cells and fibroblasts of human skin to freeze injury. *Cryobiology*, 5:262, 1969.

32. Lyne, A. C. and Hollis, D. E.: Effects of freezing the skin and plucking the fibres in sheep, with special reference to pigmentation. *Aust J Biol Sci*, 21: 981, 1968.

33. Horwitz, N. H., Goklap, H. and Randall, J.: *In situ* freezing of the common carotid artery and a sagittal sinus of the dog. *Cryobiology*, 2:233, 1966.

34. Gage, A. A., Fazekas, G., and Riley, E. E.: Freezing injury to large blood vessels in dogs. *Surgery*, 61:748, 1967.

35. Beazley, R. M., Bagley, D. H., and Ketcham, A. S.: The effect of cryosurgery on peripheral nerves. *J Surg Res, 16*: 231, 1974.

36. Torre, D.: Cryosurgery in dermatology. In Von Leden, H. and Cahan, W. G. (Eds.): *Cryogenics in Surgery*. Flushing, NY, Med Exam, 1971, p. 500.

37. Argyris, T. S.: Wound healing and control of growth of skin. In Montagna, W. and Billingham, R. E. (Eds.): *Advances in Biology, vol 5, Wound Healing*. New York, Pergamon, 1964, p. 231.

38. Argyris, T. S. and Chase, H. B.: Effect of X-radiation on differentiating hair follicles. *Anat Rec, 136*:445, 1960.

39. Johnson, B. E. and Daniels, F.: Enzyme studies in experimental cryosurgery of the skin. *Cryobiology*, 11:222, 1974.

40. Farrell, R. K. and Johnston, S. D.: Identification of laboratory animals: freeze marking. *Lab Anim Sci*, 23:107, 1973.

41. Billingham, R. F. and Medawar, P. B.: The freezing, drying and storing of mammalian skin. *J Exp Biol*, 29:454, 1952.

42. Zacarian, S. A.: *Cryosurgery of Tumors of the Skin and Oral Cavity*. Springfield, Thomas, 1973, p. 67.

43. Gill, W., Fraser, J. and Carter, D. C.: Repeated freeze-thaw cycles in cryosurgery. *Nature (Lond)*, 219:410, 1968.

44. Nell, H. B. and DeSanto, L. W.: Cryosurgical control of cancer: Effects of freeze rates, tumor temperatures, and ischemia. *Ann Otol Rhinol Laryngol*, 82:716, 1973.

45. Öhman, S.: Epinephrine induction of white hair in ACI rats. *J Invest Dermatol*, 53:155, 1969.

46. Zacarian, S. A.: *Cryosurgery of Tumors of the Skin and Oral Cavity*. Springfield, Thomas, 1973, p. 98.

47. Amoils, S. P.: *Cryosurgery in Ophthalmology*. London, Year Bk Med, 1975, p. 167.

CHAPTER NINE

The Treatment of Neoplasms of the Head and Neck With Cryosurgery

DANIEL MILLER, M.D., F.A.C.S.

THE UTILIZATION of cryosurgery for the destruction of neoplasms in the head and neck, as of 1976, is an established fact. The proper utilization of the technique of cryosurgery and its application by the oncologist depends on many factors. The technique which at first was rather imprecise has been improved upon over the past ten years, and the technical changes involved in the delivery of the freezing technique have made it a more precise tool. Its utilization requires a background knowledge of the medium used, whether it be freon, carbon dioxide, or nitrogen, and whether it be a liquid or a gas. The cryosurgeon must have a knowledge of the potential of the equipment he is using to deliver the cryogen. It also requires a knowledge of the depth of the tissue penetration resulting from the delivery of these specific heat extractors with the equipment that is being used.[1]

The therapeutic application of local cold dates back to the use of cold compresses in the treatment of compound skull fractures and infected wounds of the chest as early as 2500 BC. There have been variations of the technique over many centuries. The dermatologists in the late 1800's found it to be an effective measure for treatment of lesions of the skin. Dr. Irving S. Cooper[2-4] at St. Barnabas Hospital in New York City reestablished the value of cryosurgery as a therapeutic measure when he treated Parkinson's disease with cryosurgery to the thalamus. He also attempted to destroy localized brain tumors with this destructive tool. In 1959, Rowbotham et al.[5] attempted to eradicate tumors of the brain using circulating 90 percent alcohol through a freezing mixture of solid carbon dioxide and acetone.

The author's experience in the utilization of cryosurgery for tumors of the head and neck over the past decade includes treatment of more than 1,500 patients (Figures 9-1 and 9-2). The technique has been utilized in neoplasms of the oral cavity, sinuses, nasopharynx, middle and external ear, skin, the face, larynx, and exophytic lesions of the neck. The technique and the media used involved the freezing agent liquid nitrogen at $-196°C$ through an open spray tip as well as a closed cryoprobe. It has been found by cryobiologists that in order for the cryo-

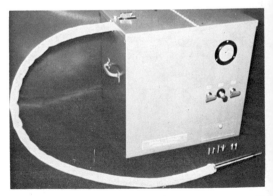

Figure 9-1. Brymill SP5 apparatus, self-pressurizing.

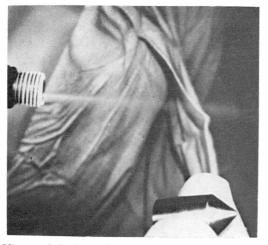

Figure 9-2. Liquid nitrogen stream, 1 mm, screw-on tip.

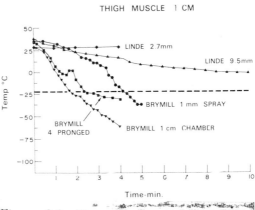

Figure 9-3. Tissue penetration studies for general section.

surgery to be effective as a destructive agent, the freezing temperature delivered to the cryotarget must reach at least −20°C. As a result of experimental evidence gained by studies of the depth of tissue penetration using various open and closed techniques with delivery of the liquid nitrogen, we foresaw a reasonably good tool for destruction of those areas desirous of being destroyed. We learned that the open spray of liquid nitrogen at −196°C penetrated much deeper and faster than the closed cryoprobe using the same medium of liquid nitrogen (Figures 9-3 and 9-4). However, the closed cryoprobe has proven to be a more precise method of application when compared with the spray.[6]

One must consider all tissues as heat-sinks and the application of the intense cold serves as a heat extractor with the resultant destruction of that tissue in which the temperature level is recorded as being below −20°C. Cryosurgery is preferably carried out with a large probe-to-tumor-ratio, if possible, approaching a 2 : 1 size relationship, or by the utilization of direct liquid nitrogen spray. Originally the closed cryoprobe was used for small tumors or in re-

gions in which the accessibility of the tumor was limited. However, direct liquid nitrogen spray has been applied in all areas of the head, oral cavity, and neck that are exposed or can be made exposed by surgery. Either the open or closed probe can be used for lesions which involve the sinuses, ear, or larynx.

Freezing may be described as the removal of pure water from solution and its isolation into biologically inert foreign bodies and ice crystals;[10] thereby the primary event is crystallization. The actual mechanisms of cell death are dehydration and concentration of electrolytes from removal of water from the solution, de-

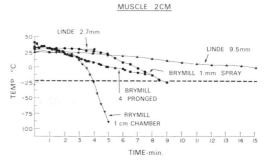

Figure 9-4. Tissue penetration studies for general section.

naturization of protein molecules, rupture of cell membrane, thermal shock, and vascular stasis. If at all possible, a thermocouple should be placed tangentially at the depth and/or the periphery of the area to be so treated as to be certain that −20°C is reached. If it is not reached, the probability of destruction of the cells despite the formation of a good ice ball is not a certainty. While thermocouples are not perfect as a monitoring system, they are still the *only tool which can tell the surgeon that he has destroyed the local tissue* without depending on the appearance of the ice ball produced.

The effect of cryosurgery on the various types of tissues confronted in the head and neck relates to the amount of heat and fluid content of the tissues. Large blood vessels are not destroyed with the application of the liquid nitrogen spray even at −50°C (recorded in the carotid artery of a dog), mainly because of the warmth of the blood passing through such large vessels. However, smaller vessels such as capillaries, veins, and arteries are readily destroyed. Bone acts as a barrier for short sprays of liquid nitrogen, but mucous membrane, periosteum, and muscle are easily and readily destroyed. There is probably as much or more destruction in the thawing process as during the rapid freeze process (Figures 9-5, 9-6, and 9-7).

It is possible to use cryosurgery for persistent tumors that have already received a full course of radiation therapy or radical surgery. It is another modality which can be used as a palliative measure for relief of pain. It has been found that sensory nerves concerned with pain located adjacent to the tumor are easily destroyed almost on contact with the freezing liquid nitrogen. However, pain is not eliminated if the nerve pathways are involved at some distance from the site of the cryolesion produced.

When the cryoprobe or cryospray produces a lesion, the ice ball forms and spreads and subsequently thaws; the resultant necrosis becomes apparent shortly thereafter and remains fairly well demarcated for from two to four weeks, depending on the size of the tumor and the amount of the tissue destroyed. There is sharp delineation of the surrounding tissue following the freeze. The cryosite becomes edematous with bleb formation about the gangrenous area produced by the freeze. The necrotic area grossly resembles the tissue response of an infarct seen with vascular ischemia. The cells look as though they have been irradiated when studied under the microscope. Usually when the slough demarcates with crust formation, it can be removed mechanically leaving a clean base that heals slowly. After a cryolesion is produced in the oral cavity or the larynx, epithelialization of the mucosa eventually occurs unless residual tumor remains, or unless there is secondary infection with a great lack of blood supply still persisting. A cryotreated skin area also epithelializes, but because melanocytes are very sensitive to freezing, the resultant cryolesion in the skin may leave a pale soft scar.

In order for a cell to function properly, there are many enzymes which are essential; some are stable, and others are relatively unstable during the freezing process. Many fast freezes and fast thaws result in injury to some enzymes but not necessarily their complete breakdown. Of course, without certain enzymes, the cell cannot function as before and, therefore, if sufficient of these enzymes can be destroyed by the cryosurgery, it is still another method for disrupting the inner chemical work-

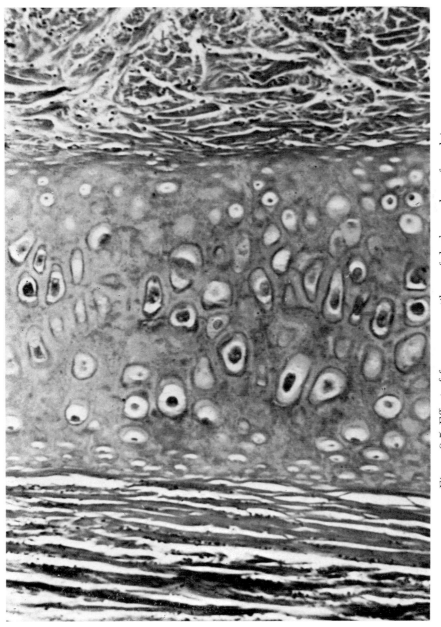

Figure 9-5. Effect of freeze on cartilage of dog's ear; loss of nuclei.

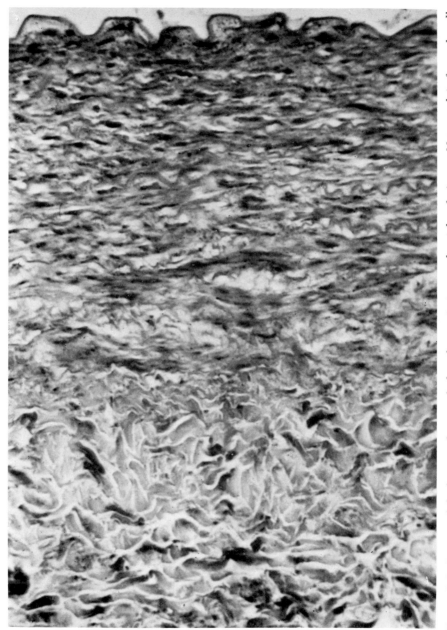

Figure 9-6. Section of dog's carotid artery before freeze; intima to the right of picture. Note nuclei of muscle cells beneath intima.

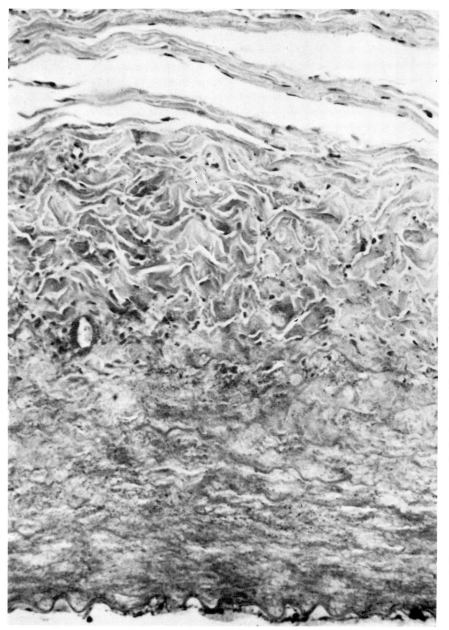

Figure 9-7. Postcryosurgery of dog's carotid artery. Note loss of muscle cell and maintenance of architecture.

ings of the cells involvement in cancer. As a result, both DNA and RNA may be affected rapidly, utilizing the modality of cryosurgery. Goldstein[7] et al. and Sherman and Kim[8] et al. have shown by electron microscopic studies that there are definitive changes in the mitochondria and chromosomes revealing these disruptive changes in the cell mechanism following freezing.

Cryobiologists are directing most of their attention towards the problem of preservation of tissues with freezing techniques rather than the effect of destruction. Their areas of investigation involving the work being done with preservation of viruses by freezing is of special concern to the otolaryngologist. Viruses are characterized by their ultramicroscopic size and their ability to propagate only within the living cells. They contain one type of nucleic acid and at least one antigenically active protein. The maintenance of viruses in a frozen viable state has become a practical procedure now used routinely in most virus laboratories. Over three hundred agents are kept at low temperatures in the Registry of Viral and Rickettsial Organisms in Washington, and can still be utilized after thawing. It is the slow freeze rather than the rapid freezing that allows the viruses to remain in a viable state. In view of the various reports of electron microscopic studies which suggest that inclusion bodies found in laryngeal papillomata may contain a virus producing these papilloma, they led us to the possibility of treating patients with viral-induced papillomata using cryosurgery. The clinical utilization of cryosurgery for treatment of papillomata viruses will be discussed later on in this chapter.[9]

Specific studies were made by the author on various tissues as to their relative response to cryosurgery. Cartilage is very easily destroyed by almost any open or closed probe in a very short time. Therefore, the utilization of cryosurgery near cartilage may involve cartilage destruction which may not be desired. Conversely, studies on the effect of liquid nitrogen on the common carotid artery have shown that the walls of the large vessels are not destroyed with intense freezing. The blood flow may be slowed within the artery temporarily. The nuclei of the muscle cells just below the intima undergo resolution, but the muscular architecture of the artery itself is maintained. However, when tumor which invades the wall of such an artery is destroyed, sufficient destruction of the wall of the artery may occur to allow for rupture of the vessel. Bone, which is more resistant to cryosurgery, can be used as a protective wall when treating a tumor over the cribriform plate of the ethmoid or in the tegmen of the mastoid. However, the destruction of a tumor involving bone, especially in a previously irradiated area, will allow for sequestration to take place over a period of time. This sequestration eventually extrudes itself and can easily be removed as long as a year or more later. Epithelium in the oral cavity or on the skull may regrow once the sequestrum has been removed. Mucous membranes very readily regrow over an alveolar ridge from which a sequestrum has been removed following tumor therapy with cryosurgery.

Studies of the cat larynx after cryosurgery and sacrifice of the animals two months later revealed adequate epithelial regeneration in all sections taken through the epithelial surfaces of the true cords. In some areas the respiratory epithelium regenerated in an epidermoid fashion. No areas remained bare as epithelialization was complete. There was some degeneration of muscle fibers with migration of the sarcolemmal nuclei to the center of the bundle with fibrosis and interstitial inflammatory infiltrates. There was frank replacement of the muscle cells in some areas. Of interest was the fact that Schwann cells were found proliferating in the nerve bundles in some areas. The cartilage remained in shape in spite of ischemic infarct type of necrosis noted in it. Studies on the dog larynx done recently will be reported later in this chapter.

TECHNIQUE OF APPLICATION

Most of the author's experience has been with utilization of the Brymill apparatus which has proven to be the most flexible unit for head and neck tumors. The large Brymill SP-5 unit contains a Dewar which is filled with liquid nitrogen and to which is attached a delivery arm. Many varied shapes and sizes, open and closed tips, can be easily screwed on to this delivery arm. It is a self-pressurizing unit and requires no electrical apparatus. The Kryospray unit is especially useful in treating tumors of the skin of the face, including the nose, eyelids, cheek, and auricle since it has varying open tip sizes ranging from 0.1 mm to 1 mm.

The Kryo laryngeal unit can be used through direct laryngoscopy with suspension, with or without a microscope. The attachment available, however, is a very small, 3.2 mm, thin, closed cryoprobe which covers about 8 sq mm of surface. Another probe is available in a 0.5 mm open spray tip which also can be utilized through a direct laryngoscope. More recently the increased square millimeter size of the probe tip was found to be necessary for greater area of destruction, but this has to be delivered through a tracheotome, observing it from above, and directing it to the vocal cord cryotarget area. A 45 sq mm surface application is now available for delivery to the larynx in this fashion.

When cryosurgery is applied in the form of a liquid nitrogen spray, the nontarget area of tissue should be protected from the target area with eight-ply petrolatum-impregnated gauze firmly pressed against the nontarget area periphery. Should the closed cryoprobe be used, only the area or tissue that might be touched with the cryoprobe as it passes to the target need be protected by the same eight-ply petrolatum-impregnated gauze or styrofoam. The Brymill tissue temperature monitor and thermocouple or the Linde temperature monitor and thermocouple should be placed in accessible areas for more precision in the application of the destructive freeze.

Depending on the amount of water content in the tissue being frozen, the ice ball may form readily. Should there be less water content, it will take longer to form. When using the closed probe, there is only an additional 20 percent increase in the size of the ice ball after the first minute. When the application of the freeze is discontinued and the cryolesion thaws, as it does within a minute or so, depending on the size of the lesion, the previously frozen area becomes red and pulpy-appearing, and then edematous with bleb formation, with a very thin reactive zone of perhaps the thickness of a few cells between the outline of the ice ball and the adjacent nontreated tissue. Utilizing between fifteen and twenty pounds of pressure on the SP-5 unit during the treatment, the duration time should not be counted until liquid nitrogen spray is applied directly to the target area; or when the closed probe is used, not until liquid nitrogen vents itself through the side of the delivery arm.

CRYOSURGERY TO THE ORAL CAVITY

Utilization of cryosurgery has been successful in many lesions of the oral cavity involving the tongue, floor of mouth, alveolar ridge, tonsillar fossa, buccal mucosa, or palate.[11] It has been particularly successful in the treatment of multicentric lesions of the oral cavity that are so common. As is well known, if a patient has a carcinoma of the palatine arch, he has a 15 percent chance of development of a second lesion in the same arch; and if a second palatine arch lesion does develop, there is about a 25 percent chance that a third primary carcinoma will develop. Because of the important fact that cryosurgery can be utilized in more than one course, it can be used repeatedly for these recurrent multicentric lesions in the oral cavity. It is especially helpful in elderly people for primary lesions or in residual lesions that have not been eliminated with radiation therapy or radical surgical resection. Oftentimes, more extensive surgery can be avoided in the elderly patients or in patients with poor medical status by the local application of cryosurgery for the primary lesion.

Therefore, cryosurgery can serve as a support for the other two better known and more often used modalities, sharp scalpel and radiation therapy. Cryosurgery has been used successfully locally for primary lymphomas of the tonsil; carcinoma of the oral cavity floor, tongue, and alveolar ridge, ameloblastoma of the alveolus; and verrucous carcinoma of the palate, tonsil and alveolar ridge.

One of the criticisms of cryosurgery is that one does not know whether tumor cells are left behind since the freeze depth is not as precise as one would like, and because one may not appreciate the exact extent of a lesion such as a carcinoma of the tongue and its frequently observed pseudopods. It is true that when surgical excision is done, histopathological studies of margins can determine whether there is or there is not residual tumor present. If the

lesion in the tongue is small, such as a T_1 lesion, it can be treated primarily by cryosurgery, local excision with scalpel, or by radiation therapy. However, small recurrent multicentric carcinomas of the tongue and the floor of the mouth can be treated successfully using cryosurgery after radiation therapy or surgical failure. These lesions can be treated with a curative goal as well as palliative measure. It is important to note that radiation when given in a full course cannot be safely used once again in a second course for the recurrent lesion. Therefore, cryosurgery may be the best follow-up modality available for postradiation failures since it can be used repetitively (Figures 9-8, 9-9, and 9-10).

A tumor such as the ameloblastoma which invades the alveolar ridge and may produce large cavities, often necessitates resection of the mandible. There is a high rate of recurrence unless the mandible is resected rather than conservatively scooping out the tumor in the cavity produced. Several patients have been treated with cryosurgery: After the conservative removal of the bulk of the tumor, the liquid nitrogen is delivered to the resultant

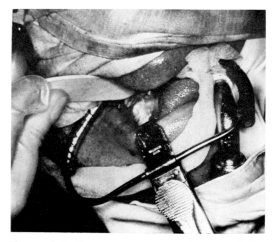

Figure 9-8. Freeze—open spray into tonsil for radiation failure of lymphosarcoma.

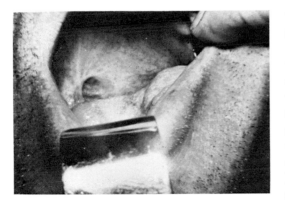

Figure 9-9. Postcryosurgery to radiated failure of lymphosarcoma tonsil. No local persistence or recurrence.

cavity through a 1 mm spray tip. The cavity subsequently fills in with new bone and fibrous tissue, and the mucous membrane regrows covering the defect. Treatment of leukoplakia in the oral cavity using cryosurgery has been found to be quite satisfactory by Goode and others utilizing superficial application of the cryosurgery with the closed or open probe, preferably

the closed probe. Mucous membrane easily regrows to cover the healed defect.

Gage[12] has reported a high rate of cure with cryosurgery for carcinoma of the oral cavity using a closed probe. However, until more experience is gained, one must consider the more proven modalities of sharp surgery or radiation or a combination of both for most carcinomas of the oral cavity before deciding on cryosurgery. However, for those patients with serious medical or logistic problems, cryosurgery can certainly be used as a primary modality in the treatment of early carcinoma of the oral cavity, and it certainly can be used effectively in radiation failure lesions or multicentric lesions.

So-called benign tumors such as lymphangioma and cavernous hemangioma can be treated successfully with cryosurgery in the oral cavity, especially since one may use the cryosurgery in more than one course. One hesitates to destroy an entire tongue in order to eradicate a cavernous hemangioma or lymphangioma, but sufficient de-

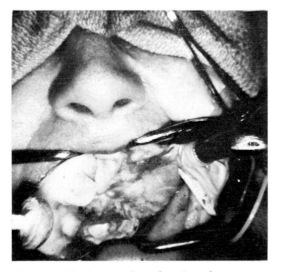

Figure 9-10. Copper disc closed probe to postradiation failure carcinoma of floor of mouth extending to mandible in elderly lady. Freezing process and beginning thaw.

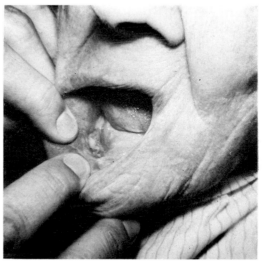

Figure 9-11. Beginning sequestration postoperative for radiation failure of carcinoma of floor of mouth and alveolus in elderly lady.

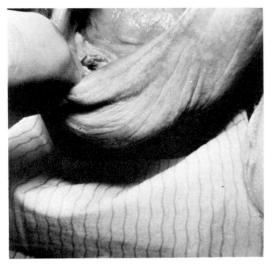

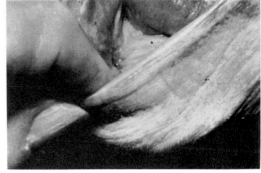

Figure 9-14. Healed mucosa over mandible and floor of mouth two and one-half years postcryosurgery of radiated failure in elderly lady.

Figure 9-12. Sequestration almost ready to be extracted postcryosurgery for radiated failure of carcinoma of floor of mouth and alveolus.

struction with subsequent fibrosis of the tissue adjacent to the tumor can be obtained by the use of the closed cryoprobe approach at intervals of many months for each course.

When treating recurrent carcinoma of

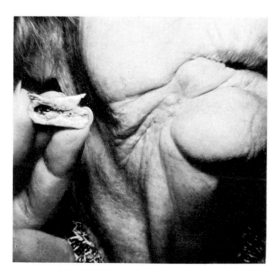

Figure 9-13. Note sequestration postcryosurgery in radiated failure of carcinoma of floor of mouth and alveolus in elderly lady.

the floor of the mouth that extends to the alveolar ridge following radiation therapy failure, one can expect a sequestration of the alveolar ridge (Figures 9-11, 9-12, 9-13, and 9-14). However, this sequestration can be removed as an office procedure many months later. There may be so much involvement of the periosteum due to the tumor that the necessity for deep penetration of the freeze may produce a pathologic fracture of the mandible later on. The patient and his family should be made aware of this possibility. However, it can be managed. Since verrucous carcinoma tends not to metastasize regionally, these are very adequately treated with cryosurgery in the oral cavity as primary management. Thus, the value of cryosurgery as a modality of treatment for tumors of the oral cavity has grown with increased experience.

CRYOSURGERY TO TUMORS OF THE NASOPHARYNX

One of the more serious tumors of the nasopharynx is that of nasopharyngeal angiofibroma. Excessive bleeding from such tumors even from simple biopsy can lead to great morbidity. Cryosurgery has been an effective modality in the removal of such tumors because of two factors:[13] (1) Many of the smaller vessels such as arteries and veins are thrombosed or undergo complete vascular stasis during the period in which a freeze is applied to the target tumor; (2) The adherent qualities of the freeze on the target area of the tumor produced by applying a closed cryoprobe allows a handle on the tumor. The tumor is usually quite rubbery and if it breaks during its delivery, profuse sudden hemorrhage usually occurs. This handle technique enables one to more easily deliver the tumor with its many lobulations via a transpalatal or transantral approach or a combination of both using finger dissection or electrocautery or even scissor dissection utilizing the freeze attached probe to tumor as a handle. Should several pseudopods still remain, the cryoprobe can be reapplied to those areas to slow up or to stop the bleeding and once again remove the residual tumor in a similar fashion. Cryosurgery of itself cannot destory an angiofibroma unless it has a very small pedicle.[14, 15] This is not the usual finding, however. The resultant reduction in loss of blood during removal of such a tumor has been a gratifying adjunctive help using this handle technique. More recently, the use of embolization of Gelfoam® through an angiographic catheter two to three days prior to surgery of the angiofibroma and the subsequent utilization of the cryosurgery handle technique after sufficient exposure of the tumor surgically, has definitely reduced the morbidity of the operative procedure.

The use of cryosurgery in nasopharyngeal cancer is limited. The recurrent primary tumor which has already undergone a full course of radiation therapy can be treated palliatively to rid the patient of gross tumor, bleeding, slough, odor, and subsequent pain. It may be used in successive courses as deemed indicated. However, should the tumor have extended through the base of the skull, cryosurgery as a modality for palliation would be greatly limited and better not applied.

CRYOSURGERY FOR TUMORS OF THE EAR

The past record of cure rates for cancer of the middle ear has been poor indeed. Most patients with ear cancer who have been referred for help with cryotherapy have already had surgery and/or radiation therapy, with facial nerve paralysis and invasion of bone, often with other intracranial involvement through the jugular foramen. Patients who have been forced to take considerable morphine for relief of pain were treated using the open spray with liquid nitrogen at −195°C. Four out of six patients with middle ear cancer have been free of disease (Figures 9-15, 9-16, and 9-17), the longest over five years by using the open spray.[16] Therefore, cryosurgery has been effective in the treatment of

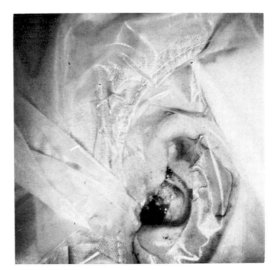

Figure 9-15. Precryosurgery for carcinoma of ear.

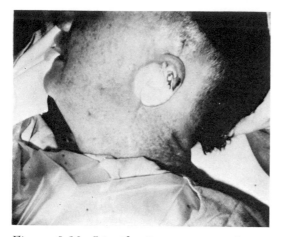

Figure 9-16. Liquid nitrogen spray, 1 mm aperture to ear cancer.

malignant tumors of the ear. One must of necessity produce a facial nerve paralysis if it is not already present. Destruction of the inner ear with loss of vestibular function also must take place unless it has already been destroyed by the tumor. The tumor area to be treated should be exposed as much as possible through conventional mastoid surgery prior to the delivery of the liquid nitrogen. However, the tegmen should be preserved whenever possible, otherwise the open spray[11] when applied through to the dura would cause brain destruction and its associated cerebral problems. A flat disc closed cryoprobe can be applied to that area of the tegmen to obtain minimal destruction of the cryotarget site.

Chemodectomas of the middle ear can be kept under control and occasionally completely destroyed using cryosurgery. Using a closed cryoprobe, the smaller probe produces less destruction but it also prevents facial nerve paralysis and labyrinthitis after its application. Several such patients have been maintained with cryosurgery given at intervals of three to five years, keeping an extensive tumor under control with a minimum of symptoms.

More recently, embolization of the feeding vessels to the chemodectoma with Gelfoam by angiocatheter, with follow up in a few days by cryosurgery of the tumor, has added to the success of control. The other alternative, of course, for treatment in these tumors is X-ray therapy and/or subtotal temporal bone resection with its high morbidity rate. Cryosurgery can be used in conjunction with either or both of them.

Recurrent carcinomas of the auricle can be treated palliatively as well as primarily with cryosurgery and may be used in repeated courses determined by the size of the regrowth of the carcinoma. Even if the tumor of the auricle extends to the scalp where it invades the cortex of the parietal bone and temporal bone, it can be eradicated with the use of cryosurgery. Subsequent regrowth of epithelium covers the denuded bone after a period of many months. One must keep in mind that cartilage is very sensitive to cryosurgery and is easily destroyed in the event that one is attempting to preserve some of the auricle during the treatment of a small lesion of the auricle with cryosurgery. The drum should also be protected with petrolatum gauze, when only the auricle is desirous of being treated, to prevent complications to

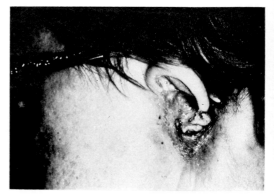

Figure 9-17. Postcryosurgery of ear with sequestrum; 5 year cure.

the middle and inner ear. Cryosurgery using the Kryospray unit has now been used successfully in more than one hundred carcinomas about the auricle on an outpatient basis, rather than the previously common use of wedge resection or radiotherapy.

CRYOSURGERY FOR TUMORS OF THE NOSE AND SINUSES

As in all areas about the ears, nose, and throat, the utilization of cryosurgery as a treatment for tumors in the nose or sinuses requires exteriorization of the target areas to be so treated. For example, if a tumor of the nasal vestibule is the cryotarget, a partial lateral rhinotomy with elevation of the alar region must be accomplished prior to the administration of the liquid nitrogen. One must also recall that cartilage is readily destroyed when utilizing destructive freezing in this area. Should maxillectomy be required for a carcinoma of the antrum, with residual disease being present in resection margins or recurring later, cryosurgery can be used. In order for cryosurgery to be utilized successfully, sufficient room is required to get to the residual tumor, as by a prior orbital exenteration. This is especially true if there is residual disease in the greater wing of the sphenoid or ethmoid region. The probability of optic nerve destruction from the cryosurgery must be considered if there is an attempt to preserve an orbit that is close to the presence of a recurrent tumor. Eight out of ten patients with recurrence in the ethmoid-sphenoid area have been free of this recurrence after cryosurgery. All patients had been previously treated with radiation, surgery or both. The sequestrated residual ethmoid bone and cribriform plate area eventually comes away easily followed by regrowth of mucous membrane covering fibrous tissue over the area

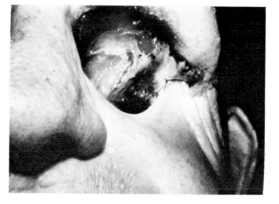

Figure 9-18. Two months postcryosurgery to greater wing of sphenoid residual carcinoma postmaxillectomy and orbital exenteration, post preoperative x-radiation.

of the dura. One such patient is now eight years post cryosurgery following recurrence after combined radiation therapy and surgery for the tumor (Figures 9-18 and 9-19). The cryosurgery can be delivered at the time of the primary surgery of orbital exenteration and maxillectomy if residual inoperable disease is found, or if discovered later, it may be treated as a sec-

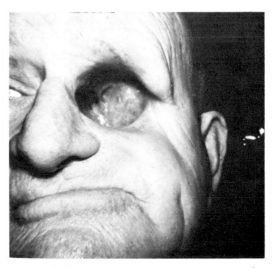

Figure 9-19. Six years postcryosurgery cure for residual carcinoma in greater wing of sphenoid postradiation, maxillectomy, and orbital exenteration.

ond procedure. Should the tumor have invaded the skull through the optic foramen or the other foramina, cryosurgery will not reach intracranially and may prove to be of very little palliative help. One should be cognizant of the proximity of the optic nerves in the region of the chiasm when utilizing liquid nitrogen spray to an open orbital-maxillectomy cavity. One can prevent complications in the remaining good eye by the use of eight-ply petrolatum-impregnated gauze as protection of the nontarget areas, an important part of the technique.

CRYOSURGERY FOR THE TREATMENT OF CARCINOMA OF THE SKIN OF THE FACE

It is possible to use the modality of cryosurgery successfully with a 98 percent chance for cure as primary treatment for squamous cell carcinoma or basal cell carcinoma of the skin about the head. Zacarian[17, 18] has reported over 1,000 such patients so treated with a similar high cure rate. The utilization of the Kryospray unit or the closed copper disc probe has been very effective in the management of these lesions. It can usually be done as an outpatient procedure with local anesthesia. Careful protection of the nontarget area is indicated using windowed styrofoam such as found in coffee cups. Cryosurgery is a particularly useful modality in patients who present with lesions near the alar region, inner canthus, eyelids, auricle, or other areas that usually would require a pedicle flap to close a large surgical defect after scalpel excision of the lesion. Recently, it has been used to deepilate lids that, due to disease such as pemphigus erratic regrowth of the tiny hairs in the presence of scarred lip, cause corneal irritation and pain.

Since cryosurgery can be used in many courses and for multiple lesions in nearby areas, and radiation can only be used one time in the area involved, it would suggest that cryosurgery is a very effective modality for primary treatment of these lesions. It often mitigates need for hospitalization and a general anesthesia, thereby reducing the expense of hospital care. Cryosurgery to skin lesions of the face mitigates the need for pedicle flaps, grafts and radiation in many such cases.

Of interest is the fact that edema of the eyelid may take place easily in face lesions treated with cryosurgery if the lesion treated is located within 6 cm of the eye. This edema takes place within a few hours and may last one to two days. It may be due to a local protein toxicity or lymphatic obstruction, temporarily, in the area of the freeze. The patient should be warned of this probability (Plates 119-122).

CRYOSURGERY OF THE LARYNX

The attempt to cure carcinoma of the larynx and yet maintain a semblance of voice production is the aim of all otolaryngologists. Various surgical procedures have been devised, as well as the utilization of radiation therapy, in an attempt to attain this goal. Cryosurgery to the larynx[21, 22] as a modality for the preservation of the voice and elimination of the tumor has reached a point of clinical application which indicates possible greater use of this

TABLE 9-I

T₁ CANCER OF THE LARYNX

Number treated with cryosurgery (1968-1973)	17
Post-X-radiated failures	14
Primary T₁ carcinomas	2
Granular cell myoblastoma recurrent surgical failures	1
Erroneous preoperative classifications	4
Larynges preserved (duration of follow up 1-5 years)	13

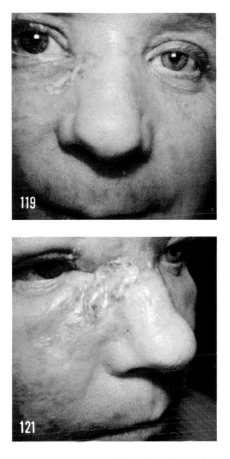

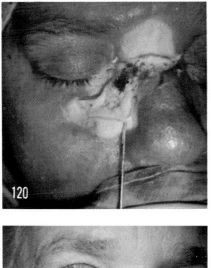

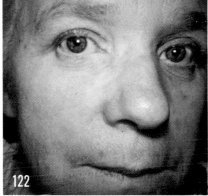

Plate 119. Post radiated basal cell carcinoma near inner canthus.
Plate 120. Thawing after freeze using nitrogen spray with 1 mm aperture. Note thermocouple.
Plate 121. Few days post cryosurgery with fibrin covering.
Plate 122. Three months post cryosurgery for basal cell carcinoma. Note some loss of pigment in skin, soft scar.

modality in the future. This might be considered as an attempt at a conservation procedure through destructive freezing. There is an 89 percent cure rate for a T_1 N_o carcinoma of the larynx with radiation, and salvage of an additional 6 percent with total laryngectomy, making a 95 percent cure rate for this disease.[19] Since most of the salvage accomplished is with a total laryngectomy, it was felt there was a possibility of preserving the larynx and eliminating the disease in the 11 percent radiation failure patients with return of persistent disease by cryosurgery (Table 9-I). The author's earlier clinical report revealed that thirteen out of seventeen patients so treated were free of disease from one to five years, with subsequent recurrence in two others necessitating total laryngectomy.

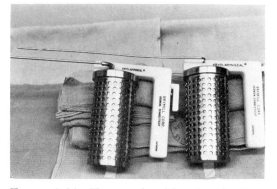

Figure 9-21. Kryo probe (closed tip). Kryo probe (open tip) for larynx via laryngoscope.

The technique used originally was through the direct laryngoscopy with Lewy suspension (Figures 9-20 and 9-21) using the small 3.2 mm Brymill cryoprobe for T_1 lesion failures. Although one could

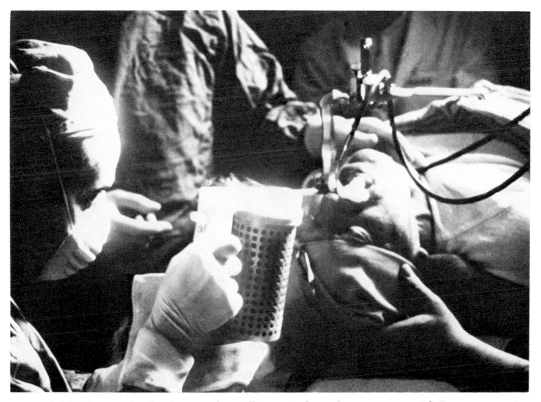

Figure 9-20. Kryo probe for laryngeal papilloma via direct laryngoscopy with Lewy suspension.

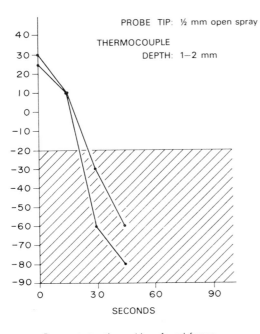

UNIT: KRYOLARYNGEAL ₜₘ

PROBE TIP: ½ mm open spray

THERMOCOUPLE
DEPTH: 1–2 mm

Demonstrates the rapid profound freeze
at least 2 mm tissue depth accomplished
with liquid nitrogen spray

Figure 9-22. Kryolaryngeal Unit freeze chart.

not desirous of destruction was not entirely satisfactory.

As a result of a 2-phase project[20] with an assessment of time (Figures 9-22 and 9-23), temperature, and freeze depth relationships with different sized closed cryoprobes via a larynx splitting operation on large dogs, the author was able to determine by thermocouple studies what would occur with specific variations in surface-sized closed cryoprobes in terms of tissue destruction. He was also able to determine the probability of the nondestructive effect of the lamina of the thyroid cartilage depending on the size of the contact probe and the duration of the application. Double freeze applications were essential to produce the most efficient destruction.

As a result of this study, it became apparent that if one were to increase the 3.2 mm probe to 5 mm it would make it 20 sq

produce a destructive freeze, the actual size of the cryolesion produced was small because of the necessity for using the thin 3.2 mm cryoprobe through the laryngoscope. From this experience it was felt that lesions larger than a T_1 lesion be attained under proper visualization. As a result of a study done in 1974, Mulvaney and Miller found evidence which solves some of the technical details necessary to adequately treat larger recurrent carcinomas of the larynx with cryosurgery. The use of more penetrating open spray in the larynx with liquid nitrogen through a laryngoscope often destroys more tissue than desired. Good vision was disturbed by the smoke vapor produced by the freeze. Petrolatum-impregnated gauze used to protect the tissue

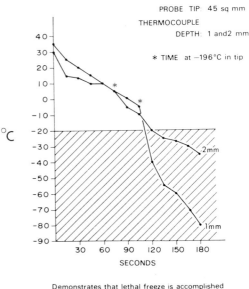

UNIT: BRYMILL SP5

PROBE TIP: 45 sq mm
THERMOCOUPLE
DEPTH: 1 and 2 mm

* TIME at –196°C in tip

°C

Demonstrates that lethal freeze is accomplished
within 1 minute of probe tip temperature
reaching –196°C to tissue depth at least 2 mm

Figure 9-23. Brymill Unit freeze chart.

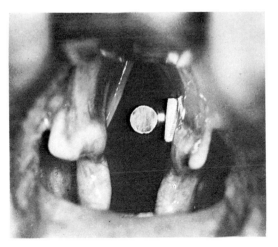

Figure 9-24. Note cryoprobe against vocal cord. Styrofoam not inserted at this point.

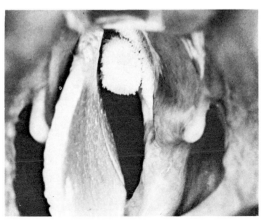

Figure 9-26. Freeze of vocal cord with cryoprobe pressed on it. Note styrofoam paddle protecting opposite nontarget vocal cord.

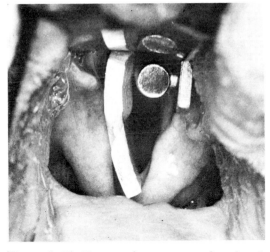

Figure 9-25. Note prefreeze cryoprobe placed against vocal cord with styrofoam paddle protecting opposite vocal cord.

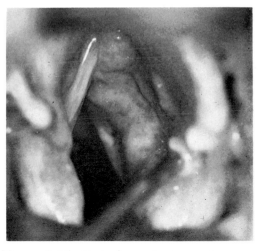

Figure 9-27. Forty-five minutes postcryosurgery freeze via tracheostomy showing edema of cord and subglottic region.

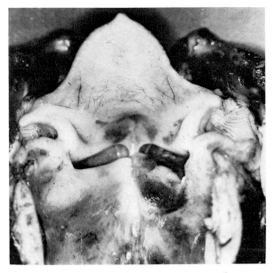

Figure 9-28. Five days post cryoprobe one minute application to vocal cord with 45 sq mm closed tip.

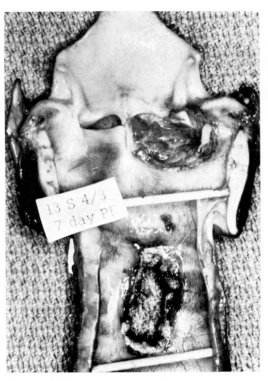

Figure 9-30. Appearance of postcryosurgery to vocal cord seven days later in canine. Note tracheostomy below 45 mm square surface closed cryoprobe used.

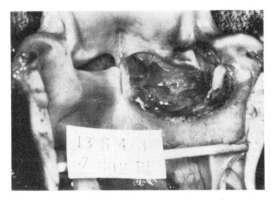

Figure 9-29. Note close up view of canine larynx seven days postcryosurgery with 45 sq mm closed probe.

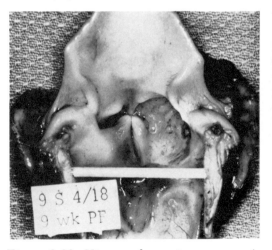

Figure 9-31. Nine weeks postcryosurgery in canine larynx; one minute application of 45 sq mm closed cryoprobe.

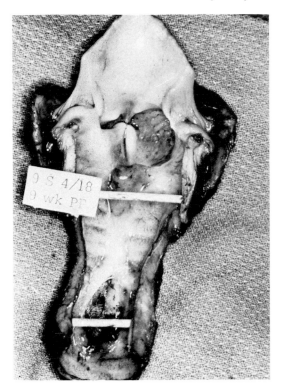

Figure 9-32. Nine weeks postcryosurgery in canine showing tracheostomy. One minute of closed cryoprobe application with 45 sq mm probe tip.

mm in surface area. The delivery area of the probe tip increases by the square of the radius. Subsequently, a 45 sq mm surface rectangular closed cryoprobe was developed and definitely extended the perimeter of the tissue desirous of destruction.

The second phase of the project to determine the practical considerations involved in creating cryolesions through a tracheostomy with good visual control via a direct laryngoscopy from above was then evaluated. This technique, which has since been successfully applied clinically, included the utilization of a tracheostomy through which the cryoprobe was passed to the proposed target area on the vocal

cord desirous of destruction, visualizing this through the direct laryngoscope with suspension. A styrofoam paddle was fashioned and inserted from above to protect the opposite nontarget vocal cord.

With this technique, an entire vocal cord down to the cartilage (Figures 9-24 through 9-32) has been destroyed and with no significant destruction of the cartilage of the lamina itself. Swallowing was not interfered with. It took about four weeks for the dog's larynx to heal. The tracheostomy can be decannulated and closed in the human patients so treated within four to five days as a rule. The liquid nitrogen is passed through the closed cryoprobe via the SP-5 Brymill unit. As a result of the studies in the dog, one can predict the amount of depth of destruction with much greater precision. This technique appears to have significant promise. A double course of one minute each of cryosurgery is used, beginning the count only when the liquid nitrogen has begun to vent from the delivery arm. The 45 sq mm surface area cryoprobe can completely destroy one vocal cord after this double freeze cycle. Time and experience will determine the size of the tumor of the larynx that can be so treated.

The use of cryosurgery for *papilloma* of the larynx has revealed its efficacy.[9] However, it is not the complete answer. A combination of excision of the papilloma-

TABLE 9-II

PAPILLOMA OF LARYNX

Number of patients treated with cryosurgery (1968-1973)	21
Adults treated	15
Children treated	6
Number of direct laryngoscopies and cryosurgeries	55
Number free of disease up to 5 years	16

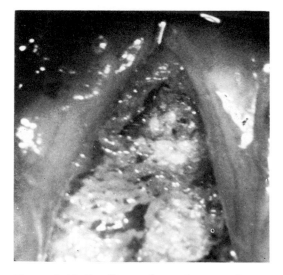

Figure 9-33. Papilloma of anterior commissure. Microlaryngoscopy showing petrolatum gauze in subglottic region to protect against liquid nitrogen spill over from Kryospray through laryngoscope.

ta, cryosurgery, and microcautery through the direct laryngoscopy at the same procedure has proven to be the best treatment to date. Laser surgery is also of great value in treating these stubborn benign tumors.

In a series of twenty-one patients so treated, it has taken about one to five such treatments to eradicate most of the patients of their papillomata (Table 9-II). Occasionally, some of the patients have needed seven to eight courses at three to eleven month intervals. What is of most importance is to not wait until a larger number of papilloma reform, but to repeat the cryosurgery to the larynx shortly after the onset of new lesions.

When treating a child with cryosurgery, tracheostomy should always be performed because of the resultant ease of edema. When an adult larynx is treated in this fashion, tracheostomy is rarely if ever necessary (Figure 9-33).

COMPLICATIONS OF CRYOSURGERY

Protection of the tissue not desirous of being destroyed involved the use of eight-ply petrolatum-impregnated gauze walling off the areas away from the tumor not to be treated. Cryosurgery using the open spray is not as precise a tool as one would desire; when treating anatomically irregular areas involving various ridges, undesired destruction of tissue may result. Therefore, the choice of the aperture size for delivery of the liquid nitrogen is important. This ranges from 0.25 to 1 cm. The 0.1 mm spray aperture is probably the most commonly used and can reach the depth desired for thin but wide tumors. Using a thermocouple inserted into the periphery of the target area desired of destruction, one can decide the duration of treatment. Usually, about two to three minutes of freezing, repeated by a second freezing after the first ice ball has thawed, is what frequently is planned. For buccal mucosa lesions, the thermocouple should be placed as close to the skin as possible within the oral cavity. Occasionally, liquid nitrogen may seep through improperly packed petrolatum gauze, and the nitrogen may slip into the oropharynx or over the lip and cause destruction of tissue which may interfere with function later on. Liquid nitrogen may leak through the protective packs on to the lip around the intratracheal tube, which may produce destruction of the skin and contracture of the lip. It is most important to pack carefully about the intratracheal anesthesia tube at the angle of the lip. Cryosurgery to lesions of the retromolar triangle in which the tumor extends up into the pterygo-palatine region may eventually cause trismus. However, the tumor itself may invade the area and cause this trismus. It is important to spend as much or more time on protecting the nontarget areas as it is to apply sufficient freeze to destroy the target areas.

CONCLUSION

The results of cryosurgery statistically cannot yet be compared to the statistical surveys of radiation therapy or scalpel surgery or combination of both. It has not been used long enough in sufficient controlled studies to make this comparison. The research studies that are ongoing by both cryobiologists and cryosurgeons have produced sufficient information at this time to state that cryosurgery is an effective modality in the treatment of tumors of the head and neck, not only for its palliative effects but also as a primary treatment. It is supportive both to scalpel and to X-ray therapy. The proper application of the closed and open cryoprobe is readily learned and easily applied. The treatment takes much less time, and the hospital stay if required is considerably lessened. It can be used in multiple courses. Its effectiveness as a palliative measure in the elimination of pain is important. The modality of cryosurgery should be a part of the armamentaria of all oncologists.

BIBLIOGRAPHY

1. Miller, D. and Metzner, D.: Tissue penetration studies using liquid nitrogen. Trans AAOO, 1969.
2. Cooper, I. S.: A cryogenic method for physiology inhibition and production of lesions in the brain. *J Neurosurg*, 9:853-858, 1962.
3. Cooper, I. S.: Cryogenic surgery: a new method of destruction of extirpation of benign or malignant tissues. *N Engl J Med*, 268:743-749, 1963.
4. Cooper, I. S.: Cryobiology as viewed by the surgeons. *Cryobiology*, 1:44-51, 1964.
5. Robowtham, G. F., Haigh, A. L. and Leslie, W. G.: *Lancet*, 1:12, 1959.
6. Neel, H. B. and DeSanto, L. W.: Cryosurgical control of cancer: effects of freeze rates, tumor temperatures, and ischemia. *Ann Otol Rhinol and Laryngol*, 82:716-723, Jan., 1973.
7. Goldstein, J. C.: Cryotherapy in head and neck cancer. *Laryngoscope*, 80:1046-1052, 1972.
8. Sherman, J. K. and Kim, K. S.: Correlation of ultrastructure before freezing, while frozen, and after thawing in assessing freeze-thaw induced injury. *Cryobiology*, 4:16, 1967.
9. Miller, D.: Does cryosurgery have a place in the treatment of papillomata or carcinoma of the larynx? *Ann Otol Rhinol and Laryngol*, 82 (5):656, 1973.
10. Amoils, S. P. and Walker, A. J.: The thermal and mechanical factors involved in ocular cryosurgery. *Proc R Soc Med*, 59:1056-1064, Nov, 1966.
11. Miller, D.: Cryosurgery for the treatment of neoplasms of the oral cavity. *Otolaryngol Clin North Am*, 5:2, June, 1972.
12. Gage, A., Koepf, S., Wehrle D. and Emmings, F.: Cryotherapy for cancer of the lip and oral cavity. *Cancer, 18:* 1646, 1965.
13. Miller, D., Wilson, W., Yules, R. and Lee, K.: Management of nasopharyngeal cancer. *Laryngoscope*, LXXXII (6):985-997, June, 1972.
14. Smith, M. F. W. and Lipson, L.: Angiofibroma: role of cryosurgery. *J Cryosurgery*, 2:12, 1969.
15. Smith, M. F. W., Boles, R. and Work, W. P.: Cryosurgery techniques in removal of angiofibromas. *Laryngoscope*, 74:1071-1080, 1964.
16. Miller, D., Silverstein, H. and Gacek, R.: Cryosurgical treatment of carcinoma of the ear. AAOO, Sept, 1972.
17. Zacarian, S. A.: Cryosurgery in dermatologic disorders and in the treatment of skin cancer. *J Cryosurgery*, 1:70, 1968.
18. Zacarian, S. A. and Adham, M. I.: Cryotherapy of cutaneous malignancy. *Cryobiology*, 2:212-218, 1966.
19. Wang, C. C.: Treatment of glottic carcinoma by megavoltage radiation therapy and results. *Am J Roentgenol Ra-*

dium Ther Nucl Med, CXX:1, Jan, 1974.

20. Mulvaney, T. and Miller, D.: *Cryosurgery as a Modality in the Treatment of Carcinoma of the Larynx—A Tracheal Approach.* Reprinted from *Arch Otol.,* 102:226-229, April, 1976.

21. Miller, D.: Management of keratosis and carcinoma in situ with cryosurgery. *Can J Otol,* 3:4, 1974.

22. Miller, D.: Cryosurgery as palliation for carcinoma of the larynx. *Can J Otol,* 4:3, 1975.

CHAPTER TEN

Evaluation of Cryosurgery for Hemangiomas

ROBERT M. GOLDWYN, M.D.

HEMANGIOMAS which are extensive or prominent cause the patient great anxiety and may jeopardize his life. For the physician confronted by a difficult hemangioma, the situation is bewildering and frustrating. The multitude of treatment methods is evidence of the inadequacy of therapy.

While it is true that most hemangiomas of infancy regress, some do not. These may rapidly grow, occasionally bleed, or remain as noticeable and grotesque deformities. For this kind of problem, albeit a small band in the hemangioma spectrum, cryosurgery may be beneficial.[1]

As noted in chapter one of this volume, employing cold to halt and eradicate blood vessel growth is not new. In the first decade of this century, liquid air, carbon dioxide snow, and liquid nitrogen were used for small malignant and benign tumors, including port-wine stains, other types of hemangiomas, and lymphangiomas. Lack of sufficient and sustained cold penetration were the drawbacks for those early techniques for treating large vascular tumors. These disadvantages were largely overcome by Cooper[2] who developed an effective cold delivery system utilizing liquid nitrogen. Encouragement for applying this method for hemangiomas came from his reported success in the treatment of vascular tumors of the brain, pharynx and liver, as well as epitheliomas of the skin.[3-5]

TYPES OF HEMANGIOMAS AND RESULTS

Controversy still exists about the proper classification of hemangiomas. Even within the same category, these tumors may vary greatly with respect to their appearance, clinical course, and microscopic findings.[6] It is crucial that each patient be evaluated and treated according to the biological pattern of his hemangioma and not be fitted falsely into a preconceived slot.

GENERAL OBSERVATION: *The type of hemangioma which has been most responsive to liquid nitrogen is cavernous, circumscribed, saccular, and superficial.*

With these characteristics in mind, let us consider various kinds of hemangiomas.

Port-Wine Stain (Nevus Flammeus)

In the author's experience, these intradermal capillary lesions have not been significantly diminished by the application of liquid nitrogen unless skin necrosis and scarring are produced—a poor exchange. In twelve patients with this type of lesion, little response was noted when test patches were frozen from one and one-half to three minutes at $-120°C$ to $-165°C$ with the Frigitronic Cryosurgery Unit C-8 and the Brymill Cryosurgery Unit Model SP-5.

In patients whose freezing stops short of full thickness necrosis, the treated area becomes anesthetic, hairless, depressed, and firm for many months. After a year or

235

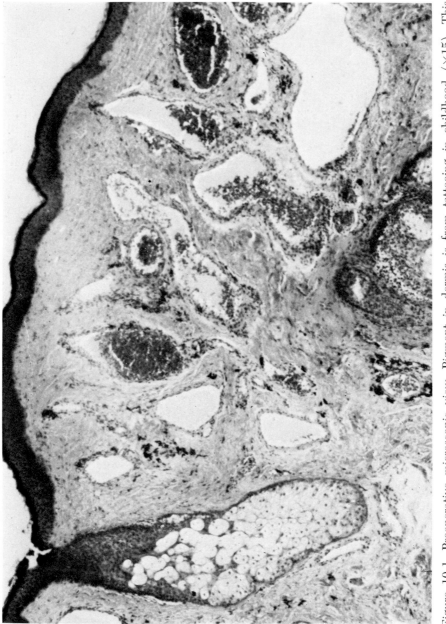

Figure 10-1. Preoperative microscopic view. Pigment in dermis is from tattooing in childhood (×15). This series, Figures 10-1 through 10-5, from R. M. Goldwyn and C. B. Rosoff, Cryosurgery for large hemangiomas in adults. *Plast Reconstr Surg, 43*:605-611, 1969. Courtesy of the Williams & Wilkins Co., Baltimore.

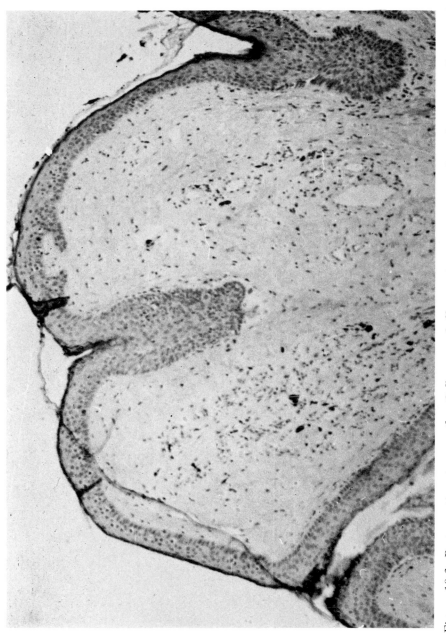

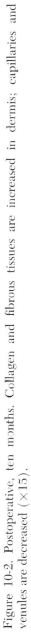

Figure 10-2. Postoperative, ten months. Collagen and fibrous tissues are increased in dermis; capillaries and venules are decreased (×15).

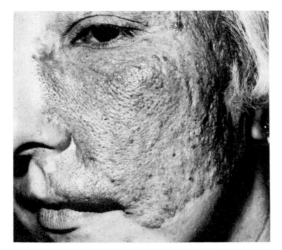

Figure 10-3. Preoperative view of thirty-year-old female with cavernous hemangioma.

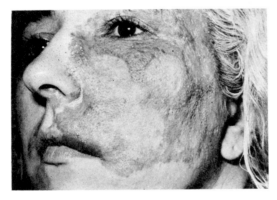

Figure 10-4. Postoperative, ten months. No regression. The lightest areas had the most freezing.

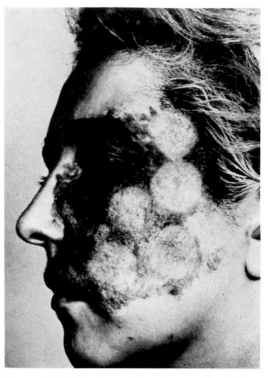

Figure 10-5. Postoperative, ten months. Infrared photograph to show areas of decreased vascularity in portions frozen. Eight years after treatment, because of a mild regrowth of the hemangioma, she again received cryotherapy.

two, the former vascular pattern may return. Presently, we are not treating this type of hemangioma with liquid nitrogen.

More encouraging results have recently been reported by Leopard,[6] who applies a flat probe ". . . site by site" and continues freezing

only two to three seconds after ice begins to form. . . . An interval of about five minutes is now allowed to elapse, during which time a triple response takes place with blanching and swelling. This effectively collapses the small vessels in the nevus, and there is a sudden ac-cumulation of extracellular fluid which happens to be conducive to rapid propagation of ice crystals during a subsequent freeze. The second freeze now begins, and at each site the probe is held for ten to fifteen seconds after ice formation. By thus shortening the freeze-thaw cycles, damage to the epidermis is avoided, whilst the subepidermal effect has been enhanced by the triple response following the preliminary freeze. . . . Treatment is repeated at fortnightly intervals, often over many weeks and the nevus gradually fades without scarring. Completed cases followed up for two years have shown only a slight tendency to deepen its colour again.

Cavernous Hemangiomas

Patients with cavernous type of hemangioma have benefited most from cryosurgery. As mentioned, the greatest gains occur when the tumor is small, saccular, and superficial. Several years ago when the author first used cryosurgery on these hemangiomas, freezing was cautious and insufficient in both depth and duration. For the well-defined, excrescent cavernous hemangioma, it is necessary to freeze *at least* three and one-half minutes at a delivery temperature of $-160°C$ to $190°C$ and usually, to repeat once or twice after thawing. Because the author believes it is important to force blood out of a bulky hemangioma prior to freezing, he prefers nitrogen delivery through copper disc attachments rather than by means of a surface spray. In general, *the greater the compression of the hemangioma, the greater the response.* It is always necessary to freeze beyond the margins of either the pure cavernous or mixed capillary-cavernous type.

Following cryosurgery, histologic findings correlate well with clinical observations. In biopsies taken in six months to a year later, the following changes have been noted: (1) The epidermis is atrophic; (2) The number and caliber of capillaries and venules in the dermis and deeper layers decrease and may resemble the pattern of a capillary hemangioma; (3) Collagen and fibrous tissue in the dermis increase.[1] (Figures 10-1 to 10-5.)

Cavernous Hemangiomas of the Oral Cavity, Pharynx, and Larynx

These difficult vascular anomalies deserve special comment. Perhaps because they involve mucous membrane and are accessible to freezing without the relative insulation of skin, they may respond very favorably. Improvement, however, is usually temporary.

Case Report (Figures 10-6 to 10-9)

S. S., a sixteen-year-old girl with a pro-

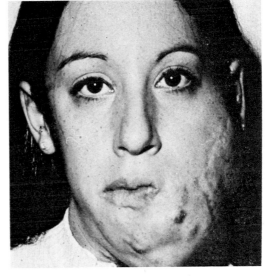

Figure 10-6. Preoperative view of sixteen-year-old girl.

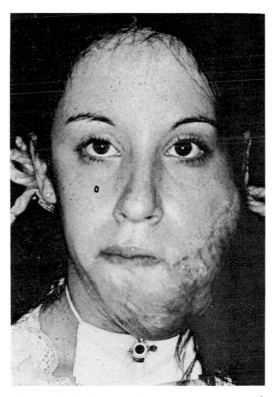

Figure 10-7. Postoperative view two years after cryosurgery with liquid nitrogen.

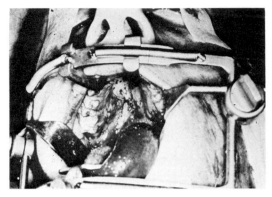

Figure 10-8. Preoperative view of same patient. Hemangioma involves base of tongue, soft palate, anterior portion of tongue and buccal areas, as well as larynx (not visualized here).

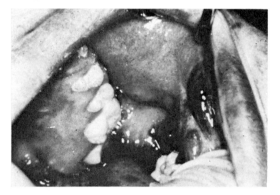

Figure 10-9. Postoperative view at twenty-two months. Marked regression of the hemangioma.

gressive, massive cavernous hemangioma of the left face and neck, soft palate, base of tongue, pharynx, and larynx presented with dyspnea and dysphagia. Because of the severity of her problem, she had been evaluated by several consultants who had advised against irradiation and extensive surgery. Examination disclosed a uvula displaced markedly to the right by the hemangioma which had almost completely replaced the soft palate and extended into the pharynx to compromise severely the airway. It did not go below the true vocal

cords and it did not involve the trachea and bronchi.

First Hospitalization (9/16/70 to 10/11/71): The patient underwent tracheostomy and then, under general anesthesia, she had a direct laryngoscopy and cryosurgical treatment of the hemangioma of the soft palate. Liquid nitrogen was delivered at −180°C for an average period of three minutes in four areas with a 2 cm copper disc attachment. Over the next few weeks and months, there was a marked diminution in the size of the vascular tumor. The soft palate began to look normal and the patient returned to finish her school year.

Second Hospitalization (6/15/71 to 6/30/71): The patient had cryosurgery externally to her face and neck in the hope that retrograde thrombosis would be induced so that the mass of vessel proliferation within the pharynx and larynx would be lessened. One area of the cheek treated at −190°C for four and one-half minutes developed skin necrosis and a depressed scar which gave the face a more normal contour.

Third Hospitalization (11/16/71 to 12/3/71): With the suspension laryngoscope and the help of Dr. Burton F. Jaffe and Dr. Marshall Strome, the patient had cryotherapy to her larynx, hypopharynx and base of tongue. The left arytenoid area involved by the hemangioma was frozen with a small caliber probe for three minutes. Care was taken to treat only one side of the larynx at this operation in order to avoid circumferential scarring.[8] It was noted that areas previously treated had regained an almost normal appearance.

At this same operation, a feeding gastrostomy was performed. However, a few weeks after the operation, the patient was able to take nourishment through her mouth by means of an Asepto® syringe with a rubber attachment. She returned to complete the remainder of her school term.

Fourth Hospitalization (2/2/72 to 2/11/72): With the patient under general anesthesia and through the still present tracheostomy tube, liquid nitrogen was directed to the areas of the larynx, hypopharynx and oral pharynx previously untreated. Where liquid nitrogen had been applied on the last hospitalization, a spectacular regression of the hemangioma was noted. The patient recovered rapidly and had improved swallowing and improved voice quality. She was able to tolerate plugging of the tracheostomy tube which was soon removed, but then had to be reinserted because the cavernous hemangioma regrew considerably in the pharynx and around the larynx and to a lesser degree in the oral cavity. She has been able to maintain her weight on a blenderized diet which she swallows fairly well. The patient is remarkable for her courage and determination and is about to graduate from college. The possibility of inducing regression of the hemangioma by embolization under angiographic control has been investigated, but because of the large number of feeding vessels and the risk, this procedure has not been undertaken. Another trial of cryosurgery would probably be of only modest and temporary value.

Her case illustrates the use of cryosurgery in a situation where no satisfactory alternative exists. The course also emphasizes the palliative yet transitory action of cryosurgery with this extensive type of hemangioma.

In patients with severe hemangiomas of the oral cavity, pharynx, and larynx, it is important to remember the need for a tracheostomy to insure an airway during the phase of postoperative edema. It is also

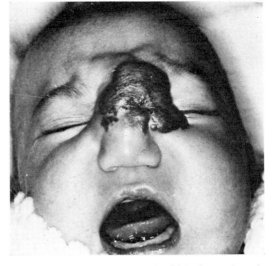

Figure 10-10. A four-month-old baby girl with a cavernous hemangioma rapidly growing on the glabella partially occluding the left eye. Cryosurgery was performed with a tissue temperature of $-70°C$ for thirty seconds. This series, Figures 10-10 through 10-13, courtesy of Dr. Luis O. Vasconez.

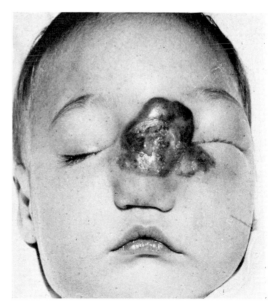

Figure 10-11. Immediately after cryosurgery.

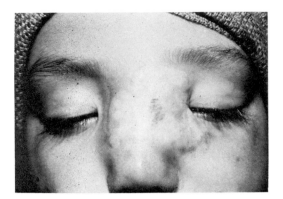

Figure 10-12. Before repeat cryotherapy three months later, followed by resolution of the hemangioma.

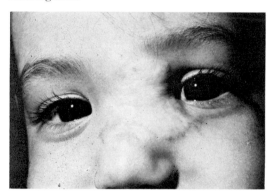

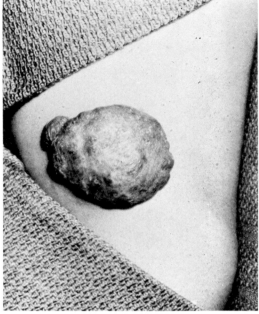

Figure 10-14. A five-month-old girl with repeated bleeding from mixed capillary-cavernous hemangioma on the left flank.

Figure 10-13. Fourteen months since first treatment, present plans are to excise the redundant tissue and to improve the scar.

advisable to stage treatment, as mentioned, in order to avoid constricting scars in tubular structures such as the pharynx and larynx,[8] and to assess precisely what changes have been produced by previous treatment.

Capillary and Mixed Hemangiomas

In addition to the port-wine nevus previously discussed, hemangiomas of the capillary type may present either in pure form or with a cavernous component. Cryosurgery should be reserved for the few instances of rapid growth or bleeding, par-

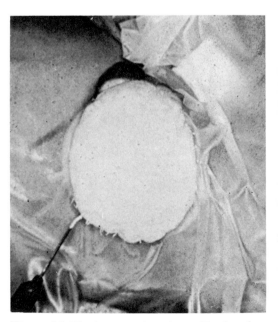

Figure 10-15. At operation, immediately after freezing.

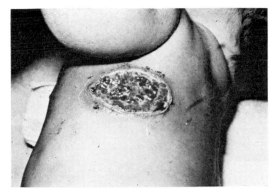

Figure 10-16. Three weeks later.

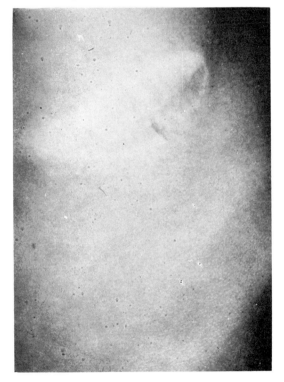

Figure 10-17. Three years later. No evidence of hemangioma but note depigmentation.

ticularly in a critical location (eyelid, Figures 10-10 to 10-13, and anus) where surgery or irradiation are the alternatives.

Case Report (Figures 10-14 to 10-17)

T. S., a five-month-old baby girl had a strawberry mark (mixed cavernous-capillary type) of her left upper flank. This area was frequently traumatized by the child during the night and several episodes of profuse bleeding had occurred.

HOSPITALIZATION (3/12/69 to 3/20/69): Under general anesthesia, and for three minutes at a tissue temperature of $-40°C$ (delivery temperature of $-130°C$) the hemangioma was treated with liquid nitrogen. The patient had minimal pain and no bleeding postoperatively.

At two weeks, the hemangioma was completely gone and by the thirty-fifty day, the wound had healed completely. Six years later there had been no evidence of the hemangioma; the scar is minimal but depigmented.

This case illustrates the use of cryosurgery in a situation which could have been endured, but jeopardized the child because of bleeding and caused the family considerable anxiety. Since most hemangiomas of this type require no treatment, cryosurgery should be considered only in an unusual circumstance such as that described above.

Occasionally, capillary hemangiomas form excrescences which do bleed. In these instances, cryosurgery can be useful since these fronds can be easily obliterated by liquid nitrogen, without anesthesia, as an office procedure.

Cavernous Hemangiomas of the Lips

This variety in this location should respond favorably because of its easy accessibility. The author's early experience was disappointing because he had not frozen sufficiently long (Figures 10-18 to 10-22). He believes that for a moderate size hemangioma at the commissure, for example, it is necessary to freeze for at least six minutes, at $-190°C$. Excellent results for

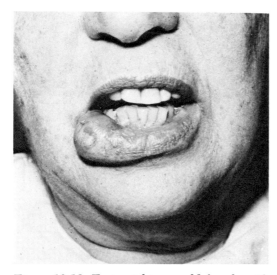

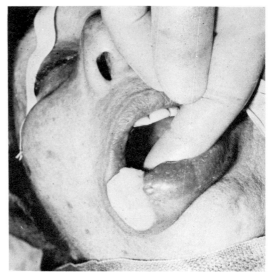

Figure 10-18. Forty-eight-year-old female with cavernous hemangioma of lower lip. Many years before, patient had excision elsewhere but this was unsuccessful.

Figure 10-20. Repeat deep freezing of longer duration than first time.

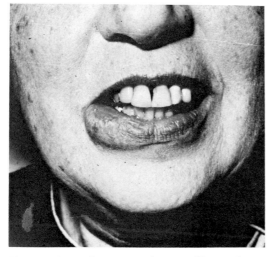

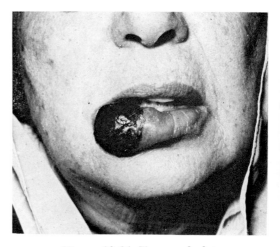

Figure 10-19. One year after insufficient freezing.

Figure 10-21. Two weeks later.

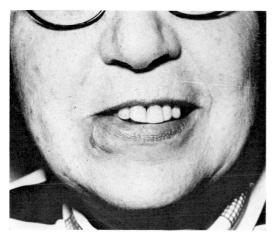

Figure 10-22. Improvement one and a half years later.

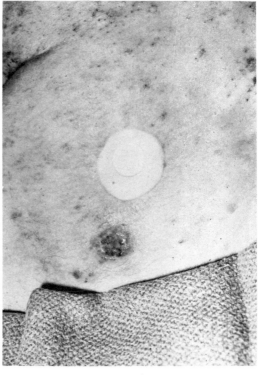

Figure 10-24. At operation.

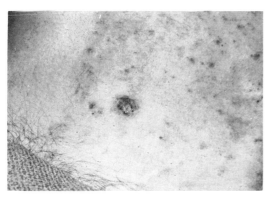

Figure 10-23. Cavernous hemangioma with periodic bleeding from projecting nodules.

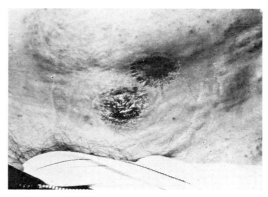

Figure 10-25. Twelve days later.

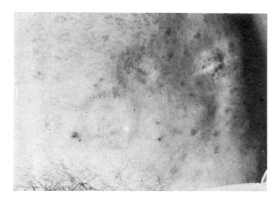

Figure 10-26. Eight years later. No further bleeding from sites treated. Note flatness and lightening.

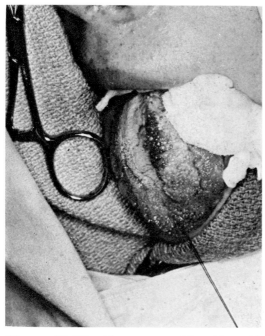

Figure 10-27. Twenty-year-old girl with lymphangioma of the tongue and episodic bleeding from excrescences in the midline, despite two operations elsewhere.

cavernous hemangiomas of the lips have been reported by Huang et al.,[9] who used ten minutes of freezing.

Other Hemangiomas

We have not employed cryosurgery for

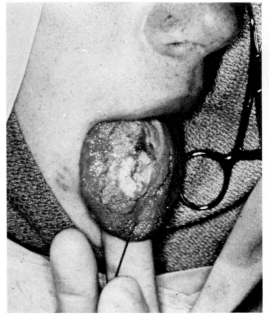

Figure 10-28. At operation, view showing lower portion just treated with liquid nitrogen. Double cycles of freezing were used for the entire lesion. There has been no recurrence after four years.

erythema-nuchae (salmon-patch capillary type) and for what has been termed *Hemangiomatous varicosities*, massive cavernous-capillary hemangiomas, often involving the upper or lower extremity with multiple arterio-venous shunts. Occasionally, projecting points of tissue bleed. One patient, a 25-year-old male (Figures 10-23 to 10-26), had periodic bleeding from multiple foci on the trunk. Liquid nitrogen on an outpatient basis with anesthesia successfully solved this annoying problem. (See also Figures 10-27 and 10-28.)

Postoperative Morbidity and Complications

The physician who uses cryosurgery for hemangiomas must be prepared to deal with undesirable sequelae:

Edema

In hemangiomas of the head and neck, marked swelling has been noted for as long as two weeks after vigorous cryosurgery. The peak usually occurs two to four days after freezing. Heavy serous exudate usually disappears by the fourth day. Because of edema, it is essential to ensure a good airway by a preparatory tracheostomy, if one is dealing with hemangioma involving a significant segment or a strategic location in the oral cavity, pharynx, or larynx.

Pain

Pain may be a prominent symptom for a few weeks. This is thought to result not only from direct nerve damage, which is usually transient, but to propagating thrombosis. In one patient, the sites of pain corresponded to areas of phlebitis at some distance from where the cold probe had been applied.

Bleeding

Only one patient, out of a total series of seventy-five, had significant bleeding. This occurred when the eschar separated at ten days from a test patch in the center of a very large cavernous hemangioma of the cheek. A through-and-through suture easily controlled the problem. Despite the infrequency of bleeding, patient and family are instructed about what to do should it occur: apply pressure, immediately call (the author) and/or go to the nearest emergency room.

Stiffness

A tight constricting feeling in the cheek, jaws, or neck may persist for weeks or months following extensive treatment of hemangiomas inside the oral cavity or on the cheek and neck. With moist hot packs, massage, and time, these complaints usually disappear.

Hoarseness

After freezing of the larynx, transient hoarseness and even aphonia may occur. Since this may take a few weeks to subside, patients should be warned about this. The author has never observed permanent vocal impairment. As a matter of fact, the timbre of the voice often improves if the hemangioma has been significantly diminished.

Scarring

Cold sufficient to cause skin necrosis inevitably produces a scar, frequently with noticeable depigmentation (refer to Figure 10-16). In some cases, the patient with a large deforming cavernous hemangioma looks better with a depressed scar which constricts the remnant hemangioma to more normal facial contour (refer to Case S. A., Figures 10-7 to 10-8). In a female, cosmetics may provide a satisfactory covering. It is the fear of scarring that has led the author to limit degree of freezing. Occasionally, a skin ulcer may form after freezing at a point of maximal skin tension and if it does not heal readily, a split-thickness graft may be necessary. This can be done on an outpatient basis, under local anesthesia.

Infection

None of the author's patients has ever developed an infection. Antibiotics are used prophylactically only when large areas are treated inside the mouth. Occasionally, the author has placed a wick loosely in the external auditory canal if he expects it to close with subsequent swelling. To prevent a middle ear infection, one must be wary about treating near the opening of the Eustachian tube.

Facial Nerve Damage

This is an *unusual* complication, since a nerve of the caliber of the facial is resistant to cold. Many patients with extensive hemangiomas already have impaired facial muscle function. This finding should be looked for in the initial examination and, if present, it should be emphasized to the patient preoperatively.

Excessive Regrowth of Hemangioma

Thus far, the author has never observed a patient developing a worse hemangioma as a result of cryosurgery. As mentioned, he has seen a return to the pretreatment state following cryotherapy for port-wine stains and cavernous hemangiomas of the pharynx and larynx.

Patient Dissatisfaction

In any list of unfavorable results, this should be mentioned. If the limitations of the procedure are thoroughly discussed before surgery, the chances for postoperative disappointment on the part of both the patient and surgeon are considerably lessened and hopefully eliminated.

CONCLUSIONS

From this brief review of a ten year experience with cryosurgery for hemangiomas, we may conclude that this technique is useful under certain circumstances; the most ideal would be a cavernous hemangioma that is small, circumscribed, saccular, and superficial. For extensive hemangiomas with multiple arteriovenous shunts involving the oral cavity, pharynx, and larynx, cryogenic surgery with liquid nitrogen may also be helpful. However, the results are less predictable and less effective than after freezing normal tissue and tumors of the brain, skin, and cervix.[4] The presence of myriads of blood-filled channels allows retention of heat and resistance to cold.[10] In the difficult situation of a massively infiltrating hemangioma, both the surgeon and the patient may have to accept the fact that at this stage in its development, cryosurgery's role is usually only palliative.

REFERENCES

1. Goldwyn, R. M. and Rosoff, C. B.: Cryosurgery for large hemangiomas in adults. *Plast Reconstr Surg, 43:*605-611, 1969.
2. Cooper, I. S. Cryogenic cooling or freezing of basal ganglia. *Clin Neurol, 22:* 336, 1962.
3. von Leden, H. and Rand, R.: Cryosurgery of the mouth, nose, and throat. *Trans Am Acad Ophthalmol Otolaryngol, 70:* 890-896, 1966.
4. Rand, R. W., Rinfret, A. P. and von Leden, H. (Eds): *Cryosurgery.* Springfield, Thomas, 1968.
5. Zacarian, S. A.: *Cryosurgery of Skin Cancer and Cryogenic Techniques in Dermatology.* Springfield, Thomas, 1969.
6. MacCollum, D. W. and Martin, L. W.: Hemangiomas in infancy and childhood, a report based on 6479 cases. *Surg Clin North Am, 36:*1647-1663, 1975.
7. Leopard, P. J.: Cryosurgery for Facial Skin Lesions. *Proc R Soc Med, 68:* 606-608, 1975.
8. Strome, M.: Cryosurgery: the effect on the canine endolaryngeal structures. *Laryngoscope, 81:*1057-1065, 1971.
9. Huang, T. T., Lynch, J. B., Doyle, J. E. and Lewis, S. R.: Cryosurgery of hemangiomas. Presented at 41st Annual Meeting of the American Society of Plastic Reconstructive Surgeons. Las Vegas. Sept. 20, 1972.
10. Miyasaki, A., Ervin, F. R., Siegfried, J., Richardson, R. P. and Mark, V. H.: Localized cooling in the central nervous system, Part II, Histopathological Results. *Arch Neurol, 9:*392-399, 1963.

CHAPTER ELEVEN

Current Concepts in Cryosurgery and Cryoimmunology

H. Bryan Neel, III, M.D., Ph.D. and Alfred S. Ketcham, M.D.

James Arnott (1797-1883) was the first physician to advocate the use of cold in the treatment of cancer.[1, 2, 9] On the basis of an extensive experience in more than 2,000 applications for analgesia in various benign disorders such as erysipelas, headache, and neuralgia, he was impressed with the antiphlogistic and anodyne properties of cold. He believed that inflammation accompanying cancer was reduced and controlled and that perhaps the viability of the cancer cell was compromised.

Modern cryosurgery employs profoundly low temperatures, those below 0°C, to destroy tissues in selected target sites. It is well known that the freezing process induces coagulation necrosis and is confined to the tissues within the region of probe application and the iceball.[4-7, 10, 33-35] The degree and extent of tissue destruction depend largely on the size of the iceball and the temperatures within it. Profound cold not only can destroy benign or malignant neoplasms but it also induces local anesthesia and hemostasis by injury to sensory nerve fibers and small blood vessels and capillaries.[35]

Various types of equipment and probes are now commercially available for cryosurgery, but it was after the development of a reliable, versatile closed cryosurgical system[6] using liquid nitrogen that numerous applications for cryosurgery were suggested, including therapy for cancer. Cryo-surgery is considered by many to be an acceptable alternative to extirpative surgery, particularly in patients with accessible neoplasms of the head and neck and the integument where classic resections produce losses of cosmetically important tissue.[4, 5, 7, 10, 33, 34]

The full theoretical potential of cryosurgery has not been realized because many early endeavors were largely clinical and lacked methodical observation of the temporal and physical factors important to success with this modality. Although clinical trials have yielded results that encouraged application of cryosurgery for the treatment of cancer in many medical and surgical specialties, the reports are largely anecdotal. Little information is available delineating the parameters necessary to ensure therapeutic success in either the clinical cases or the standardized animal-tumor systems. Therefore, over the past several years studies have been conducted in the laboratories of the Surgery Branch of the National Cancer Institute and of the Mayo Clinic to evaluate the effects on tumor control in syngeneic tumor-host systems of several variables commonly encountered in clinical cryosurgery: (1) probe-tip surface area, (2) probe-tip and tumor temperatures, (3) number of freezes, (4) freeze rates versus temperatures within the tumor, (5) local epinephrine-induced ischemia and temporary clamp-induced ischemia, and (6) selective temporary ischemia during freezing alone and thawing alone as compared with temporary ischemia during the entire freeze-thaw cycle.[20, 21, 23, 24]

Other experiments in the same tumor-host systems were designed to test the hypothesis that in situ tumor necrosis by a variety of means including cryosurgery increased host response against tumor by immunologic mechanisms.[22, 24, 25] It has been clearly established that malignant tumors in animals have cell surface antigens different from those of the tissue from which they arise—hence the term tumor-specific antigens.[29] Their presence has been demonstrated in tumors induced by chemicals and viruses as well as in tumors arising spontaneously.[13] Largely responsible for this discovery was the development and use of syngeneic, or genetically identical, animals for tumor transplantation studies. One of the most important recent advances in cancer biology is the demonstration that tumor-specific transplantation immunity (TSTI) to experimental tumors can be induced by a variety of means.[27, 29] Accordingly, TSTI was assessed (1) after complete excision and (2) after cryosurgery, ligation-release, and electrocoagulation. Comparison of TSTI was made with appropriate controls.

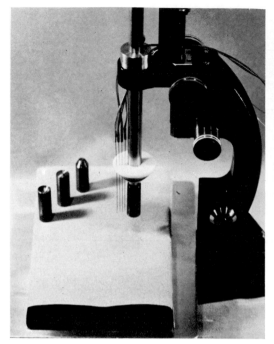

Figure 11-1. Probe stabilized in modified microscope. Teflon ring holds needle thermocouples around probe tip. Other tips, manufactured from copper rod stock, are shown on platform.

MATERIALS AND METHODS

Materials and methods used in the experiments have been described in previous publications.[19-21, 23-26] Briefly, three typical mouse tumor-host systems were used: a virus-induced mammary adenocarcinoma in adult C3H/HeN female mice and two methylcholanthrene-induced sarcomas in adult BALB/cAnN × DBA/2N F_1 (CDF$_1$) and C57BL/6N female mice. Tumors were in the second through the eighth transplant generations. In any one experiment all mice received the same transplant generation. Tumor cell suspensions were prepared by a mild enzymatic digestion method previously reported.[13] Inocula of 10^5 or 10^6 viable tumor cells were injected subcutaneously in the flank of each animal.[18, 24] When tumors reached 1.0 ± 0.2 cm in longest diameter, they were subjected to freezing through the intact overlying skin under light ether anesthesia (Figure 11-1). Mice were housed in small groups with free access to food and water and observed for tumor recurrence during the eight weeks after freezing. By this time all local recurrences had become apparent and most of these mice were dead from progressive tumor growth. Tumor control data were analyzed statistically by the Chi-square test.

In the immunologic experiments, mice were divided into three to five groups before tumor inoculation, depending on the comparisons to be made in any single experiment.[25] The number of animals in each group ranged from nine to nineteen. One group was set aside for later use as challenge controls, and the other groups received inoculations in the right flank of 10^6 viable tumor cells. About seven days later, depending on the tumor-host system, tumors were 0.9 ± 0.1 cm in longest diameter. One group of tumor-bearing animals was set aside without treatment for later challenge. In the other groups, tumor was treated in one of the following ways: (1) completely excised, (2) frozen through the intact overlying skin with standard cryosurgical equipment and technique, or (3) infarcted by placing a 1.0 mm ID rubber 0-ring for eight hours around a pedicle developed by outward gentle traction on tumor and overlying skin.

In cured mice, tumor was gradually absorbed, and slough of eschar occurred one and one-half to two and one-half weeks after cryosurgery or after ligation-release infarction. Animals developing local recurrences after cryosurgery were set apart for subsequent challenge as a separate group. At the time of challenge, recurrences measured 1.5 ± 0.3 cm and untreated tumors measured 2 to 4 cm in the largest diameter. All groups were challenged five weeks after primary tumor inoculation. Groups to be compared were all inoculated on the same day with appropriate dilutions of a single-cell suspension (Figure 11-2). The cumulative incidence of palpable tumor at the challenge site in the left flank was recorded every three to four days. From the long (a) and short (b) diameters, evenly bisecting the tumor at right angles, individual tumor volumes were cal-

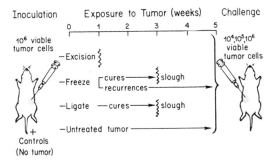

Figure 11-2. Overall experimental design. In early experiments, only portions were performed concurrently. From H. B. Neel, III, A. S. Ketcham and W. G. Hammond: Experimental evaluation of in situ oncocide for primary tumor therapy: comparison of tumor-specific immunity after complete excision, cryonecrosis and ligation. *Laryngoscope, 83:* 376-387, 1973. By permission.

culated with the formula $V = 0.4ab^2$.[3] The The significance of the observed differences comparing mean tumor volumes in various groups was tested by means of Student's one-tailed t test.

A liquid-nitrogen cryosurgical unit was used in all experiments. The probe was stabilized in a microscope stand to ensure constancy of probe-tip position and minimal pressure on the tumors (Figures 11-1). The rate and depth of congelation were varied by using probe tips with tip-to-tumor contact surface areas of 20 and 80 mm² and constant tip temperatures of $-60°$ or $-180°C$. The commercially available cryogenic probe tip is conical and has a surface area of 20 mm², so a sleeve with a concave tip (80 mm² surface area) was made from copper rod stock to fit tightly over the commercial probe. The concave surface conformed to the surface of the spheroidal subcutaneous tumors, ensuring maximal heat extraction from the tumors (Figure 11-3).

High-speed-response microminiature thermocouples with a time constant of 0.1 sec-

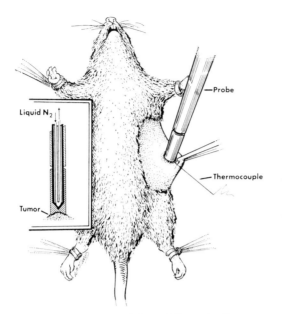

Figure 11-3. Tumors 1.0 ± 0.2 cm in diameter are frozen through overlying skin. Concave surface of 80 mm² probe tip conforms to tumor surface and ensures maximal heat extraction. From H. B. Neel, III and L. W. DeSanto: Cryosurgical control of cancer: effects of freeze rates, tumor temperatures, and ischemia. *Ann Otol Rhinol Laryngol,* 82:716-723, 1973. By permission of Annals Publishing Company.

ond were used to detect temperature changes within the tumor and in adjacent normal tissues.[26]

To ensure comparability of technique with that generally employed in clinical cryotherapy, the endpoint of each freeze was taken as the achievement of a standard cryolesion (iceball) extending 5 mm beyond the medial border of the tumor. Cryolesion size was measured with a Vernier caliper, and the time required to produce the standard lesion was determined with a stopwatch.

CELL DEATH BY FREEZING

Biologists have known for many years that repeated cycles of freezing and thaw-ing produce a series of events that are lethal to cell suspensions in vitro. These events are (1) temperature change (thermal shock), (2) formation of extracellular and intracellular ice crystals, (3) concentration of extracellular and intracellular solutes and pH change, and (4) cell shrinkage. Cells in vivo respond similarly to profound cold, but the circulation of blood, a continuous source of heat to the target area, variably and inconsistently changes the amount of cold required for cell death.

In clinical cryosurgery for cancer, the time required to destroy tumor is determined largely by the size of the tumor. The iceball must extent well beyond the tumor into grossly normal tissues if all of the tumor is to be destroyed. Tumor margins must be accurately estimated to ensure that temperature sensors are placed beyond the tumor, including the deep side. A *wide margin* of normal tissue must be included within the target area, just as a wide margin of normal tissue must be included in the specimen in the classic excision.

Effects of Repeated Freezing and Spontaneous Thawing

Two and three freezes (repetitive cycles of freezing and *spontaneous* thawing) of the same tumor are far more effective than one freeze.[21, 24] If the temperature of the probe tip approaches the boiling point of liquid nitrogen ($-196°C$), tumor control increases from approximately 50 percent after one freeze to between 83 and 100 percent after three freezes, depending on the tumor-host system.[21, 24] These differences are significant ($P < 0.01$) (Table 11-I). In the CDF_1 system, one freeze yields a 35 percent cure rate, two freezes 60 percent, and *three freezes* 100 percent, with the large probe tip at $-170°$ to $-180°C$. With an

TABLE 11-I

COMPARISON OF TUMOR CONTROL
FOLLOWING REPETITIVE FREEZING
WITH PROBE TIP AT –60° OR –180°C*

No. of	No. of Mice		
Freezes	Treated†	Cured	% Cured
at –180°C			
1	56	28	50
2	79	49	62
3	78	65	83‡
at –60°C			
1	15	1	7
2	35	9	26
3	38	16	42

* Data pooled for both 20 and 80 mm² surface area probe tips.

† Data pooled for all three tumor-host systems.

‡ 100% cure in C57BL/6N and CDF₁, using 80 mm² tip.

From H. B. Neel, III, A. S. Ketcham, and W. G. Hammond, Requisites for successful cryogenic surgery of cancer. *Arch Surg, 102*:45-48, 1971. Courtesy of American Medical Association.

increase in the number of freezes, there is a definite trend toward better tumor control; the differences between one and three freezes and between two and three freezes are significant ($P < 0.01$). With the same probe tips at $-60°C$, one freeze cures 7 percent of animals whereas three freezes cure 42 percent. Therefore, cryosurgical systems that employ cooling agents other than liquid nitrogen probably would be ineffective for cancer therapy.

Repetitive freezing can simply enlarge the iceball.[11] However, in the mouse-tumor studies, the endpoint of freezing was determined by extension of the visible iceball 0.5 cm beyond the margins of the tumor into grossly normal tissues. Hence, the size of the iceball was constant and determined the duration of freezing. Tumor control was dependent not on the size of the iceball but on the conditions of freezing within the frozen mass. However, it can be seen that the time required for the

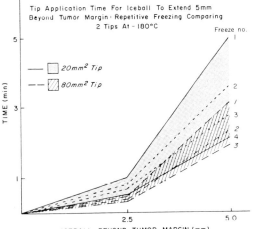

Figure 11-4. Cryoprobe tip application time for ice ball to enlarge is progressively reduced with addition of two and three freezes, allowing for complete thaw between freezing.

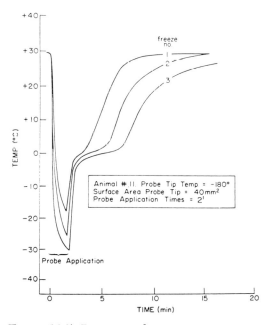

Figure 11-5. Repetitive freezing increases rate and depth of freezing and prolongs thawing. From H. B. Neel, III, A. S. Ketcham and W. G. Hammond: Cryonecrosis of normal and tumor-bearing rat liver potentiated by inflow occlusion. *Cancer, 28*:1211-1218, 1971. By permission of J. B. Lippincott Company.

iceball to extend 5 mm beyond the tumor margin was reduced with the addition of two and three freezes (repetitive freezing) with either probe tip (Figure 11-4).

In studies of normal liver, local temperature measurements show that depth of freezing and duration of thawing are both increased by repetitive freezing (Figure 11-5). Rapid freezing and *slow thawing* encourage recrystallization and formation of larger, more stable ice crystals. These effect cell destruction and ischemia, resulting in necrosis of tissues within the target site.

Probe Contact With the Tumor

When the surface of the probe tip makes contact with most of the exposed surface of the tumor, all other conditions of freezing being equal, tumor control is most effective. At $-180°C$, the 80 mm² probe tip with a tip-tumor contact ratio of about 1 : 1 produced cures in 82 percent of animals studied, whereas a tip-tumor ratio of

TABLE 11-II

TUMOR CONTROL COMPARING LARGE AND SMALL PROBE TIPS AT -60° AND -180°C

Surface Area Tip-Tumor Contact (mm²)	No. of Mice Treated*	Cured	% Cured
at 180°C			
80	95	78	82†
20	118	64	54†
at -60°C			
80	43	19	44†
20	45	7	16

* Pooled data for three tumor-host systems after one, two, and three freezes.
† No significant difference.

From H. B. Neel, III, A. S. Ketcham, and W. G. Hammond, Requisites for successful cryogenic surgery of cancer. *Arch Surg,* 102:45-48, 1971. Courtesy of American Medical Association.

one fourth that size produced cures in only 54 percent[24] (Table 11-II).

TEMPERATURES REQUIRED FOR CRYONECROSIS

It has often been stated that freezing to about $-20°C$ is adequate for complete necrosis of all tissues within the target area, but differential cell sensitivities to cold or variations in blood supply (or both) make that a marginal temperature at best. Because size of tumor, size of probe tip, and probe temperature remained constant in individual experiments, any differences in tumor control would be due to other factors, such as depth of freeze, duration of freeze, rates of freezing, and duration of thawing. In addition, when the large (80 mm²) probe tip was employed, the possibility that changes in tumor boundary were induced by movement of tumor cells in the advancing ice front was excluded because the probe tip-to-tumor ratio was approximately 1 : 1. (Whether or not tumor cells move with the advancing ice front is speculative.)

Freezing three times to tumor temperatures of $-18°C$ and $-44°C$, removing the probe from the tumor when that temperature was reached, and allowing *complete* thaw between freezes generally failed to control tumor; freezing to temperatures below $-60°C$ controlled the tumor in more than 80 percent of animals studied.[24] Freezing three times to temperatures of $-100°C$ or below led to 100 percent tumor control in the CDF_1 system.[21, 24] Similarly, whether the tumor was frozen very rapidly (260°C/min) or less rapidly (100°C-min), one freeze to $-90°C$ was far more effective than one freeze to $-30°C$.[21] At either rate of freezing, freezing to $-90°C$ increased cure rates and delayed recurrence as compared with freezing to $-30°C$. This difference was significant at $-100°C/min$ ($P < 0.01$).[21] Tumor control was best in the group of mice in which tumors were more rapidly frozen to $-90°C$ (Figure 11-6).

Duration of probe application appears to have less bearing on tumor control because the time required to freeze to either terminal tumor temperature at the slower rate was two to four times that at the more rapid rate. Optimally, tumors should be frozen rapidly to temperatures of at least $-60°C$. These data are consistent with those

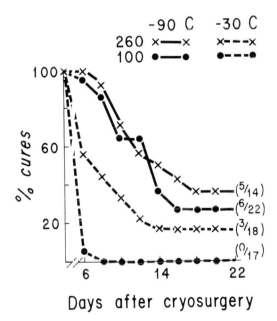

Figure 11-6. Effect of freezing one time at two different tumor temperatures ($-90°C$ and $-30°C$) achieved at two different freeze rates (260° and $100°C/min$). Rapid freezing to lower tumor temperature increased tumor control (number cures/total number treated) and delayed reappearance of palpable tumor in mice that eventually developed recurrences. From H. B. Neel, III and L. W. DeSanto: Cryosurgical control of cancer: effects of freeze rates, tumor temperatures, and ischemia. *Ann Otol Rhinol Laryngol*, 82:716-723, 1973. By permission of Annals Publishing Company.

of Zacarian,[34] who compared viability of cell suspensions of human skin, human foreskin, and human epidermoid carcinoma from the larynx in vitro, using trypan blue exclusion as the criterion of cell survival. In all groups, freezing to $-44°C$ and below at rates of about $100°C/min$, as would be employed in clinical practice, resulted in cell survival below 10 percent in all groups, and malignant cells appeared to be slightly more cryosensitive than normal cells.

In clinical situations where rapid freezing is not possible, as with large tumors, freezing to low temperatures is a satisfactory alternative. In his studies of freezing cell suspensions, Zacarian[34] has shown that freezing sustained in the range of $-40°C$ is more damaging than simply lowering the temperature and allowing immediate thawing. Because the time required to induce adequate freezing increases with tumor size, the freeze rate is reduced, but longer applications of the probe will eventually reduce the temperature to the desired level.

EFFECTS OF ISCHEMIA IN CRYOSURGERY

Because blood is a continuous source of heat to the target area, limitations or exclusion of blood flow should potentiate cryonecrosis. Temporary ischemia, induced in the liver by clamping the porta hepatis, quadruples the volume of cryonecrosis and assures death of all cell types within the target.[19, 23] The effects of ischemia on the freeze-thaw cycle are shown in Figure 11-7. Compared with congelation without ischemia, inflow occlusion produces greater depth of freezing and more prolonged thaw times. One probe application with inflow occlusion approximates the effects of between two and three freezes without ischemia.[19, 23] With temporary ischemia, tu-

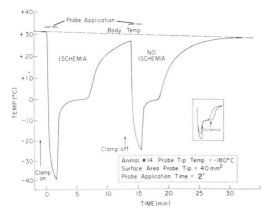

Figure 11-7. One freeze with ischemia has effect of between two and three freezes without ischemia. From H. B. Neel, III, A. S. Ketcham and W. G. Hammond: Cryonecrosis of normal and tumor-bearing rat liver potentiated by inflow occlusion. *Cancer,* 28:1211-1218, 1971. By permission of J. B. Lippincott Company.

mor implants in the livers of syngeneic rats were successfully eradicated by repetitive cryoprobe applications.[23]

Clamping is impractical and often not feasible in many anatomic regions. Therefore, the authors evaluated tumor control after local injection of pharmacologic doses of epinephrine.[20, 21] Subcutaneous fi-

TABLE 11-III

EFFECT OF REPETITIVE FREEZING WITH
AND WITHOUT TEMPORARY ISCHEMIA

No. of Freezes	Group	No. of Mice Treated	Cured	% Cured
1	No ischemia . . .	17	6	35
	Epinephrine . . .	17	8	47
	Clamp	11	6	55
2	No ischemia . . .	15	9	60
	Epinephrine . . .	11	10	91
	Clamp	10	10	100
3	No ischemia . . .	16	16	100

From H. B. Neel, III and L. W. DeSanto, Cryosurgical control of cancer: effects of freeze rates, tumor temperatures, and ischemia. *Ann Otol Rhinol Laryngol,* 82:716-723, 1973. Courtesy of Annals Publishing Company.

brosarcomas in CDF_1 mice were frozen after local infiltration of epinephrine around the tumor and clamping of the tumor vascular pedicle with a serrefine clamp during freeze-thaw cycles. Tumor control in these two groups was compared with controls. No significant differences were observed between the two groups that were treated in the presence of ischemia. Compared with the nonischemia groups, tumor control was increased after cryosurgery in the presence of temporary ischemia, whether ischemia was induced by epinephrine or by clamping. Comparing the nonischemia group and the clamp-induced ischemia group, the difference in tumor control after two freezes is significant ($P < 0.03$). Clamping appears to have a greater effect than epinephrine, but these differences were not significant whether one or two freezes were used. Tumor control after two freezes with ischemia was equivalent to that observed after three freezes without ischemia, indicating economy of effort when ischemia is used (Table 11-III). This represents not only a significant conservation of effort but also a marked potentiation of heat extraction, all other conditions being the same.

With evidence that ischemia improved

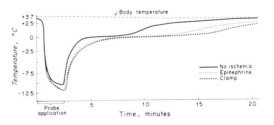

Figure 11-8. Effect of epinephrine and clamping on thawing time. From H. B. Neel, III and L. W. DeSanto: Cryosurgical control of cancer: effects of freeze rates, tumor temperatures, and ischemia. *Ann Otol Rhinol Laryngol,* 82:716-723, 1973. By permission of Annals Publishing Company.

tumor control, studies were undertaken to determine the effects on tumor control of ischemia induced during selected portions of the freeze-thaw cycle.[21] Whereas small increases in depth of freezing were produced by ischemia, thaw time was clearly prolonged (Figure 11-8). Clamp-induced ischemia during freezing alone had no effect on tumor control and was similar to that observed in the groups treated cryosurgically without ischemia, whether tumors were frozen once or twice. Tumor control was significantly improved after freezing with clamping during the entire freeze-thaw cycle and was virtually identical to that seen with clamping during thawing alone. Therefore, the effects of ischemia are mediated primarily during thawing (Table 11-IV).

Passy and associates[28] found that injecting epinephrine in saline beneath the oral mucosa of dogs before cryoprobe application significantly enhanced cryonecrosis of these tissues. Indeed, all data indicate that *local administration of epinephrine* before cryosurgery markedly *potentiates* the effects of cryosurgery and may be a useful

TABLE 11-IV

EFFECT OF CLAMP-INDUCED ISCHEMIA

No. of Freezes	Clamp Application	No. of Mice Treated	Cured	% Cured
1	Freeze and thaw*	11	6	55
	Freeze only	6	2	33
	Thaw only	6	3	50
2	Freeze and thaw*	10	10	100
	Freeze only	8	5	63
	Thaw only	8	7	88

* From Table 11-III.
From H. B. Neel, III and L. W. DeSanto, Cryosurgical control of cancer: effects of freeze rates, tumor temperatures, and ischemia. *Ann Otol Rhinol Laryngol,* 82:716-723, 1973. Courtesy of Annals Publishing Company.

adjunct to cryogenic treatment of neoplasms in patients.

IMMUNOLOGIC CONSIDERATIONS

Cryosurgery and cryonecrosis produce a *definite* and specific antibody response to normal tissues and tumor.[30] This has led to the term cryoimmunization. Among normal tissues, the coagulating gland of the rabbit has been extensively studied. After cryonecrosis in situ, circulating antibody specifically directed against components of that origin has been detected by passive hemagglutination and gel-diffusion techniques. This autoantibody is species- and tissue-specific. The antibody is detected in the serum within four days after cryotherapy, and the titers reach a maximal level by seven to ten days. Antibody titers decline thereafter. Antibody activity was predominantly 19S early in the postoperative period; later, 7S activity was detected. This corresponds to the pattern observed after antibody induction in general. Subsequent cryotherapy of the same tissue led to a booster effect, with production of higher and more prolonged elevations of 7S antibody.

Evidence now accumulating suggests that many human tumors—for example sarcomas,[8] melanomas,[15, 17] neuroblastomas,[14] and colon carcinomas[12]—contain tumor-specific transplantation antigens. This has led to a resurgence of interest and investigation concerning the possibility of effective immunologic therapy for cancer. Although the existence of tumor-specific transplantation antigens (TSTA) in rodents and humans has been clearly demonstrated, little is known about the relationship between the nature and duration of exposure to tumor antigen and the subsequent effectiveness of the host immune response. Strauss and associates[32] were the first to propose that destruction of tumor

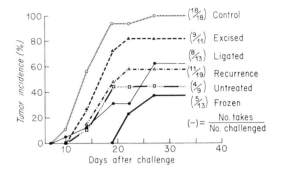

Figure 11-9. Cumulative tumor incidences after challenge with 10^4 viable tumor cells in CDF$_1$-SA system. From H. B. Neel, A. S. Ketcham and W. G. Hammond: Experimental evaluation of in situ oncocide for primary tumor therapy: comparison of tumor-specific immunity after complete excision, cryonecrosis, and ligation. *Laryngoscope,* 83:376-387, 1973. By permission.

in situ augmented host resistance to tumors to a greater degree than did excision. They found that partial electrocoagulation of human rectal tumors was followed by regression and disappearance of residual tumor in some cases, and they suggested that both local and systemic effects were induced by prolonged absorption of nonviable tumor tissue, presumably including TSTA. Immunologic mechanisms for these results in man were adduced from tumor challenge data in rabbits after electrocoagulation of Brown-Pearce tumors; however, this tumor-host system is not syngeneic, the tumor is not of recent origin, and immunogenicity was not demonstrated.

Using a different modality for in situ necrosis, Neel, Ketcham, and Hammond[22, 24, 25] demonstrated consistently greater tumor-specific transplantation immunity to subsequent challenge with tumor after cryosurgery as compared with tumor excision. In those studies, two syngeneic murine systems were employed using viral and chemically induced tumors with demonstrable tumor-specific immunogenicity. Moore and

associates[16] reported that cryosurgical treatment of several different human tumors induced an immune response not seen after surgical excision. Soanes and associates[31] reported roentgenographic regression of metastatic pulmonary prostatic carcinoma after repeated cryotherapy of the primary tumor. These data further suggest that in situ necrosis augments host resistance to tumor.

The differential immunity may be due to more prolonged exposure to TSTA as compared with complete excision.[25] Consistently greater immunity is seen after tumor necrosis in situ by cryosurgery or by ligation of tumor than by tumor excision, and the magnitude of the immune response was the same after treatment by

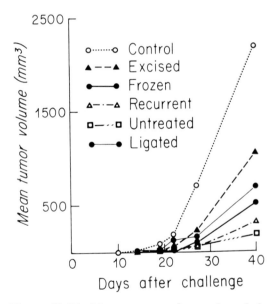

Figure 11-10. Mean tumor volume after challenge with 10^4 viable tumor cells in CDF$_1$-SA system. Numbers of mice are those developing tumor as shown in Figure 11-9. From H. B. Neel, III, A. S. Ketcham and W. G. Hammond: Experimental evaluation of in situ oncocide for primary tumor therapy: comparison of tumor-specific immunity after complete excision, cryonecrosis and ligation. *Laryngoscope,* 83:376-387, 1973. By permission.

either method. Animals bearing untreated tumors or recurrences and therefore also having continued exposure to tumor antigen(s) were similarly immune (Figure 11-9 and 11-10). This suggests that cryosurgery does not significantly alter tumor antigen(s) and that the immunologic effects are induced by mechanisms that involve rapid tumor kill in situ and subsequent absorption of tumor-specific antigen(s). More recent data (Neel, unpublished data) show that electrocoagulation has an effect similar to that seen after cryosurgery or ligation-release.

The mechanisms of so-called cryoimmunization are not clear, but because cryosurgery, ligation and electrocoagulation appear to have equivalent effects, duration of host exposure to tumor-specific transplantation antigens appears to be a factor. These techniques lead to ischemic necrosis and delayed slough of tumor one and one-half to two and one-half weeks after treatment (Figure 11-2). Necrosis may produce molecular changes in antigen or may liberate normally sequestered antigen(s) into blood, lymph, or both. Antigen release can be induced by immune complex formation and cell lysis in the presence of complement.

It has been generally impossible to produce regression of established tumors by immunologic means alone, but in the near future immunotherapy may become an important adjunct to surgery. Because tumor-specific antigens have been demonstrated in many human tumors, the immunologic response of patients to cryotherapy of cancer should be studied.

SUMMARY

If malignant disease is to be consistently controlled by cryosurgery, it is important to utilize low probe-tip temperatures approaching the boiling point of liquid nitrogen; large probe tip-to-tumor contact surfaces or liquid nitrogen sprays, which are more difficult to control; repetitive probe applications to the tumor; *spontaneous* thaw between freezes; freezing to tumor temperatures well below $-30°C$ and, better, to below $-60°C$; and rapid rates of freezing. In experimental tumor-host systems, ischemia induced either by local administration of pharmacologic doses of epinephrine or by temporary clamping markedly potentiates the effects of freezing and thawing. A definite tumor-specific transplantation immune response which exceeds the immune response seen after excision of tumor, follows cryonecrosis and other forms of in situ necrosis.

REFERENCES

1. Arnott, J.: Practical illustrations of the remedial efficacy of a very low or anaesthetic temperature. I. In cancer. *Lancet,* 2:257-259, 1850.
2. Arnott, J.: *On the Treatment of Cancer, by the Regulated Application of an Anaesthetic Temperature.* London, J Churchill, 1851.
3. Attia, M. A. M. and Weiss, D. W.: Immunology of spontaneous mammary carcinomas in mice. V. Acquired tumor resistance and enhancement in strain A mice infected with mammary tumor virus. *Cancer Res,* 26:1787-1800, 1966.
4. Cahan, W. G.: Cryosurgery of malignant and benign tumors. *Fed Proc,* 24 (Suppl 15):S241-S248, 1965.
5. Chandler, J. R. and Hiott, C.: Cryosurgery in the management of tumors of the head and neck. *South Med J,* 64:1440-1445, 1971.
6. Cooper, L. S. and Lee, A. S.: Cryothalamectomy—hypothermic congelation: a technical advance in basal ganglia surgery; preliminary report. *J Am Geriatr Soc,* 9:714-718, 1961
7. DeSanto, L. W.: The curative, palliative, and adjunctive uses of cryosurgery in the head and neck. *Laryngoscope,* 82:1282-1291, 1972.

8. Eilber, F. R. and Morton, D. L.: Immunologic studies of human sarcomas: additional evidence suggesting an associated sarcoma virus. *Cancer, 26:*588-596, 1970.

9. Fell, J. W.: *A Treatise on Cancer and Its Treatment.* London, J Churchill, 1857.

10. Gage, A. A.: Cryosurgery for oral and pharyngeal carcinoma. *Am J Surg, 118:*669-672, 1969.

11. Gill, W., Fraser, J. and Carter, D. C.: Repeated freeze-thaw cycles in cryosurgery (letter to the editor). *Nature, 219:*410-413, 1968.

12. Gold, P., Gold, M. and Freedman, S. O.: Cellular location of carcinoembryonic antigens of the human digestive system. *Cancer Res, 28:*1331-1334, 1968.

13. Hammond, W. G., Fisher, J. C., and Rolley, R. T.: Tumor-specific transplantation immunity to spontaneous mouse tumors. *Surgery, 62:*124-133, 1967.

14. Hellström, L. E., Hellström, K. E., Pierce, G. E. and Bill, A. H.: Demonstration of cell-bound and humoral immunity against neuroblastoma cells. *Proc Natl Acad Sci USA, 60:*1231-1238, 1968.

15. Lewis, M. G., Ikonopisov, R. L., Nairn, R. C., Phillips, T. M., Fairley, G. H., Bodenham, D. C., and Alexander, P.: Tumour-specific antibodies in human malignant melanoma and their relationship to the extent of the disease. *Br Med J, 3:*547-552, 1969.

16. Moore, F. T., Blackwood, J., Sanzenbacher, L. and Pace, W. G.: Cryotherapy for malignant tumors: immunologic response. *Arch Surg, 96:*527-529, 1968.

17. Morton, D. L., Malmgren, R. A., Holmes, E. C. and Ketcham, A. S.: Demonstration of antibodies against human malignant melanoma by immunofluorescence. *Surgery, 64:*233-239, 1968.

18. Myers, R. S., Hammond, W. G. and Ketcham, A. S.: A method for cryosurgical investigation of mouse tumors. *Int Surg, 52:*232-233, 1969.

19. Neel, H. B., III, Ketcham, A. S. and Hammond, W. G.: Ischemia potentiating cryosurgery of primate liver. *Ann Surg, 174:*309-318, 1971.

20. Neel, H. B., III and DeSanto, L. W.: Ischemia potentiating cryosurgery of tumor. *Surg Forum, 23:*484-486, 1972.

21. Neel, H. B., III and DeSanto, L. W.: Cryosurgical control of cancer: effects of freeze rates, tumor temperatures, and ischemia. *Ann Otol Rhinol Laryngol, 82:*716-723, 1973.

22. Neel, H. B., III, Ketcham, A. S., and Hammond, W. G.: Comparison of tumor immunity after complete excision, cryonecrosis, and in the presence of persistent tumor. *Surg Forum, 21:*120-122, 1970.

23. Neel, H. B., III, Ketcham, A. S., and Hammond, W. G.: Cryonecrosis of normal and tumor-bearing rat liver potentiated by inflow occlusion. *Cancer, 28:*1211-1218, 1971.

24. Neel, H. B., III, Ketcham, A. S. and Hammond, W. G.: Requisites for successful cryogenic surgery of cancer. *Arch Surg, 102:*45-48, 1971.

25. Neel, H. B., III, Ketcham, A. S. and Hammond, W. G.: Experimental evaluation of in situ oncocide for primary tumor therapy: comparison of tumor-specific immunity after complete excision, cryonecrosis and ligation. *Laryngoscope, 83:*376-387, 1973.

26. Neel, H. B., III, Riggle, G. C., Myers, R. S., Ketcham, A. S. and Hammond, W. G.: Apparatus modifications for experimental cryogenic surgery of cancer. *Cryobiology, 8:*501-505, 1971.

27. Oettgen, H. F., Old, L. J. and Boyse, E. A.: Human tumor immunology. *Med Clin North Am, 55:*761-785, 1971.

28. Passy, V., d'Ablaing, G., Turnbull, F. M., Jr. and von Leden, H.: Cryosurgery: a comparison of the clinical and histological response to epinephrine. *Laryngoscope, 81:*1917-1925, 1971.

29. Ritts, R. E., Jr. and Neel, H. B., III: An overview of cancer immunology. *Mayo Clin Proc, 49:*118-131, 1974.

30. Shulman, S. and Zappi, E.: Cryoimmunology: an aspect of cryobiology. In von Leden, H. and Cahan, W. G. (Eds.): *Cryogenics in Surgery.* Flushing, NY, Med Exam, 1971, pp. 42-79.

31. Soanes, W. A., Ablin, R. J. and Gonder,

M. J.: Remission of metastatic lesions following cryosurgery in prostatic cancer: immunologic considerations. *J Urol, 104:*154-159, 1970.

32. Strauss, A. A., Appel, M., Saphir, O. and Rabinovitz, A. J.: Immunologic resistance to carcinoma produced by electrocoagulation. *Surg Gynecol Obstet, 121:*989-996, 1965.

33. Von Leden, H. and Rand, R. W.: Cryo- surgery of the head and neck. *Arch Otolaryngol, 85:*93-98, 1967.

34. Zacarian, S. A.: *Cryosurgery of Tumors of the Skin and Oral Cavity.* Springfield, Thomas, 1973.

35. Zacarian, S. A., Stone, D. and Clater, M.: Effects of cryogenic temperatures on microcirculation in the golden hamster cheek pouch. *Cryobiology,* 7:27-39, 1970.

Author Index

Subject Index